MANUAL OF
NERVE CONDUCTION VELOCITY AND
CLINICAL NEUROPHYSIOLOGY

THIRD EDITION

Manual of Nerve Conduction Velocity and Clinical Neurophysiology

THIRD EDITION

Joel A. DeLisa, M.D., M.S.

Professor and Chairman
Department of Physical Medicine and Rehabilitation
UMD-New Jersey Medical School, Newark, New Jersey;
Senior Vice President and Chief Medical Officer
Kessler Rehabilitation Corporation and Other Kessler Affiliates
West Orange, New Jersey; and Chairman,
Department of Physical Medicine and Rehabilitation
St. Barnabas Medical Center, Livingston, New Jersey

Hang J. Lee, M.D.

Associate Professor
Department of Physical Medicine and Rehabilitation
UMD-New Jersey Medical School
Newark, New Jersey

Ernest M. Baran, M.D., M.S.B.M.E.

Associate Professor
Department of Rehabilitation Medicine
Jefferson Medical College
Thomas Jefferson University; and Medical Director
Lafayette Hill Medical Center
Lafayette Hill, Pennsylvania, and Department of Physical Medicine and Rehabilitation
Nazareth Hospital
Philadelphia, Pennsylvania

Ka-Siu Lai, M.D.

Jefferson Pain and Rehabilitation Center
Pittsburgh, Pennsylvania

Neil Spielholz, PH.D.

Associate Professor
Department of Orthopaedics and Rehabilitation
University of Miami School of Medicine, Miami, Florida

Keith Mackenzie, M.D.

Rehabilitation Associates
St. Luke's Rehabilitation Institute
Spokane, Washington

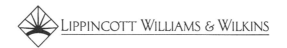

Made in the United States of America

Library of Congress Cataloging in Publication Data

Manual of nerve conduction velocity and clinical neurophysiology /
   Joel A. DeLisa . . . [et al.].—3rd ed.
      p.   cm.
      Rev. ed. of: Manual of nerve conduction velocity and somatosensory
   evoked potentials / Joel A. DeLisa, Keith Mackenzie, Ernest M.
   Baran. 2nd ed. c1987.
      Includes bibliographical references and index.
      ISBN 0-7817-0138-4 : $48.00 (approx.)
      1. Neural conduction—Measurement—Handbooks, manuals, etc.
   2. Somatosensory evoked potentials—Handbooks, manuals, etc.
   3. Evoked potentials (Electrophysiology)—Handbooks, manuals, etc.
   I. DeLisa, Joel A.   II. DeLisa, Joel A.   Manual of nerve conduction
   velocity and somatosensory evoked potentials.
      [DNLM: 1. Electrodiagnosis—handbooks.   2. Neural Conduction—
   handbooks.   3. Evoked Potentials, Somatosensory—handbooks. WL 39
   M294   1994]
   RC349.N48M28   1994
   616.8'047547—dc20
   DNLM/DLC
   for Library of Congress   93-21370
                                                                      CIP

   The material contained in this volume was submitted as previously unpublished material, except in the instances in which some of the illustrative material was derived. The Appendix, a glossary of terms in clinical electromyography, is reprinted from *Muscle & Nerve,* Vol. 10, No. 8S, Supplement 1987, with permission by the American Association of Electrodiagnostic Medicine. Approval for inclusion of the glossary in this book in no way implies review or endorsement by the American Association of Electromyography and Electrodiagnosis (AAEM) of material contained in this book. The authors thank the members of the AAEM Nomenclature Committee, who compiled this glossary: Drs. Charles K. Jablecki, Charles F. Bolton, Walter G. Bradley, William F. Brown, Fritz Buchthal, Roger Q. Cracco, Ernest W. Johnson, George H. Kraft, Edward H. Lambert, Hans O. Lüders, Dong M. Ma, John A. Simpson, and Erik V. Stålberg.

   Great care has been taken to maintain the accuracy of the information contained in the volume. However, neither Raven Press nor the authors can be held responsible for errors or for any consequences arising from the use of the information contained herein.

   Materials appearing in this book prepared by individuals as part of their official duties as U.S. Government employees are not covered by the above-mentioned copyright.

9 8 7 6 5

Contents

Preface

This manual will help physicians who are in electrodiagnosis training and electromyographers who are in practice to develop consistent techniques for performing motor and sensory nerve conduction velocity and latency studies, as well as repetitive stimulation of motor nerves. It provides ready access to standardized values for these studies and serves as a reference when studying nerves not commonly tested. The manual is developed for use in the electrodiagnosis laboratory and is not intended to replace standard tests and literature references.

Descriptions of each nerve conduction technique follow the same sequence, beginning with the placement site for the active electrode, and the stimulating cathode and anode. Typical electromyography equipment settings (frequency, sweep speed, and gain) are noted, as these sensitivity values may affect the normal values.

Specific normal values and comments that pertain to that particular nerve, or the referenced study, are also included. The normal values reported are taken from the articles referenced at the beginning of each nerve conduction technique. In order to use these normal values as standards, it is essential to follow each technique exactly as described. We present studies that use a standardized distance and that document skin temperature. When these potential sources of error are not noted, it is so indicated.

Illustrations demonstrating the electrodiagnostic setup have been included to supplement the descriptions of nerve conduction technique. These are intended to show the location of the active, reference, ground, and stimulating electrodes, as described in the text.

The book is organized beginning with an introduction, followed by chapters on the cranial nerves and cervical plexus, and continuing with nerves of the upper extremity (proximal to distal), the intercostal nerves, and the nerves of the lower extremities (proximal to distal).

These topics are followed by those on reflexes, late waves and long latencies, as well as conduction and repetitive stimulation studies in premature infants, infants, and children. In the above section 22 new studies have been added.

In the chapter on somatosensory evoked potentials, the sections on transbrachial plexus and movement-related potentials have been added. The five new chapters in this edition are entitled: Intraoperative Monitoring Using Somatosensory Evoked Potentials, Auditory and Visual Evoked Potentials, Magnetoelectric Stimulation, Motor Unit Action Potential Analysis, Single Fiber Electromyography, and Anatomy. This edition also features an appendix of the official terminology of electrodiagnosis terms of the American Association of Electrodiagnostic Medicine, and a bibliography.

Joel A. DeLisa
Hang J. Lee
Ernest M. Baran
Ka-Siu Lai
Neil Spielholz

Acknowledgments

We want to thank our many colleagues and trainees who let us know how helpful the first two editions were in their practice and in their training. We tried to incorporate their suggestions into this edition.

Thanks are due to Raven Press and to Dr. Sheela Jain, who encouraged us to write this third edition.

Joel A. DeLisa
Hang J. Lee
Ernest M. Baran
Ka-Siu Lai
Neil Spielholz
Keith Mackenzie

CHAPTER 1

Introduction

Nerve conduction studies are technical procedures used to assess objectively the functional status of the peripheral neuromuscular system. The reliability of the studies is increased when the technical procedures are standardized. The standardized procedures presented in this manual represent the consensus opinion of experts who routinely perform nerve conduction studies and whose studies have been published in peer-reviewed journals.

BASIC NERVE CONDUCTION STUDIES: GENERAL INFORMATION

The study of nerve conduction assumes that when a nerve is stimulated electrically, a reaction should occur somewhere along the nerve. The reaction of the nerve to stimulation can be monitored with appropriate recording electrodes. Direct recording can be made along sensory or mixed nerves. Indirect recording from a muscle can be used for motor conduction studies. Both orthodromic and antidromic conduction can be studied because stimulus propagation occurs proximally to and distally to the point of stimulation. Orthodromic conduction is the action potentials or stimuli eliciting action potentials propagated in the same direction as physiological conduction (e.g., sensory conduction toward the spinal cord and motor conduction away from the spinal cord). Antidromic conduction is propagation in the opposite direction. The response of the nerve to stimulation can be identified using appropriate recording electrodes. The time relationship between the stimulus and the response can be displayed, measured, and recorded.

For a glossary of terms in clinical electromyography, see the Appendix on pp. 393–465.

Electrodes:

Active (recording) and reference electrodes: The type of metal surface electrodes used is determined by the type of nerve response being studied.

Motor Response:

Peripheral nerves may be stimulated by passing electrical currents through the skin, resulting in a synchronized muscle contraction. When recorded by surface electrodes, this is called the compound muscle action potential (CMAP). Motor responses are recorded over the muscle being studied. The active (recording) electrode should be placed over the motor point of the muscle so that a clear negative deflection (upward) is recorded when electrostimulation is applied to the nerve supplying that muscle. The reference electrode should be placed off the muscle on a nearby tendon or bone. Recording and reference electrodes used for motor responses are surface disc electrodes about 0.5 to 1.0 cm in diameter. The surface disc electrodes may be separate discs or fixed 2.0 to 3.0 cm apart in a plastic bar (Figures 1.1, 1.2).

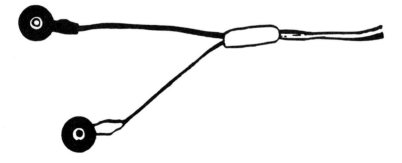

Figure 1.1. Surface recording disc electrodes.

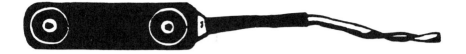

Figure 1.2. Surface recording bar electrodes.

Sensory Response:

A compound nerve action potential (CNAP) produced by electrical stimulation of the afferent nerve may be recorded over peripheral sensory nerves in a number of areas. The reference electrode usually is the same type as the recording electrode and in antidromic study it is placed distal to the recording electrode. Recording and reference electrodes used for sensory responses usually are surface electrodes with spring rings or clips (Figures 1.3, 1.4).

Note: Disc, bar, clip, and ring electrodes may be used interchangeably for recording and stimulating.

INTRODUCTION

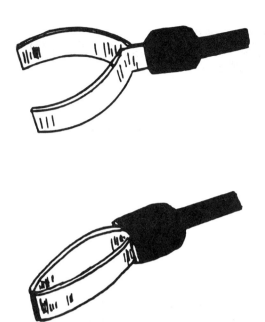

Figure 1.3.   Clip electrodes for sensory recording.

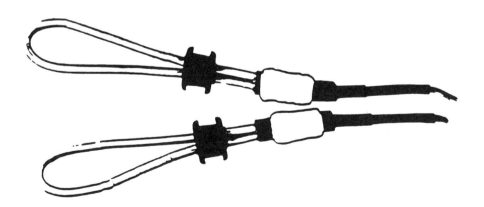

Figure 1.4.   Sensory ring electrodes.

Ground Electrodes:

The ground electrode is a metal plate that provides a large surface area of contact with the patient (Figure 1.5). It usually is larger than the recording and reference electrodes. The ground electrode is placed *between* the stimulating electrode and the recording electrode.

Stimulating Electrodes:

Surface stimulating electrodes usually are two metal or felt pad electrodes placed 1.5 to 3.0 cm apart (Figure 1.6). The use of this stimulator is standard in conventional nerve conduction studies. However, the monapolar needle electrode also can be used for nerve stimulation. Its use has certain advantages: (a) a smaller stimulus intensity is required, (b) the nerve can be stimulated more selectively than with a surface stimulating electrode, and (c) nerves that lie anatomically deep to the surface can be stimulated (e.g., the spinal nerve roots or sciatic nerve in the sciatic notch).

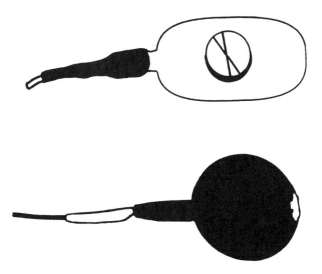

Figure 1.5.   Ground electrodes.

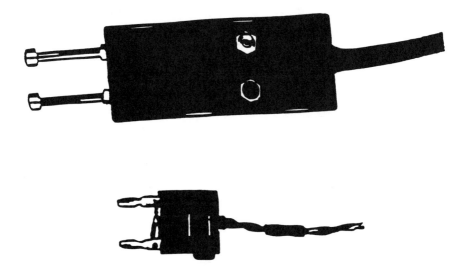

Figure 1.6.   Stimulators.

TECHNIQUES: GENERAL CONSIDERATIONS

A few general rules make nerve conduction velocity studies easy to perform and greatly reduce the number of examiner errors. Be sure that:

1. All recording, reference, ground, and stimulating electrodes are cleaned after each use by washing them with warm soapy water. Each electrode should then be dried completely.
2. All electrodes are electrically tested for broken wires or defective contact points. If a defect is noted, repair or replace the electrode.
3. A thin film of electrode gel is used on each electrode to maximize conductivity.
4. The electrode site on the patient's skin is clean and free of oil, grease, and soil. The site should be cleaned and abraded, as necessary, to reduce impedance at the electrode/skin interface.
5. All electrodes are fastened securely to the patient with tape or straps.
6. All recording and stimulating points are marked clearly with visible ink.
7. Distances are measured with a metal tape measure that is closely apposed to the skin and anatomic course of the nerve.
8. The cathode (negative pole) of the stimulating electrode is positioned toward the active (recording) electrode for the majority of the studies presented in this manual.
9. The stimulus is adequate to evoke a motor or sensory response. In general, a stimulus is defined as any external agent, state, or change that is capable of influencing the activity of a cell, tissue, or organism. In clinical nerve conduction studies, an electric stimulus is generally applied to a nerve or muscle. The electric stimulus may be described in absolute terms or with respect to the evoked potential of the nerve or muscle. In absolute terms, the electric stimulus is defined by a duration in milliseconds, a waveform, and a strength or intensity measured in voltage or current (milliamps). With respect to the evoked potential, the stimulus may be graded as subthreshold, threshold, submaximal, maximal, or supramaximal. The

"threshold" stimulus is that stimulus sufficient to produce a detectable response. Stimuli less than the threshold stimulus are termed "subthreshold." The "maximal" stimulus is the stimulus intensity after which a further increase in the stimulus intensity causes no increase in the amplitude of the evoked potential. Stimuli of intensity below this level but above threshold are "submaximal." Stimuli of intensity greater than the maximal stimulus are termed "supramaximal." Ordinarily, supramaximal stimuli are used for nerve conduction studies. By convention, an electric stimulus of approximately 20% greater voltage/current than required for the maximal stimulus should be used for supramaximal stimulation. The frequency, the number, and the duration of a series of stimuli should be specified on the reporting form.

10. Latency time in milliseconds (msec) for motor responses is measured from the shock artifact to the initial negative deflection (upward) of the response from the isoelectric baseline of the video display apparatus (Figure 1.7).

Figure 1.7. Motor nerve conduction velocity (NCV) technique. The reference and ground electrodes are placed over electrically inactive areas. The active electrode is placed over the abductor pollicis brevis. The median nerve is stimulated supramaximally with bipolar surface electrodes placed distally at the wrist and proximally at the cubital fossa. The latencies from stimulus artifact to the initial negative deflection of the M response (T_A and T_B) are noted. The distance between the two sites of stimulation (D) is measured. The NCV in meters per second is calculated by dividing D by $T_A - T_B$.

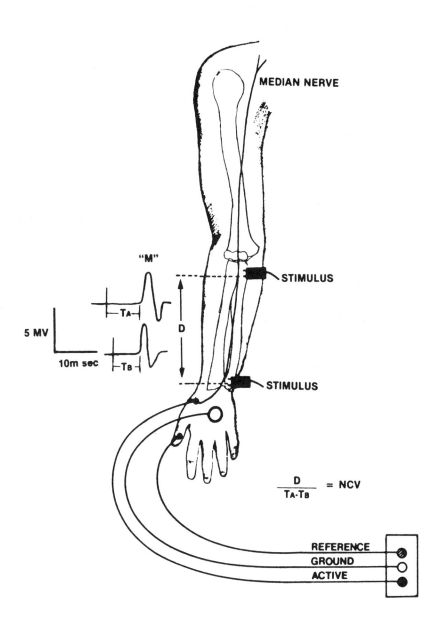

11. Latency time in milliseconds (msec) for sensory responses is measured from the shock artifact to the peak of the negative phase or the initial positive dip of the sensory response (Figure 1.8).

12. The amplitude in millivolts (mV) of the motor response is measured from the isoelectric baseline to the peak of the negative phase of the motor response.

13. The amplitude in microvolts (μV) of the sensory response usually is measured from the peak of the negative phase to the peak of the positive phase of the sensory response.

14. The duration in milliseconds (msec) of the motor and sensory responses is measured from the initial deflection of the negative phase of the response from the isoelectric baseline to the return of the positive phase of the response to the isoelectric baseline.

15. Conduction velocity (m/s) of a nerve is calculated by measuring the distance (mm) between two stimulation sites and dividing by the difference in latency (msec) from the more proximal stimulus and the latency (msec) of the distal stimulus. The equation is as follows:

$$\text{Conduction velocity (m/s)} = \frac{\text{Distance (mm)}}{\text{Proximal latency} - \text{Distal latency (msec)}}$$

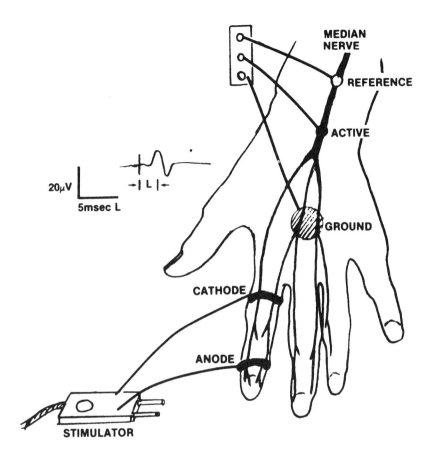

Figure 1.8. Sensory latency techniques. In the orthodromic technique, stimulating ring electrodes are placed on the digit with the negative (cathode) electrode placed proximally. Recording electrodes are placed over the medial nerve at a standard distance from the stimulating electrodes. The latency (*L*) from the stimulus artifact to the initial point of the first negative deflection of the evoked nerve action potential is recorded.

TECHNICAL PROCEDURES

The technical procedures for testing each motor and sensory peripheral nerve presented in this manual are divided into five parts. They are:

1. electromyograph instrument settings
2. patient position
3. electrode placement
4. electrostimulation
5. technical comments.

The upper extremity nerves are presented first. The motor component of the nerve is described and is followed by a description of the sensory component of that same nerve. The lower extremity nerves comprise the second half of the technical section and they are presented in the same format as those nerves in the upper extremity. Illustrations showing appropriate electrode placement, anatomic landmarks, and stimulation sites accompany each test description.

Electromyograph Instrument Settings:

Filters: The filter settings for each technical procedure allow adequate instrument response to record the motor and sensory potentials being studied. The filter settings are 10 Hz to 10,000 Hz for the motor potentials and 20 Hz to 2000 Hz for the sensory potentials.

Sweep Speeds: The sweep speeds for each technical procedure allow for display of the motor and sensory potential waveform.

The sweep speed settings are 2 to 5 msec for the motor potentials and 1 to 2 msec for the sensory potentials per horizontal division on the video display apparatus.

Sensitivity/Gain: Sensitivity or gain settings for each technical procedure are general guidelines for recording the motor and sensory potentials. *Increasing or decreasing the sensitivity or gain settings may be necessary to accommodate very low or very high amplitude motor or sensory responses.* Sensory sensitivity begins at 5 to 10 μV whereas motor sensitivity is 1,000 to 5,000 μV per vertical division on the video display apparatus.

These are general guidelines and should serve as starting points for basic evaluation procedures. These settings should be modified to meet unusual or difficult evaluation settings.

Patient Position:

The recommended patient position provides a comfortable, resting position for the patient. It also allows the examiner easy access to the extremity and nerve segment being studied.

Electrode Placement:

The active (recording) electrode is placed over the muscle or nerve segment being studied. The reference electrode for motor responses is positioned *off* and distal to the muscle being studied on a nearby bone or tendon. The reference electrode for sensory responses is placed distal to and on the nerve segment being studied.

The ground electrode for both the motor and sensory responses is placed on a bony prominence *between* the stimulating and active (recording) electrodes.

Electrostimulation:

Percutaneous electrostimulation is performed with surface electrodes at appropriate anatomic locations along the course of the nerve segment being studied. For all techniques presented in this manual, the cathode (negative pole) of the stimulating electrode is positioned toward the active (recording) electrode. Stimulation sites are designated as S1, S2, etc., to identify the location and sequence of stimulation.

Technical Comments:

Information that is considered useful for conducting an adequate and efficient evaluation is provided for each nerve. Cautions, special concerns, and recommendations for using the technical procedures also are included.

Illustrations:

Medical illustrations showing electrode placement, stimulation sites, pertinent anatomic structures, and surface anatomy accompany each technical description.

TROUBLESHOOTING

When performing nerve conduction velocity studies sometimes one cannot obtain a response. Because such nonresponse can result from many causes, a careful step-by-step analysis of the nerve stimulation technique is necessary.

Motor Nerve Stimulation But No Response Is Seen:

1. Check to be sure the stimulator is delivering an impulse. Most patients will feel the stimulus, but you can check it with your finger while turning up the voltage. If no stimulus is being delivered, then check the switches to see if they are set properly; remove the stimulator wires from their sockets and reinsert them properly. Next, check the stimulator wires for a defect, first visually and then electrically with an ohmmeter to determine whether the wire has electrical continuity. If after following these steps you find nothing amiss, then the problem lies within the stimulator. It must be tested by an electronics specialist.

2. If the stimulator is found to be working, then check the anatomical location of the stimulation electrodes. Occasionally a beginner will place the electrodes in the wrong area or over the wrong nerve.

3. If the stimulating electrodes are in the proper position, then check the amount of gel under the anode and cathode. Too much gel or sweating will create an anode–cathode bridge and

will render nerve stimulation impossible. Little or no gel will deliver a submaximal stimulus strength.

4. If the stimulating electrodes are in the proper position, then gradually raise the stimulus strength to the full output of the stimulator. If there still is no response, increase the pulse width duration of the stimulus slowly. This procedure often is necessary in extremely obese persons or in those patients with edema or severe nerve disease.

Muscle Contraction But No Evoked Response:

1. Check the switch controlling the input on the preamplifier to be sure it is in the "ON" position.
2. Confirm that the recording electrodes are over the motor-point area of the muscle being studied.
3. Remove excessive gel that can cause a bridge between the active and reference electrodes. This gel bridge will result in either a very small or no response. Add gel wherever it is insufficient under the recording electrodes. (Insufficient gel can have the same effect as too much gel.)
4. Check the recording electrodes and connecting wires with an ohmmeter to ensure electrical continuity.
5. On a multichannel electromyography (EMG) machine, if you still get no response, check the connections between the preamplifier and amplifier to ensure proper channel connections.
6. Check the ground lead. When the ground is not in contact with the patient, the trace on the video display apparatus will be off the screen.
7. Assure that the evoked response trace is centered on the video display screen.
8. Set the video display screen sweep speed so that the expected response is on the screen. (Try using a slower sweep speed, 5 or 10 msec/div, to see if the response is off the screen.)
9. In the event that the evoked response is of low voltage, increase the sensitivity by decreasing the gain on the amplifier to display the evoked response trace adequately on the video display apparatus.

Stimulus Artifact:

If the record shows a large stimulus artifact, look into these possibilities:

1. The ground is not functioning. Be sure that the ground electrode gel is adequate. Ensure that the ground is in contact with the patient. Be sure that the ground electrode is located *between* the stimulating and recording electrodes. Test the electrode wire with an ohmmeter to ensure its electrical continuity.
2. A recording electrode is defective. Again, be sure the electrode gel is adequate, the electrodes are on tightly, and the electrode and wire are checked with an ohmmeter for a defect. Defective electrodes should be repaired or replaced.
3. Check the stimulating electrodes to ensure that there is no electrode gel bridge between the anode and cathode electrodes.
4. Make sure recording and stimulating electrode connection cables are not crossed and touching.

Abnormal Recorded Potential:

If the recorded potential voltage is abnormal, follow these steps:

1. Move the stimulating electrodes in small increments until the best response is obtained. Be sure that the stimulus strength is supramaximal (submaximal stimulus may appear to give a decremental type of response, especially if the stimulator is not directly over the nerve).
2. Check the recording electrodes to ensure they are over the appropriate muscle and that the amount of electrode gel is adequate.

Initial Positive Deflection:

If the evoked response seen on the display screen has an initial positive deflection, do the following, except for the posterior tibial nerve, where recording from the abductor hallucis usually results in an initial positive deflection.

1. Move the active recording electrode until it is over the motor point of the muscle.

2. Make sure that the appropriate nerve is being stimulated and that there is no volume conduction (crossover) to another, faster conducting nerve (which can be checked by stimulating that other nerve).
3. Consider whether a crossover is present that would stimulate more remote muscles sooner than the one being tested.
4. Check for reverse electrode connections to preamplifier input jacks.

TEMPERATURE EFFECTS ON NERVE CONDUCTION VELOCITIES AND LATENCIES

Factors affecting nerve conduction velocity (NCV) and temperature:

1. Distal extremities are constantly exposed to environmental temperature changes.
2. There is a wide range of individual variation in response to environmental temperature changes.
3. The elderly have reduced adequate response to cold exposure. They have lower tissue temperatures than young adults when exposed to the same environment temperature.
4. Patients with impaired circulation may have reduced tissue temperature and additional reduced NCV.
5. Hemiplegic patients may have a lower skin temperature and motor NCV on the affected side when compared with unaffected side.
6. Boderline abnormal distal latency (DL) and NCV in patients with cool extremities may lead to erroneous diagnosis, such as peripheral neuropathy or entrapment neuropathy.

Halar EM, DeLisa JA, Brozovich FV: Nerve conduction velocity: Relationship of skin, subcutaneous, and intramuscular temperature. *Arch Phys Med Rehabil* 61:199–203, 1980.
Halar EM, DeLisa JA, Brozovich FV: Peroneal nerve conduction velocity: The importance of temperature correction. *Arch Phys Med Rehab* 62:439–443, 1981.
Halar EM, DeLisa JA, Soine TL: Nerve conduction studies in upper extremities: Skin temperature corrections. *Arch Phys Med Rehabil* 64:412–416, 1983.

Correlation of skin temperature and NCV:

1. It is practical, painless, and quick.
2. Since the skin temperature varies among sites in the parts of the extremities, a specific location for temperature measurement for each nerve has to be determined to standardize temperature correction to NCV.

Temperature and NCV correlation factors:

Temperature and NCV correlation factors vary for the same type of peripheral nerve in the literature. This variation is partially due to different tissue temperature sites, depth of thermester needle, wider range to cooling, and species variation.

Suggested NCV correlation factors:

We use skin temperature measurements (range, 26–32°C) to improve accuracy of NCV studies:

Nerve	NCV (m/sec/1°C) skin temperature change	Skin temperature recording site
Tibial motor	1.1	15 cm above medial malleolus
Sural sensory	1.7	15 cm above medial malleolus
Peroneal motor	2.0	15 cm above lateral malleolus
Median motor	1.5	Distal groove volar midwrist
Median sensory	1.4	Distal groove volar midwrist
Ulnar motor	2.1	Distal groove volar midwrist
Ulnar sensory	1.6	Distal groove volar midwrist

continues

Nerve	DL (msec)	Skin temperature recording site
Median motor	−0.2	Distal groove volar midwrist
Median sensory	−0.2	Distal groove volar midwrist
Ulnar motor	−0.2	Distal groove volar midwrist
Ulnar sensory	−0.2	Distal groove volar midwrist

Equations:

Tibial motor NCV corrected = 1.1 (skin temperature, 32°C) + NCV (m/sec).

Sural NCV corrected = 1.7 (skin temperature, 32°C) + NCV (m/sec).

Peroneal motor NCV corrected = 2.0 (skin temperature, 32°C) + NCV (m/sec).

Median motor or sensory NCV or DL corrected = $CF(T_{st} - T_m)$ + obtained NCV or DL, where T_{st} = 33°C for wrist, T_m is the measured skin temperature, and CF is the correction factor of the tested nerve.

Ulnar motor or sensory NCV or DL corrected = $CF(T_{st} - T_m)$ + obtained NCV or DL, where T_{st} = 33°C for wrist, T_m is the measured skin temperature, and CF is the correction factor of the tested nerve.

OTHER VARIABILITY IN NERVE CONDUCTION VELOCITIES AND COMMON SOURCES OF ERROR

1. Sensory and motor conduction velocities are slower in the legs than in the arms, ranging from 7 to 10 m/sec.
2. Longer nerves conduct slower than shorter nerves.
3. Conduction velocity is faster in the proximal than distal nerve segments.
4. Age:
   a. full-term infants: approximately half the adult values
   b. adult range obtained by age 3 to 5 years
   c. conduction velocities begin the decline at about age 40 years, but the decrease is less than 10 m/sec by the 80th year.

Common Sources of Error:

1. Spread of stimulation current to adjacent nerves must be avoided or you will elicit unintended potentials. This can be a particular problem with the peroneal and tibial nerves at the knee and the median and ulnar nerves above the elbow.
2. You must use supramaximal nerve stimulation or erroneously prolonged latencies with small amplitudes will be recorded.

Goodgold J, Moldaver J: Changes in electromyographic wave forms in relation to variation in type and position of electrode. *Arch Phys Med Rehabil* 36:627–630, 1955.

Gassel MM: Sources of error in motor nerve conduction studies. *Neurology* 14:825–835, 1964.

Simpson JA: Fact anf fallacy in measurement of conduction velocity in motor nerve. *J Neurol Neurosurg Psychiatry* 27:381–385, 1964.

Guld C, Rosenfalck A, Willison RG: Report of the committee on EMG instrumentation: Technical factors in recording electrical activity of muscle and nerve in man. *Electroencephalogr Clin Neurophysiol* 28:399–413, 1970.

Gutmann L: Atypical deep peroneal neuropathy in presence of accessory deep peroneal nerve. *J Neurol Neurosurg Psychiatry* 33:453–456, 1970.

Maynard FM, Stolov WC: Experimental error in determination of nerve conduction velocity. *Arch Phys Med Rehabil* 53:362–372, 1972.

Campbell WW, Ward LC, Swift RR: Nerve conduction velocity varies inversely with height. *Muscle Nerve* 4:520–523, 1981.

Kimura J: Principles and pitfalls of nerve conduction studies. *Ann Neurol* 16:415–429, 1984.

3. Excessive shock intensity can cause an unusually short latency by enlarging the electrical field and depolarizing the nerve segment away from the stimulating cathode.
4. Measuring the nerve surface length commonly overstimates or underestimates the conduction distance. Errors of measurement are amplified as the nerve segment shortens. Minimally, a 10-cm segment should be used.
5. Poorly defined takeoff will result in errors in reading the beginning of the evoked response.
6. Anomalies:
    a. Martin–Gruber anastomosis: 15% to 20% of persons have an anomalous communication from the median to the ulnar nerve at the forearm.
    b. accessory deep peroneal nerve (20–28% of persons): the anomalous branch of the superficial peroneal nerve supplies the lateral half of the extensor digitorum brevis.

CHAPTER 2

Cranial Nerves

FACIAL NERVE DISTAL MOTOR LATENCY TO THE NASALIS MUSCLE

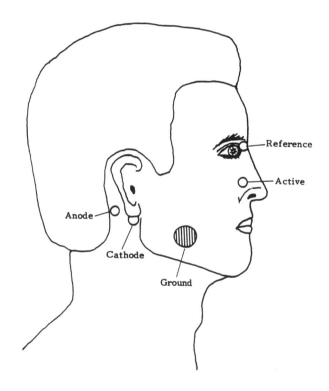

Figure 2.1. Facial nerve distal motor latency to the nasalis muscle.

Figure 2.1

Pickup: The surface active recording electrode can be placed over the following muscles: nasalis, mentalis or levator labii superioris, orbicularis oculi, and frontalis.

Reference: The reference is over the tip of the nose.

Ground: The ground is placed on the chin, cheek, or forehead.

Stimulation: Bipolar surface stimulating electrode is placed at the stylomastoid foramen or just anterior to the ear.

Normal values:
Latency: 3.4 ± 0.8 msec
Amplitude: 2–4 mV

Comments: Avoid placing the recording electrode around the mouth or cheek since the compound muscle action potential (CMAP) of the masseter may interfere. The CMAP amplitude depends on the muscle recorded; contralateral unaffected muscle should be compared.

Kraft GH, Johnson EW: *Proximal motor nerve conduction and late responses*. An American Association of Electromyography and Electrodiagonsis Workshop, September 1986.

FACIAL NERVE DISTAL MOTOR LATENCY TO THE ORBICULARIS ORIS

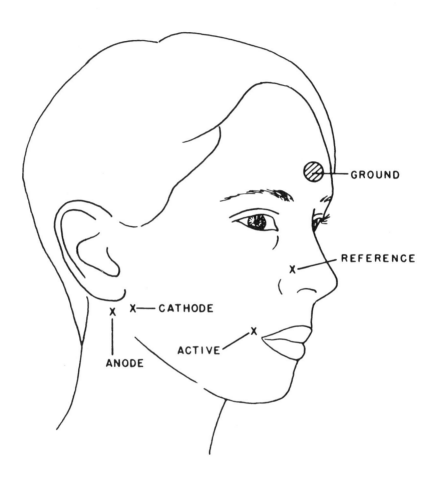

Figure 2.2. Facial nerve distal motor latency to the orbicularis oris.

Figure 2.2

Pickup: The coaxial needle is placed in the orbicularis oris just superior to the corner of the mouth (a monopolar needle can be used in the same spot). Taylor et al. found that the coaxial needle gave a slightly better end point than the monopolar needle, although both gave satisfactory results. A surface electrode often did not give the desired sharp takeoff. If a monopolar needle is used, then a reference electrode is placed on the side of the nose.

Ground: The ground is placed on the contralateral forehead.

Stimulation: Waylonis and Johnson recommended that stimulation be applied just below the ear and anterior to the mastoid process (angle of the mandible). Taylor et al., however, suggested applying it directly over the stylomastoid foramen.

Electromyograph settings:
- Frequency: 8 Hz to 8 kHz
- Sweep speed: 2 msec/div
- Gain: 250 μV

Normal values: ($N = 78$)
Latency (to onset of the negative deflection of the evoked potential) according to Waylonis and Johnson:

Waylonis GW, Johnson EW: Facial nerve conduction delay. *Arch Phys Med Rehabil* 45:539–547, 1964.

Taylor N, Jebsen RH, Tenckhoff HA: Facial nerve conduction latency in chronic renal insufficiency. *Arch Phys Med* 51:259–263, 1970.

Kimura J, DeLisa JA, Hallet M: *Cranial Nerve Testing*. An American Association of Electromyography and Electrodiagnosis Workshop, May, 1984.

Age	Mean (msec)	Range (msec)
Newborn–1 month	10.1	6.4–12.0
1 Month–1 year	7.0	5.0–10.0
1–2 Years	5.1	3.6–6.3
2–3 Years	3.9	3.8–4.5
3–4 Years	3.7	3.4–4.0
4–5 Years	4.1	3.5–5.0
5–7 Years	3.9	3.2–5.0
7–16 Years	4.0	3.0–5.0

Waylonis and Johnson report normal values in adults as 3.4 ± 0.8 msec (mean ± 1 SD). Taylor et al. report normal values in adults as 4.0 ± 0.5 msec (mean ± 1 SD). Both measure from the stimulus artifact to the onset of the negative deflection of the evoked potential.

Comments:

1. Temperature and distance were not reported in either of these studies. Evoked potential often is ragged and prolonged and does not necessarily indicate temporal dispersion.
2. In the assessment of a proximal lesion, as in Bell's palsy, the latency of the direct response rarely is useful. Even with substantial axon degeneration, the onset latency can be determined by the remaining axons to be normal or only slightly increased.
3. In contrast, the amplitude of the direct response provides useful information with regard to the prognosis by elucidating the degree of axonal loss.
4. The amplitude of the direct response varies substantially from one patient to the next. The comparison between the sides in the same individual is more meaningful than the absolute value.
5. An amplitude reduction to one-half that of the response on the normal side suggests distal degeneration.
6. Serial determinations reveal progressive amplitude changes as an increasing number of axons degenerate. Distal excitability remains normal for a few days, even after complete separation of the nerve at a proximal site, but is lost by the end of the first

week coincident with the onset of nerve degeneration. Prognosis is generally good if excitability remains normal during the first week after injury.

7. With shocks of very high intensity, stimulating current also may activate the masseter at its motor point. A volume-conducted potential from this muscle may erroneously suggest a favorable prognosis when in fact the facial nerve has already degenerated.

HYPOGLOSSAL MOTOR NERVE CONDUCTION LATENCY

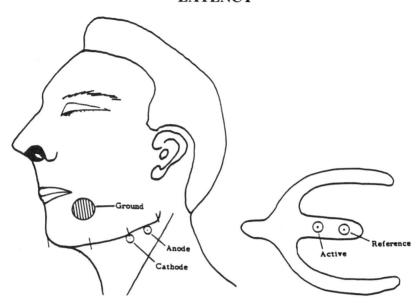

Figure 2.3. Hypoglossal motor nerve conduction latency.

Figure 2.4. Specially designed orthoplast bite for recording CMAP.

Figures 2.3 and 2.4

Pickup: The surface disc electrodes (10 mm) are placed on the anterior aspect of the tongue with the active and reference embedded in the specially designed orthoplast mouthpiece. The recording electrodes are separated by 2 cm and arranged to contact over the anterior surface of the tongue in the midline.

Ground: The ground electrode is placed over the lateral aspect of the mandible.

Redmond MD, DiBenedetto M: Electrodiagnostic evaluation of the hypoglossal nerve. *Arch Phys Med Rehabil* 65:633, 1984.
Redmond MD, DiBenedetto M: Hypoglossal nerve conduction in normal subjects. *Muscle Nerve* 11:447–452, 1988.

Stimulation: The stimulation is applied at the point determined by intersecting lines one-third the distance from the angle of the jaw to the mental tuberance, along the base of the mandible. It is also 1 cm medial to the inner aspect of the mandible.

Electromyograph settings:
- Frequency: 2–10 kHz
- Sweep speed: 2 msec/div
- Stimulus duration: 0.2 msec
- Sensitivity: 2 mV/div

Normal values:
($N = 30$; 20 men, 10 women)
Stimulation on both sides.
Age, 19–56 years (mean, 32 years)

Latency (msec)	Mean	SD	Range	Mean +2 SD
Left	2.1	0.4	1.3–3.2	2.9
Right	2.2	0.4	1.4–3.2	3.0
Amplitude (mV)				Mean −2 SD
Left	3.8	1.6	1.0–8.0	0.6
Right	3.9	1.6	1.0–7.0	0.7

Comments: Distance was not standardized. The test was performed in a sitting position. The tongue was dried with a sterile gauze before inserting the mouthpiece. Patients with carotid sinus syndrome or a cardiac pacemaker should not be tested.

CHAPTER 3

Cervical Plexus

GREATER AURICULAR NERVE CONDUCTION

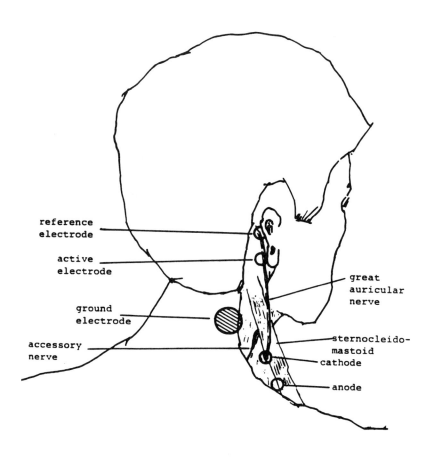

Figure 3.1. Greater auricular nerve conduction latency.

Figure 3.1

Palliyath

Pickup: The active recording electrode is placed on the back of ear lobe.

Reference: The reference is placed 2 cm distal to the active electrode on the back of ear lobe.

Ground: The ground is placed over the back of neck.

Stimulation: The nerve is stimulated antidromically at the lateral border of the sternocleidomastoid muscle (cathode distal), at a point 8 cm proximal to the active electrode.

Electromyograph settings:
- Sweep speed: 1 msec/div
- Gain: 20 μV/div

Normal values: (N = 35) Age, 21–66 years
Nerve conduction velocity: 46.8 ± 6.6 m/sec
Latency (to the negative peak): 1.7 ± 0.2 msec
Amplitude (baseline to negative peak): 12.7 ± 4.1 μV

Comments: Skin temperature was maintained between 33° and 35°C. The nerve may be injured during rhytidectomy.

Kimura et al.

The methods are similar to those previously described (Palliyath).

Normal values: (N = 64) Age, 14–88 years (mean, 45.7 years)
Latency: 1.34 ± 0.15 msec (onset)
1.89 ± 0.21 msec (peak)
Amplitude: 22.4 ± 8.93 uV
Comments: Electrodiagnostic evaluation of the great auricular nerve may be valuable in differenciating between the pre- and the postganglionic lesions of the second and third cervical roots.

Palliyath SK: A technique for studying the greater auricular nerve conduction velocity. *Muscle Nerve* 7:232–234, 1984.

Kimura I, Seiki H, Sasao SI, Ayyar DR: The greater auricular nerve conduction study: A technique, normative data and clinical usefulness. *Electromyogr Clin Neurophysiol* 27:39–43, 1987.

SPINAL ACCESSORY NERVE MOTOR LATENCY

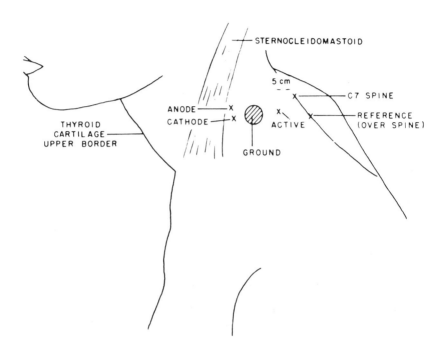

Figure 3.2.   Spinal accessory nerve motor latency.

Figure 3.2

Cherrington

Pickup: The active surface electrode is placed over the motor end plate of the upper trapezius muscle, approximately 5 cm lateral to the seventh cervical spinous process.

Reference: The reference is placed over a thoracic spinous process.

Ground: The ground is placed between the stimulus and the recording points.

Stimulation: The stimulation is applied about 1–2 cm posterior to the border of the sternocleidomastoid muscle at the level of the upper margin of the thyroid cartilage.

Electromyograph settings:
- Frequency: 8 Hz to 8 kHz
- Sweep speed: 2 msec/div
- Gain: 500 μV

Normal values: (N = 25) Age, 10–60 years
Latency: 1.8–3.0 msec

Comments: The temperature is not indicated. The distance between the stimulating and recording electrodes varied from 5.0 to 8.5 cm. The technique of measuring is not indicated, but probably represents a straight line.

Cherrington M: Accessory nerve. Conduction studies. *Arch Neurol* 18:708–709, 1968.
Kraft GH, Johnson EW: Proximal motor nerve conduction and late responses. An American Association of Electromyography and Electrodiagnosis Workshop, September 1986.
Green RF, Brien M: Accessory nerve latency to the middle and lower trapezius. *Arch Phys Med Rehabil* 66:23–24, 1985.
Shankar K, Means KM: Accessory nerve conduction in neck dissection subjects. *Arch Phys Med Rehabil* 71:403–405, 1990.

Kraft et al.

Recording technique is similar to that of the previous.

Normal values:
Latency: 1.8–3.0 msec
Amplitude: 3–4 mV

Comments: This nerve can be affected in following situations: Radical neck dissection, shoulder girdle neuropathy, space-occupying lesions, peripheral neuropathy, etc.

Green et al.

Pickup: The active recording electrode is placed over the upper (5 cm lateral to the C-7 spinous process), middle (half between the midpoint of the scapular spine and the spinous process of the thoracic vertebra at the same level), and lower trapezius (two fingerbreadths from the spinal column at the level of the scapular inferior angle). A plastic bipolar block is used as the recording electrode.

Electromyograph settings:
• Frequency: 8 Hz to 8 kHz
• Sweep speed: 2 msec/div
• Gain: 0.5 mV/div

Normal values: (N = 21) age, 18–65 years
Latency (msec):
to the upper trapezius: 2.1 ± 0.2 (1.5–2.9)
to the middle trapezius: 3.0 ± 0.2 (2.2–3.8)
to the lower trapezius: 4.6 ± 0.3 (3.9–5.6)

Shankar et al.
The recording methods are similar to those of Green et al.

Normal values: (N = 16) Age, 56–65 years

	Upper	Middle	Lower
Latency (msec)	2.1 ± 0.6	2.7 ± 0.6	5.6 ± 0.8
Amplitude (mV) (baseline to peak)	1.4 ± 0.5	2.7 ± 1.5	1.2 ± 0.2

PHRENIC NERVE MOTOR LATENCY

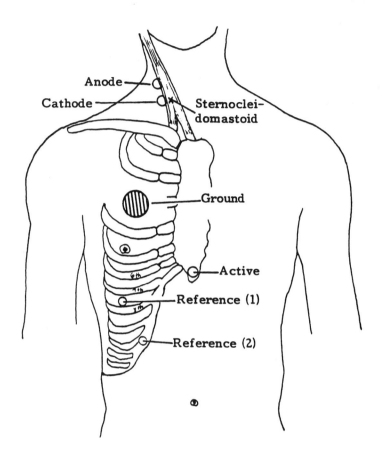

Figure 3.3. Phrenic nerve motor latency [Markand et al. (1) and Bolton (2)].

Figure 3.3

Markand et al.

Pickup: The recording electrodes were placed at the seventh intercostal space (reference) and xiphoid process (active).

Stimulation: The cathode (surface) was placed at the posterior border of the sternocleidomastoid muscle at the level of thyroid cartilage.

Normal values: (N = 50) Age, 31–72 years (mean, 50 years)
   Latency: 9.75 msec = mean + 2.5 SD
   Amplitude: >0.4 mV

Bolton

Pickup: The active surface electrode (G1) is placed at the xiphoid process and the reference surface electrode is placed over the chest wall, 16 cm apart.

Stimulation: The surface stimulating electrodes are placed at the posterior border of the sternocleidomastoid, approximately 3 cm above the clavicle. The duration of electric stimuli is used, 0.1–0.5 msec.

Normal values:
   Latency: 6.3 ± 0.8 msec
   Amplitude: 597 ± 139 μV

Comments: It is easier to stimulate the nerve with the neck in a neutral or slightly extended position. The distance between the stimulating and active electrodes is measured. This measurement does not vary the latency in adults, but it would have considerable effects in children.

Markand ON, Kincaid JC, Pourmand RA, et al.: Electrophysiologic evaluation of diaphragm by transcutaneous phrenic nerve stimulation. *Neurology* 34:604–614, 1984.
Bolton CF: AAEM minimonography #40: Clinical neurophysiology of the respiratory system. *Muscle Nerve* 16:809–818, 1993.

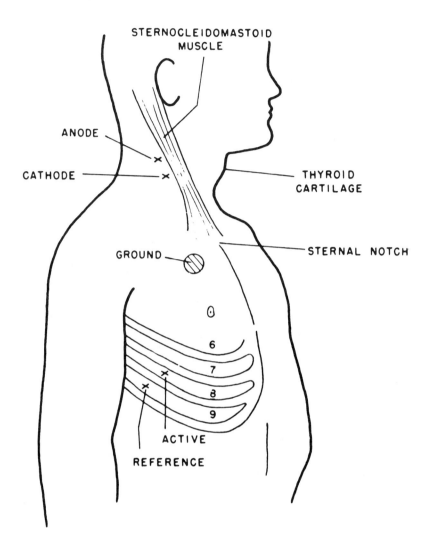

Figure 3.4. Phrenic nerve motor latency (Davis).

Figure 3.4

Davis

Pickup: The active surface electrode is placed in the eighth intercostal space in the anterior axillary line.

Reference: The reference is placed 3.5–5.0 cm from the active, either in the ninth intercostal space or posteriorly in the eighth intercostal space.

Ground: The ground is placed on the chest wall over the upper pectoral region.

Stimulation: Stimulation is applied at the posterior border of the sternocleidomastoid muscle at the level of the upper margin of the thyroid cartilage.

Electromyograph settings:
- Frequency: 8 Hz to 8 kHz
- Sweep speed: 5 msec/div
- Gain: 250 μV

Normal values: ($N = 18$ normal adults; 4 were tested bilaterally)
Latency: 7.7 ± 0.8 msec (mean $\pm$ 1 SD)
Amplitude: 160–500 μV

Comments: Care must be taken to avoid concurrently stimulating the brachial plexus. Distance was not indicated, and temperature apparently was not measured.

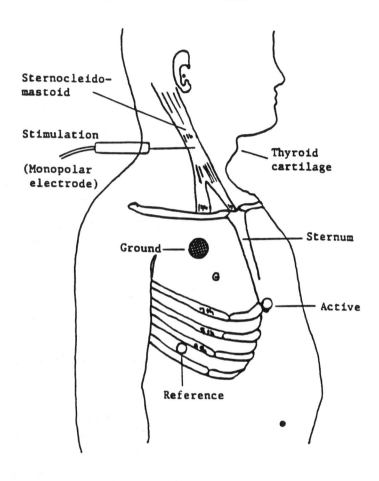

Figure 3.5. Phrenic nerve motor latency (MacLean and Mattioni).

Figure 3.5

MacLean et al.

Pickup: Active surface electrode was placed over the xiphoid process.

Reference: Reference electrode was placed on the right and left eighth intercostal space at the costochondral junction.

Stimulation: The cathode was a monopolar needle. The needle was inserted near the posterior margin of the sternocleidomastoid muscle at the level of cricoid cartilage.

Normal values: (N = 60 in 30 normal persons)

	Mean ± SD
Latency (msec)	7.44 ± 0.59 (6.0–9.5)
Amplitude (μV)	845 ± 405 (200–2,000)

Davis JN: Phrenic nerve conduction in man. *J Neurol Neurosurg Psychiatry* 30:420–426, 1967.

MacLean IC, Mattioni TA: Phrenic nerve conduction studies: A new technique and its application in quadriplegic patients. *Arch Phys Med Rehabil* 62:70–72, 1991.

CHAPTER 4

Upper Extremity Nerves

LONG THORACIC NERVE MOTOR LATENCY

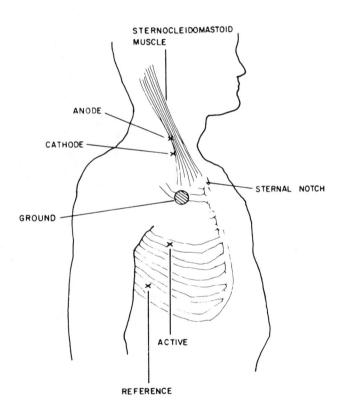

Figure 4.1. Long thoracic nerve motor latency.

Figure 4.1

Pickup: The active surface electrode is a monopolar needle electrode placed into the digitation of the serratus anterior muscle at the fifth thoracic rib level in the midaxillary line.

Reference: The reference is placed 20 mm caudally to the active electrode.

Stimulation: The cathode of the surface stimulation electrode is placed at Erb's point (above the upper margin of the clavicle, lateral to the clavicle head of the sternocleidomastoid muscle). The anode is located above and medially.

Electromyograph settings:
- Frequency: 8 Hz to 8 kHz
- Sweep speed: 5 msec/div
- Gain: 500 μV

Distance: Distance is measured with obstetric calipers. The range of distance from the point of stimulation to the point of recording is 170–230 mm.

Normal values: (N = 25 normal adults)
Latency: 3.9 ± 0.6 msec (mean ± 1 SD)

Comments: No skin temperature was taken.

Kaplan PE: Electrodiagnostic confirmation of long thoracic nerve palsy. *J Neurol Neurosurg Psychiatry* 43:50–52, 1980.

Alfonsi E, Moglia A, Sandrini G, Pisoni MR, Arrigo: Electrophysiological study of the long thoracic nerve conduction in normal subjects. *Electromyogr Clin Neurophysiol* 26:63–67, 1986.

Alfonsi et al.

Pickup and reference electrodes: The active surface electrode is placed on the digitation of the serratus anterior along the mid axillary line on the fifth rib and the reference electrode in front of the active electrode at the fixed distance of 3 cm.

A concentric needle can be inserted at the same level as the surface active electrode.

Stimulation: Erb's point with a bipolar surface electrode.

Normal values:

Age (years)	Latency (msec)	Amplitude (mV)
20–35	3.2 ± 0.3	4.3 ± 3.0 (*N* = 16)
36–50	3.3 ± 0.3	3.8 ± 2.4 (*N* = 16)
51–65	3.3 ± 0.3	2.7 ± 1.2 (*N* = 12)

Recording with a concentric electrode:

Age (years)	Latency (msec)	Amplitude (mV)
20–35	3.6 ± 0.3	7.1 ± 6.0 (*N* = 16)
36–50	3.8 ± 0.4	5.7 ± 3.8 (*N* = 16)
51–65	4.0 ± 0.4	5.6 ± 4.5 (*N* = 12)

Comments: The distance between the recording and stimulation electrodes were measured using an obstetric caliper. The authors believe the measurement of compound muscle action potential using surface electrodes could be unreliable because of a great variability.

DORSAL SCAPULAR NERVE MOTOR LATENCY

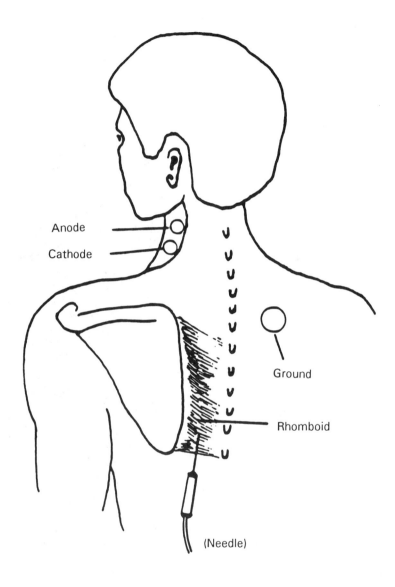

Figure 4.2.   Dorsal scapular nerve motor latency.

Figure 4.2

Pickup: The concentric needle is inserted into the rhomboid major muscle at the medial edge of the inferior angle of the scapula.

Ground: The ground is placed between the stimulating and recording electrodes.

Stimulation: A bipolar surface electrode is placed at Erb's point. The duration required is 0.2–0.5 msec.

Normal values: (N = 21) Age, 19–73 years, mean age, 42.3
　　Latency: 5.2 ± 0.7 msec
　　Mean distance: 19.9 cm (16.5–21.5 cm)

Comments: The distance was measured using an obstetric caliper and from the cathode to the recording needle electrode. The room temperature was maintained at 22°C or more. Other nerves, accessory, long thoracic, and thoracodorsal nerves were simultaneously tested. The amplitude of responses was not measured.

Lo Monaco M, Di Pasqua PG, Tonali P: Conduction studies along the accessory, long thoracic, dorsal scapular, and thoracodorsal nerves. *Acta Neurol Scand* 68:171–176, 1983.

SUPRASCAPULAR NERVE MOTOR LATENCY TO
SUPRASPINATUS AND INFRASPINATUS

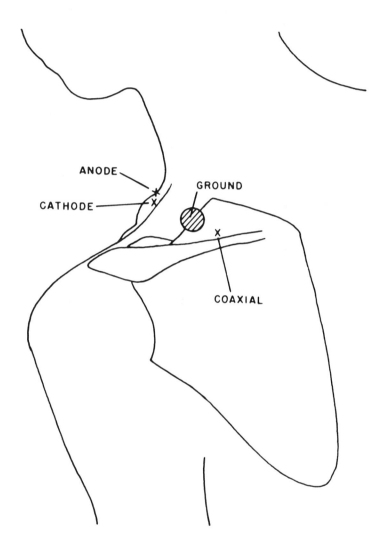

Figure 4.3. Suprascapular nerve motor latency to supraspinatus muscle.

Figure 4.3

Stimulation: The cathode is slightly above the upper margin of the clavicle and lateral to the clavicular head of the sternocleidomastoid muscle. The anode is superior medially.

Electromyograph settings:
- Frequency: 8 Hz to 8 kHz
- Sweep speed: 2 msec/div
- Gain: 500 μV

To supraspinatus (N = 62)

Pickup and Reference: The coaxial needle is inserted medial to the midpoint of the scapular spine and just above the spine. It is inserted in a downward and forward direction until the scapula is touched, then the needle is withdrawn several millimeters. Shoulder abduction confirms the needle placement. The study is done with the patient sitting with arms at their side.

Ground: The ground is placed between the stimulation and pickup sites.

Distance: A measuring tape is used with the arm at the side; the range is 7.4–13.8 cm.

Normal values:
Latency: 2.7 ± 0.5 msec (mean ± 1 SD); normal range, 1.7–3.7 msec. The M wave recorded with a coaxial needle electrode is polyphasic and of large amplitude.

Amplitude: 5 mV or more. Highly variable with small needle movement.

Kraft GH: Axillary, musculocutaneous and suprascapular nerve latency studies. *Arch Phys Med Rehabil* 53:383–387, 1972.
Kraft GH, Johnson EW: Proximal motor nerve conduction and late responses. An American Association of Electromyography and Electrodiagnosis Workshop, September, 1986.

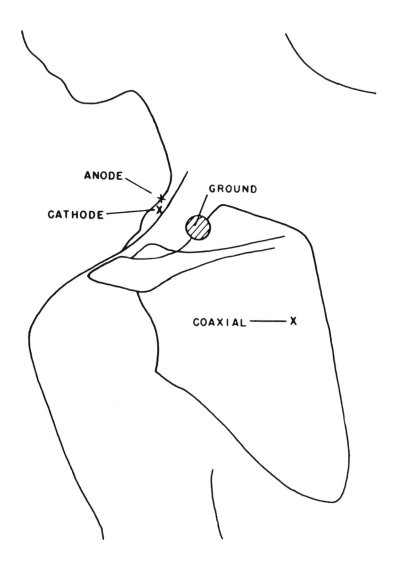

Figure 4.4. Suprascapular nerve motor latency to infraspinatus muscle.

Figure 4.4

To infraspinatus ($N = 62$)

Pickup and Reference: The coaxial needle is inserted into the infraspinatus muscle several centimeters lateral to the medial border of the scapula and several centimeters below the scapular spine. It is inserted until it touches the scapular periosteum, and then withdrawn several millimeters. The study is done with the patient sitting with arms at their side. External rotation of the shoulder confirms placement of the needle electrode.

Ground: The ground is placed between stimulation and pickup sites.

Distance: A measuring tape is used with arms at side, and the range is 15.0–19.5 cm. The distance is measured directly from the point of stimulation to the pickup using the shortest distance possible, rather than following the course of the nerve.

Normal values:

Latency: 3.3 ± 0.5 msec (mean ± 1 SD); normal range, 2.4–4.2 msec

Amplitude: 5 mV or more. It is highly variable with small needle movement

Comment: Studies were done in a room in which the temperature ranged from 75–84°F.

AXILLARY NERVE MOTOR LATENCY TO THE DELTOID

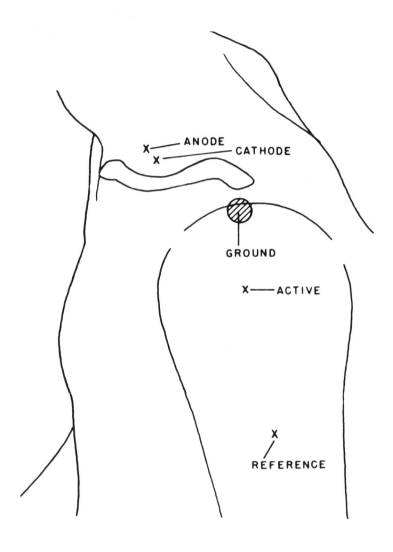

Figure 4.5. Axillary nerve motor latency to the middle deltoid muscle.

Figure 4.5

Pickup: The active surface disk electrode (8–9 mm) is placed over the most prominent portion of the middle deltoid muscle, in the region containing the motor end plate band.

Reference: The reference is over the junction of the deltoid muscle and its tendon of insertion.

Ground: The ground is between the stimulating and pickup sites.

Stimulation: The cathode is placed slightly above the upper margin of the clavicle and lateral to the clavicular head of the sternocleidomastoid. The anode is superior medially.

Electromyograph settings:
- Frequency: 8 Hz to 8 kHz
- Sweep speed: 2 msec/div
- Gain: 500 μV

Distance: Distance is measured using a flexible tape with the arm at the side, and ranges between 14.8 and 26.5 cm. Distance is measured from the point of stimulation directly to the pickup, taking the shortest distance possible, rather than following the course of the nerve.

Normal values: (N = 62)
Latency: 3.9 ± 0.5 msec (mean ± 1 SD); normal range, 2.8–5.0 msec

Comments: Studies were done in a room in which the temperature ranged from 75–84°F.

Kraft GH: Axillary, musculocutaneous and suprascapular nerve latency studies. *Arch Phys Med Rehabil* 53:383–387, 1972.

MUSCULOCUTANEOUS MOTOR LATENCY TO THE BICEPS BRACHII

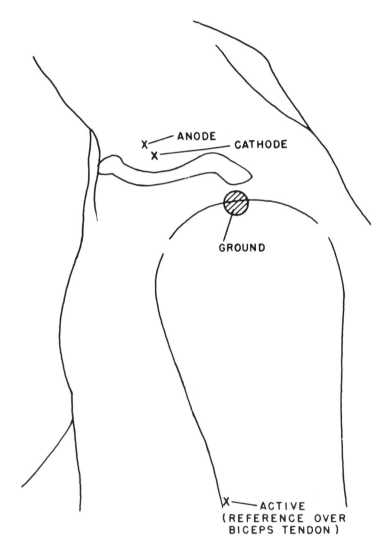

Figure 4.6. Musculocutaneous motor latency to the biceps brachii muscle.

Figure 4.6

Pickup: The active surface electrode is placed just distal to the midportion of the biceps brachii muscle.

Reference: The reference is placed proximal to the antecubital fossa, in the region of the junction of the muscle fibers and the biceps brachii tendon.

Ground: The ground is over the deltoid muscle.

Stimulation: The active cathode is slightly above the upper margin of the clavicle and lateral to the clavicular head of the sternocleidomastoid. The anode is superiorly medially.

Electromyograph settings:
- Frequency: 8 Hz to 8 kHz
- Sweep speed: 2 msec/div
- Gain: 500 μV

Distance: When a measuring tape with the arm at the side is used, the range is 23.5–41.5 cm. Distance is measured from the point of stimulation directly to the pickup site, taking the shortest distance possible, rather than following the course of the nerve.

Normal values: (N = 62)
Latency: 4.5 ± 0.6 msec (mean ± 1 SD); normal range, 3.3–5.7 msec

Comments: Studies were done in a room in which the temperature ranged from 75°F to 84°F. The initial negative deflection of the evoked compound muscle action potential is less vertical and the amplitude generally lower than that seen in the axillary nerve motor latency to the deltoid muscle.

Kraft GH: Axillary, musculocutaneous and suprascapular nerve latency studies. *Arch Phys Med Rehabil* 53:383–387, 1972.

MUSCULOCUTANEOUS SENSORY LATENCY AND NERVE CONDUCTION VELOCITY

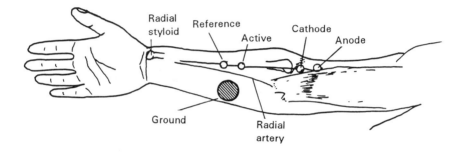

Figure 4.7. Musculocutaneous sensory latency and nerve conduction velocity.

Figure 4.7

Pickup: The active surface electrode is placed over the anterior branch of the nerve. A line is drawn between the stimulating point and the radial artery at the wrist. The active electrode is placed along this line 12 cm from the cathode.

Reference: The reference is 4 cm distal.

Ground: The ground is placed between the points of stimulation and recording.

Stimulation: The cathode is at the elbow crease just lateral to the biceps tendon, and antidromic stimulation is used.

Electromyograph settings:
- Frequency: 2 Hz to 2 kHz
- Sweep speed: 2 msec/div
- Gain: 10 μV

Normal values: (60 nerves in 30 normal adults)
Latency to *onset* of the negative phase of the compound sensory nerve action potential: 1.8 ± 0.1 msec (mean ± 1 SD); range, 1.6–2.1 msec
Latency to *peak* of the negative phase of the compound sensory nerve action potential: 2.3 ± 0.1 msec (mean ± 1 SD); range, 2.2–2.6 msec

$$\text{Conduction velocity} = \frac{12 \text{ cm}}{\text{latency to onset in msec}}$$

$$= 65 \pm 3.6 \text{ msec (mean} \pm 1 \text{ SD)}$$

Amplitude: 24 ± 7.2 μV (mean ± 1 SD); range, 12–50 μV
Right and left arm latency difference: <0.3 msec (mean ± 2 SD)

Comments: Temperature was not indicated, although all of the examinations were done at a room temperature of 23.9°C.

Spindler HA, Felsenthal G: Sensory conduction in the musculocutaneous nerve. *Arch Phys Med Rehabil* 59:20–23, 1978.

RADIAL MOTOR NERVE CONDUCTION VELOCITY

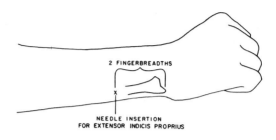

Figure 4.8. Needle electrode pickup in the extensor indicis proprius muscle for radial nerve motor nerve conduction velocity.

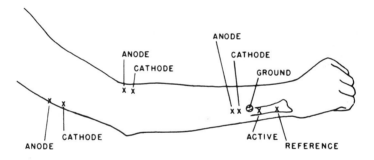

Figure 4.9. Radial nerve motor nerve conduction velocity.

Figures 4.8 and 4.9

Pickup: The active electrode is a monopolar needle inserted into the extensor indicis proprius muscle, which is located about two fingerbreadths proximal to the ulna styloid, just radial to the ulna at a depth of about 0.5 inch. Placement of the needle can be confirmed by extension of the second finger.

Reference: The reference is placed over the fifth finger.

Ground: The ground is between the pickup and stimulation sites.

Stimulation: (Testing distal to proximal segments)
1. To test the branch to the extensor indicis proprius muscle, the nerve is stimulated 3–4 cm proximal to the site of the active electrode.
2. To test the forearm portion of the radial nerve, it is stimulated in the lateral antecubital space, approximately 5–6 cm proximal to the lateral epicondyle of the humerus, between the brachialis and brachioradialis muscles.
3. To test the upper arm segment of the radial nerve in the region of the spiral groove, the nerve is stimulated just posterior to the deltoid muscle insertion. (*Note:* If the nerve is deep, increased stimulus duration may be necessary.)
4. To test the entire radial nerve distal to Erb's point, it is stimulated in the supraclavicular fossa (at the angle of the clavicle and posterior aspect of the sternocleidomastoid muscle).

Distance: The distance is measured using a tape between the above-elbow and forearm sites. An obstetrical caliper is used for a straight line measurement from Erb's point to the above-elbow site. The arm is abducted 10°, the elbow flexed 10–15°, and the forearm pronated. The head is rotated away from the stimulation site.

Electromyograph settings:
- Frequency: 8 Hz to 8 kHz
- Sweep speed: 5 msec/div
- Gain: 500 μV

Normal values: (N = 49)
   Erb's point to above elbow: 72 ± 6.3 m/sec (mean ± 1 SD); range, 56–93 m/sec
   Above elbow to the extensor indicis proprius: 61.6 ± 5.9 m/sec (mean ± 1 SD); range, 48–75 m/sec

Comments: No limb temperatures were measured.

Jebsen RH: Motor conduction velocity in proximal and distal segment of the radial nerve. *Arch Phys Med Rehabil* 47:597–602, 1966.
Trojaborg W, Sindrup EH: Motor and sensory conduction in different segments of the radial nerve in normal subjects. *J Neurol Neurosurg Psychiatry* 32:354–359, 1969.

RADIAL MOTOR NERVE CONDUCTION TO EXTENSOR DIGITORUM COMMUNIS

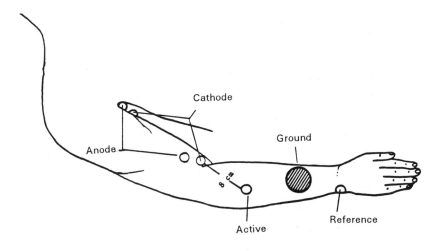

Figure 4.10.   Radial motor nerve conduction to extensor digitorum communis.

Figure 4.10

Pickup: The active surface recording electrode is placed over the extensor digitorum communis 8 cm from the stimulation point in the antecubital fossa.

Reference: The reference is placed over the ulnar styloid.

Ground: The ground is between the active and stimulating electrodes.

Stimulation: The bipolar surface stimulating electrode is applied at the antecubital fossa lateral to the biceps tendon and axilla.

Electromyograph settings:
- Gain: 5 mV/div
- Sweep speed: 5 msec/div
- Frequency: 5 Hz to 10 kHz

Normal values: (N = 30; 8 women, 22 men) Age, 21–49 years
Latency (msec): 2.6 ± 0.44
Conduction velocity (m/s): 68 ± 7.0
Amplitude (mV): 11.24 ± 3.5

Comments: Skin temperature measured over the forearm was at or above 34°C.

Young AW, Redmond MD, Hemler DE, Belandres PV: Radial motor nerve conduction studies. *Arch Phys Med Rehabil* 71:399–402, 1990.

RADIAL NERVE DISTAL SENSORY LATENCY

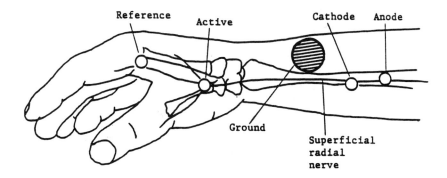

Figure 4.11. Radial nerve distal sensory latency.

Figure 4.11

Pickup: The active surface electrode is placed over the major branch of the sensory nerve as it crosses the extensor pollicis longus tendon. The nerve crosses about 1 cm distal to the extensor retinaculum. It can be palpated over the tendon when the thumb is extended.

Reference: The reference is placed on the lateral side of the head of the second metacarpal.

Ground: The ground is placed between the stimulating site and the pickup.

Stimulation: The superficial radial nerve courses along the lateral border of the radius and can be palpated. Antidromic stimulation is applied at 10, 12, or 14 cm, with the cathode played distally. Distance is measured with the wrist neutral and the thumb lightly adducted.

Electromyograph settings:
- Frequency: 8 Hz to 8 kHz
- Sweep speed: 2 or 5 msec/div
- Gain: 10 μV

Normal values: (to peak of the negative phase of the compound sensory nerve action potential: $N = 49$)

Distance (cm)	2 msec/div (mean ± 2 SD)(msec)	5 msec/div (mean ± 2 SD)(msec)
10	2.3 ± 0.4	2.4 ± 0.3
12	2.6 ± 0.4	2.8 ± 0.4
14	2.9 ± 0.4	3.1 ± 0.4

Comments: Skin temperature was measured adjacent to the pickup electrode. The values reported are for a temperature range of 31–35°C. For colder hands, if the latency is outside the range of 2 SDs, hot packs are applied to warm them, and then the study repeated.

Mackenzie K, DeLisa JA: Determining the distal sensory latency of the superficial radial nerve in normal adult subjects. *Arch Phys Med Rehabil* 62:31–34, 1981.

ANTERIOR INTEROSSEOUS NERVE MOTOR LATENCY TO THE PRONATOR QUADRATUS

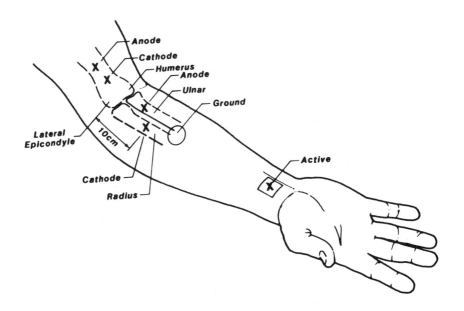

Figure 4.12. Anterior interosseous nerve motor latency to the pronator quadratus.

Figure 4.12
Nakano et al.

Pickup: A concentric needle electrode is placed in the pronator quadratus muscle. If the initial waveform deflection is not negative (upward), then the needle electrode is moved until the negative initial deflection occurs.

Reference: The reference is placed on the phalanx of the thumb.

Ground: The ground is placed in the volar surface of the forearm between the stimulation and pickup sites.

Stimulation: *Above elbow:* surface stimulation on the ventromedial aspect of the arm, medial to the biceps brachii. *Below elbow:* 10 cm below the level of the lateral epicondyle, over the flexor digitorum superficialis muscle.

Electromyograph settings:
- Frequency: 20 Hz to 2 kHz
- Sweep speed: 5 msec/div
- Gain: 20 μV to 1 kV

Normal values: (N = 84) Age, 9–67 years; mean age, 40.2
Proximal latency to onset of potential: 5.1 ± 0.9 msec (mean ± 1 SD)
Distal latency to onset of potential: 3.6 ± 0.8 msec (mean ± 1 SD)
Duration of compound motor action potential (first negative deflection to the isoelectric point of the negative spike): 3.6 ± 1.1 msec

Comments: Skin temperature was not measured. No fixed distance was used, nor was a range of distances reported. In their study of seven patients with anterior interosseous syndrome, Nakano et al. found that all had a prolonged duration of the compound motor action potential, whereas five (70%) had a prolonged latency from the elbow.

Nakano KK, Lundergan C, Okihiro MM: Anterior interosseous nerve syndromes. *Arch Neurol* 34:477–480, 1977.
Mysiw WJ, Colachis SC III: Electrophysiologic study of the anterior interosseous nerve. *Am J Phys Med Rehabil* 67:50–54, 1988.

Mysiw et al.

Pickup: The active surface recording electrode is placed over the dorsum of the forearm 3 cm proximal to the ulnar styloid.

Reference: The reference is attached to the ulnar styloid.

Ground: The ground is placed between the stimulating and recording electrodes.

Stimulation: Using conventional median nerve stimulation technique, the stimulation is applied at the elbow.

Electromyograph settings:
* Frequency: 20–10,000 Hz
* Gain: 500 μV/div
* Sweep speed: 2 msec/div

Normal values: (N = 52, S = 26) Age, 24–63 years (mean age, 30.2 years)

	Right	Left
Latency (msec)	3.6 ± 0.4	3.5 ± 0.4
Amplitude (mV)	3.1 ± 0.8	3.1 ± 0.8
Distance: 17.5–28 cm (mean, 23 cm)		

Comments: The skin temperature was measured at the volar aspect of the midforearm and controlled to 32–34°C. In a sitting position, the elbow was flexed to 90° and the forearm was pronated.

MEDIAN MOTOR NERVE CONDUCTION VELOCITY AND LATENCY

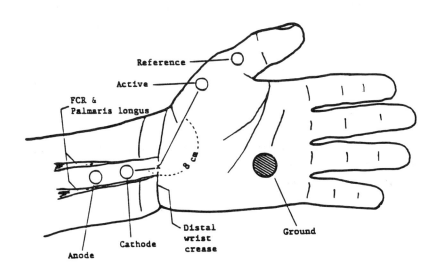

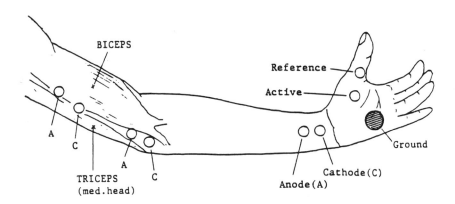

Figure 4.13.   Median motor nerve conduction velocity and latency.

Figure 4.13

Pickup: The active surface electrode is placed one-half the distance (prominence of abductor pollicis brevis) between the metacarpophalangeal joint of the thumb and the midpoint of the distal wrist crease.

Reference: The reference is placed on the distal phalanx of the thumb.

Ground: The ground is between the pickup electrode and the stimulating electrode.

Stimulation: Stimulation is applied with the cathode 8 cm proximal to where the active electrode is placed, as shown in Figure 4.15, between the flexor carpi radialis and the palmaris longus tendons. Proximal stimulation is applied in the medial aspect of the antecubital space, just lateral to the brachial artery.

Electromyograph settings:
- Frequency: 8 Hz to 8 kHz
- Sweep speed: 5 msec/div
- Gain: 1,000 μV

Normal values: (N = 47)

Distal latency: 3.7 ± 0.3 msec (mean ± 1 SD); range, 3.2–4.2 msec

Velocity: 56.7 ± 3.8 m/sec (mean ± 1 SD); range, 50.0–67.3 m/sec

Amplitude of the evoked potential at the wrist: 13.2 mV ± 5.0 (mean ± 1 SD); range, 5–25 mV

Amplitude of the evoked potential at the elbow: 13.5 mV ± 4.1 (mean ± 1 SD); range, 5–23 mV

Comment: Skin temperature was not recorded.

Melvin JL, Harris DH, Johnson EW: Sensory and motor conduction velocities in the ulnar and median nerves. *Arch Phys Med Rehabil* 47:511–519, 1966.

Melvin JL, Schuchmann JA, Lanese RR: Diagnostic specificity of motor and sensory nerve conduction variables in the carpal tunnel syndrome. *Arch Phys Med Rehabil* 54:69–74, 1973.

Buchthal F, Rosenfalck A, Trojaborg W: Electrophysiological findings in entrapment of the median nerve of wrist and elbow. *J Neurol Neurosurg Psychiatry* 37:340–360, 1974.

MEDIAN NERVE DISTAL SENSORY LATENCY

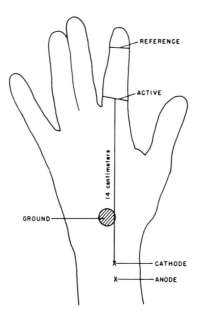

Figure 4.14. Median nerve distal sensory latency (palmar surface with antidromic technique).

Melvin JL, Harris DH, Johnson EW: Sensory and motor conduction velocities in the ulnar and median nerves. *Arch Phys Med Rehabil* 47:511–519, 1966.

Johnson EW, Melvin JL: Sensory conduction studies of median and ulnar nerves. *Arch Phys Med Rehabil* 48:25–30, 1967.

Melvin JL, Schuchmann JA, Lanese RR: Diagnostic specificity of motor and sensory nerve conduction variables in the carpal tunnel syndrome. *Arch Phys Med Rehabil* 54:69–74, 1973.

Figure 4.14

Pickup: Ring recording electrodes are placed on digits 2, 3, or both. The active and reference electrodes are placed 4 cm apart, mounted in a plastic bar, with the active proximal at the base of the digits.

Ground: The ground is placed between the pickup and stimulation electrodes.

Stimulation: Stimulating cathode is applied 14 cm proximal (straight line) from the active ring electrode, over the median nerve between the tendons of the palmaris longus and flexor carpi radialis. Stimulation also may be applied medial to the biceps tendon. The anode is proximal.

Orthodromic:

Pickup: The active and reference electrodes are 4 cm apart, mounted in a plastic bar with the active placed distally 14 cm from the cathode, over the median nerve between the tendons of the palmaris longus and flexor carpi radialis.

Ground: The ground is placed between the pickup and stimulating electrodes.

Stimulation: Stimulation is applied with ring electrodes, 4 cm apart, around digits 2 and 3 with the cathode at the base of the digits.

Electromyograph settings:
- Frequency: 8 Hz to 1.6 kHz
- Sweep speed: 5 msec/div, measure on 2 msec/div
- Gain: 10 μV

Normal values: (N = 24)
Latency to peak: 3.2 ± 0.2 msec (mean ± 1 SD), for both the orthodromic and the antidromic techniques.
Forearm sensory conduction velocity: 56.9 ± 4.0 m/sec (mean ± 1 SD); range, 48–64.9 m/sec
Amplitude of potentials: 41.6 ± 25 μV (mean ± 1 SD); range, 10–90 μV

Comment: Skin temperature was not reported.

MEDIAN NERVE SENSORY CONDUCTION: SHORT SEGMENT STIMULATION AT THE WRIST

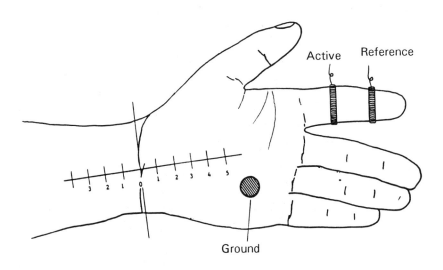

Figure 4.15. Median nerve sensory conduction: short segment stimulation at the wrist.

Figure 4.15

Recording: The ring electrodes are placed around the proximal (G1) and distal (G2) interphalangeal joints of the second digit.

Ground: The ground is placed around the forearm.

Stimulation: The stimulation is applied at 1-cm intervals along the 12 cm of median nerve. The "0" point is assigned at the distal wrist crease. A negative sign is designated distal stimulation point from the distal wrist crease.

Normal values: (N = 122) Age, 15–50 years (mean age, 43 years)

Stimulation points	Latency (msec) change
−5 to −4	0.17 ± 0.08
−4 to −3	0.22 ± 0.10
−3 to −2	0.20 ± 0.09
−2 to −1	0.19 ± 0.08
−1 to 0	0.16 ± 0.08

Comments: Skin temperature was measured over the forearm and maintained at 34°C or greater. The latency was measured from the stimulus artifact to the onset of the initial negative peak.

Kimura J: The carpal tunnel syndrome: Localization of conduction abnormalities within the distal segment of the median nerve. *Brain* 102:619–635, 1979.

MEDIAN AND ULNAR ANTIDROMIC SENSORY
LATENCIES TO THE RING FINGER

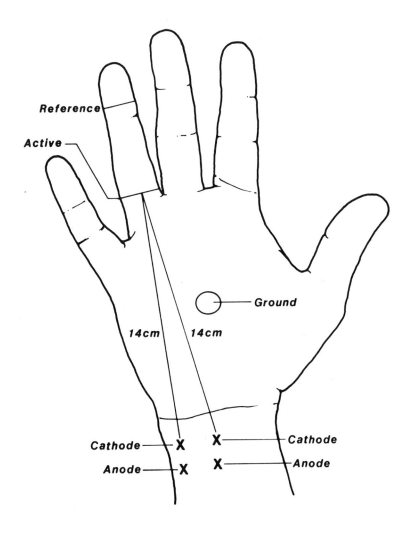

Figure 4.16.   Median and ulnar antidromic sensory latencies to the ring finger.

Figure 4.16

Pickup: Ring active and reference electrodes are placed on the fourth (ring) digit with at least a 4-cm separation. The active is proximal at the base of the digit.

Ground: The ground is between the stimulating and pickup electrodes.

Stimulation: Stimulation was done over the median and ulnar nerves at the wrist 14 cm proximal to the recording electrodes.

Electromyograph settings:
- Frequency: 8 Hz to 1.6 kHz
- Sweep speed: 1 msec/div
- Gain: 20 μV

Normal values: (N = 37; 18 women, 19 men)

Numbers in parentheses are mean ± 2 SD (msec):

Patients (N)	Age range (years)	Sex		Dominant hand	
		F	M	Median IV	Ulnar IV
10	20–29	5	5	3.12 ± 0.18 (3.5)	3.11 ± 0.15 (3.4)
10	30–39	4	6	2.96 ± 0.15 (3.3)	2.89 ± 0.20 (3.3)
7	40–49	4	3	3.19 ± 0.27 (3.7)	3.04 ± 0.20 (3.4)
10	50–59	5	5	3.30 ± 0.23 (3.8)	3.08 ± 0.23 (3.5)
37		18	19	3.14 ± 0.24 (3.6)	3.03 ± 0.21 (3.5)

Johnson EW, Kukla RD, Wongsam PE, Piedmont A: Sensory latencies to the ring finger: Normal values and relation to carpal tunnel syndrome. *Arch Phys Med Rehab* 62: 206–208, 1981.

Subjects (N)	Age range (years)	Sex		Nondominant hand	
		F	M	Median IV	Ulnar IV
10	20–29	5	5	3.15 ± 0.18 (3.5)	3.06 ± 0.16 (3.4)
10	30–39	4	6	2.96 ± 0.22 (3.4)	2.91 ± 0.20 (3.3)
7	40–49	4	3	3.19 ± 0.30 (3.8)	3.19 ± 0.29 (3.8)
10	50–59	5	5	3.28 ± 0.24 (3.8)	3.12 ± 0.24 (3.6)
37		18	19	3.11 ± 0.32 (3.7)	3.01 ± 0.32 (3.6)

Comment: Skin temperature was not reported.

MEDIAN AND ULNAR ORTHODROMIC SENSORY CONDUCTION WITH THE RING FINGER STIMULATION

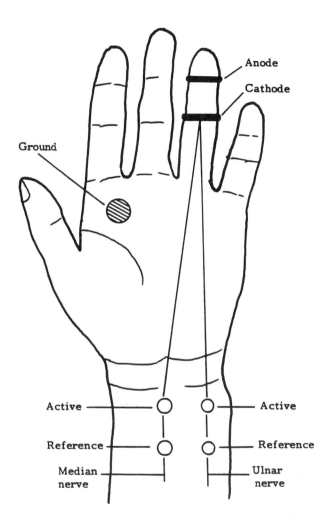

Figure 4.17. Median and ulnar orthodromic sensory conduction with the ring finger stimulation.

Figure 4.17

Pickup: The active surface electrode is placed at the same distance over the median and ulnar nerves at the wrist.

Reference: The reference surface electrode is placed proximal to the active electrode.

Ground: The ground is placed on the palm.

Stimulation: The stimulating ring electrodes are placed on the fourth digit. The cathode is placed proximal to the anode.

Electromyograph settings:
• Frequency: 10 Hz to 2 kHz

Normal values: (N = 43)

Latency:	Onset (msec)	Peak (msec)	Amplitude (μV)
Median	2.4 ± 0.2 (1.9–2.9)	2.9 ± 0.3 (2.4–3.3)	14.7 ± 5.5
Ulnar	2.3 ± 0.2 (1.9–2.8)	2.8 ± 0.3 (2.3–3.3)	10.2 ± 4.4

Distance: 130 ± 11.2 mm

Comments: This is a useful screening test for carpal tunnel syndrome. The double peak appearance of sensory potentials recorded over the median nerve at the wrist after fourth digit stimulation is suspicious for an early carpal tunnel syndrome.

Uncini A, Lange DJ, Solomon M, et al.: Ring finger testing in carpal tunnel syndrome: A comparative study of diagnostic utility. *Muscle Nerve* 12:735–741, 1989.

MEDIAN PALMAR CUTANEOUS NERVE CONDUCTION: ORTHODROMIC AND ANTIDROMIC STUDIES

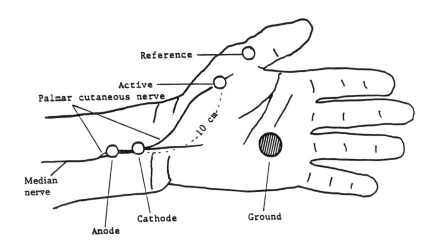

Figure 4.18. Median palmar cutaneous nerve conduction: orthodromic and antidromic studies.

Figure 4.18
Chang et al.

Pickup: The active electrode is placed 10 cm proximal to the stimulating electrode along the median nerve at the wrist.

Stimulation: The stimulating electrode is placed over the thenar eminence.

Normal values: (N = 40) Age, 22–60 years (mean age, 38.6 years)
NCV: 43.34 ± 3.52 m/sec (39.16–52.18)
Latency: 2.24 ± 0.18 msec (1.92–2.56)

Comments: Orthodromic study. Sensory nerve conduction in palmar cutaneous branch and digit I sensory nerves was compared.

Lum et al.

Pickup: The active surface electrode is placed on the midthenar eminence.

Reference: The reference is placed 3 cm distally to the active electrode on the thumb.

Ground: The ground is placed between the active and the stimulating cathodes.

Stimulation: The stimulating electrode is placed 10 cm proximal to the active electrode along the median nerve at the wrist.

Electromyograph settings:
• Frequency: 20 Hz to 2 kHz
• Sweep speed: 2 msec/div
• Gain: 5 μV/div

Normal values: (N = 50)
Latency: 2.6 ± 0.2 msec
Amplitude: 12 ± 4.6 μV

Comments: The study was performed at a room temperature of 25–27°C.

Chang CW, Lien IN: Comparison of sensory nerve conduction in the palmar cutaneous branch and first digital branch of the median nerve: A new diagnostic method for carpal tunnel syndrome. *Muscle Nerve* 14:1173–1176, 1991.
Lum PB, Kanakamedala R: Conduction of the palmar cutaneous branch of the median nerve. *Arch Phys Med Rehabil* 67:805–806, 1986.

C-8 AND T-1 NERVE ROOT STIMULATION

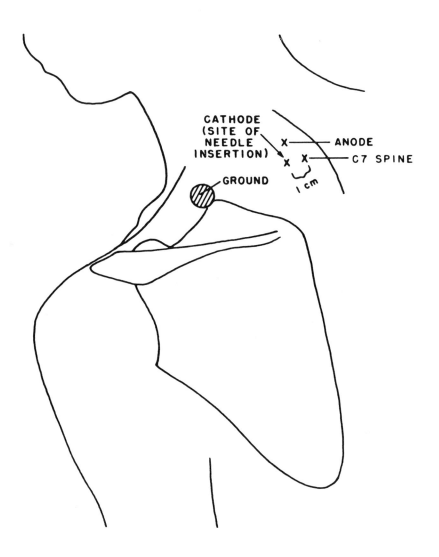

Figure 4.19. C-8 and T-1 nerve root stimulation.

Figure 4.19

Pickup: The active surface electrode is placed in the hypothenar eminence (abductor digiti minimi) on a point midway between the distal wrist crease and the crease at the base of the fifth digit, at the junction of dorsal and palmar skin.

Reference: The reference is placed on the distal fifth digit.

Ground: The ground is over the lateral neck, back of the lateral neck, or over the back.

Stimulation: The active cathode is 1–2 cm lateral and slightly caudal to the seventh cervical spinous process. A 2-inch monopolar needle is inserted perpendicular to the skin surface in a sagittal plane until the tip rests directly over the vertebral transverse process. If the needle is not at this depth, the current intensity required to depolarize the nerve roots greatly increases. The anode is placed over the bony scapula, close to the stimulating electrode.

Electromyograph settings:
- Frequency: 8 Hz to 8 kHz
- Sweep speed: 3 msec/div is best for takeoff and 5 msec/div is best for entire M response
- Gain: 500 μV
- Duration of stimulus: 0.1–0.2 msec
- Stimulus intensity: approximately 100–150 V

Normal values: A 0.4-msec difference from side to side = 1 SD. A 1-msec difference between the sides is abnormal, but problems must be ruled out at the wrist and elbow.

Comments:
- 1. The *C-8 and T-1 roots* are used to measure across the lower trunk and medial cord of the brachial plexus.

MacLean IC: Nerve root stimulation to evaluate conduction across the brachial and lumbosacral plexus. Recent advances in clinical electromyography. *American Association of Electromyography and Electrodiagnosis Third Annual Continuing Education Course* 51–55. September 1980.

2. The *C-5 and C-6 roots* can be stimulated together as a pair to measure the conduction across the upper trunk and lateral cord of the brachial plexus. The stimulating needle electrode is placed 1–2 cm lateral to the C-5 spinous process with the surface recording electrode over the middle of the biceps brachii muscle.

3. The posterior cord can be evaluated by stimulating the *C-6, C-7, and C-8 roots*. The stimulating cathode electrode is put between the sites for the C-5 and C-6 and the C-8 and T-1 stimulation. The surface recording electrode is over the middle of the triceps brachii muscle.

ELECTRODIAGNOSTIC VALUES THROUGH THE THORACIC OUTLET USING C-8 ROOT NEEDLE STUDIES, F WAVES, AND CERVICAL SOMATOSENSORY EVOKED POTENTIALS

C-8 Nerve Root Stimulation:

Pickup: The active electrode is placed on the medial midhumerus, 35 cm from the C-7 spinous process, between the flexor and extensor muscle compartments, over the ulnar nerve.

Reference: The bar surface electrode is placed at the 35-cm medial midhumerus position.

Ground: The ground is over the lateral neck, back of the lateral neck, or over the back.

Stimulation: The active cathode is placed 1.5 cm laterally from the midline and just caudally to the C-7 vertebral spinous process. The needle anode electrode was placed approximately 2 cm inferior to the stimulating needle cathode.

Livingston EF, DeLisa JA, Halar EM: Electrodiagnostic values through the thoracic outlet using C-8 root needle studies, F waves, and cervical somatosensory evoked potentials. *Arch Phys Med Rehabil* 65:726–730, 1984.

Electromyograph settings:
- Frequency: 10 Hz to 2 kHz
- Sweep speed: 5 msec/div
- Gain: 50 μV

Normal values: (N = 20 normal adults, both arms)
Latency measured to onset, the amplitude from the takeoff to the negative peak.

C-8 Root Needle Stimulation: Midhumerus Pickup:

	Latency (msec) (mean ± SD)	Velocity (m/sec) (mean ± SD)	Amplitude (μV) (mean ± SD)
Bilateral	4.9 ± 0.2	71.4 ± 2.2	22.7 ± 10.7
Right	4.9 ± 0.2	71.4 ± 2.4	22.2 ± 10.5
Left	4.9 ± 0.1	71.5 ± 1.9	23.2 ± 11.2
Range:	4.7–5.3	63.3–74.5	6.1–39.4

Comment: The 35-cm distance is marked by using a caliper and measuring from the C-7 spinous process, with the patient seated, head in neutral position, shoulders abducted 60° and internally rotated 45°, and elbows flexed to 65°. The 35 cm is the distance marked on the medial midhumerus between the flexor and extensor compartments.

Midhumerus Stimulation:

Opposite technique from above; reverse stimulation and recording sites, ground electrode, and distance remain the same.

Pickup: The needle electrode is the active electrode and is placed over the C-8 root.

Normal values: (N = 20 normal adults, both arms)
Latency measured to the negative peak and amplitude from takeoff to the negative peak.

	Latency (msec), negative peak (mean ± SD)	Amplitude (μV), takeoff to negative peak (mean ± SD)
Bilateral	5.1 ± 0.4	2.0 ± 0.6
Right	5.1 ± 0.4	2.0 ± 0.6
Left	5.2 ± 0.4	1.9 ± 0.6
Range:	4.4–5.9	1.0–3.3

Comment: Each series of stimulation was an average trace of 256 stimulations. Three or four series were then averaged for each upper extremity to verify reproductive waveforms.

Ulnar F-Wave Stimulation at the 35-cm Mark (Midhumerus):

Pickup: The active surface electrode is over the abductor digiti quinti.

Reference: The reference is on the fifth digit.

Ground: The ground is between the stimulation and pickup sites.

Stimulation: The midhumeral F wave was obtained with stimulation at this 35-cm mark, using collision technique with simultaneous countershock applied at the wrist.

Electromyograph settings:
- Frequency: 10 Hz to 2 kHz
- Sweep speed: 5 msec/div
- Gain: 250 μV

Normal values: (N = 20 normal adults, both arms)

	Latency (msec) (mean ± SD)	Velocity (m/sec) (mean ± SD)
Minimal F wave		
Bilateral	21.8 ± 1.2	59.7 ± 2.4
Right	21.7 ± 1.1	59.9 ± 2.4
Left	21.8 ± 1.3	59.5 ± 2.6
Range:	19.9–24.4	55.2–64.9
Maximal F wave		
Bilateral	23.4 ± 1.2	
Right	23.0 ± 1.1	
Left	23.1 ± 1.3	
Range:	20.9–26.0	
F-wave latency, mean of 10		
Bilateral	22.3 ± 1.1	
Right	22.3 ± 1.1	
Left	22.3 ± 1.2	
Range:	20.4–25.2	

	Latency (msec) (mean ± SD)	Velocity (m/sec) (mean ± SD)
Difference minimal–maximal F-wave latency		
Bilateral	1.4 ± 0.4	
Right	1.4 ± 0.3	
Left	1.4 ± 0.4	
Range:	0.6–2.5	
F-wave duration		
Bilateral		9.7 ± 0.6 msec
Right		9.7 ± 0.5 msec
Left		9.7 ± 0.6 msec
Range:		8.5–10.8 msec

Comment: The minimal and maximal onset latencies of 10 F waves, as well as the average onset of 10 F waves, were obtained and the velocity calculated.

ULNAR MOTOR NERVE CONDUCTION VELOCITY

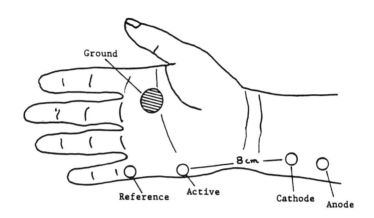

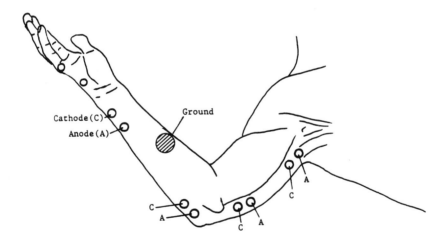

Figure 4.20. Ulnar motor nerve conduction velocity.

Figure 4.20

Pickup: The active surface electrode is placed on the abductor digiti minimi on a point midway between the distal wrist crease and the crease at the base of the fifth digit, at the junction of the dorsal palmar skin.

Reference: The reference is on the fifth digit.

Ground: The ground is between the stimulation and pickup sites.

Stimulation: Stimulation is applied (a) 8 cm proximal to the active recording electrode and just over the flexor carpi ulnaris tendon, (b) just distal to the ulnar groove, and then (c) proximal to the ulnar groove.

Electromyograph settings:
- Frequency: 8 Hz to 8 kHz
- Sweep speed: 5 msec/div
- Gain: 1,000 μV

Distance: Measurement across the elbow is done with the elbow flexed to 70° (elbow straight is 180°). The arm may be tested in the straight position and flexed for measurements.

Normal values: (N = 31 nerves in 18 adults)
Distal latency to onset: 3.2 ± 0.5 msec (mean ± 1 SD)
Motor forearm segment velocity: 61.8 ± 5.0 m/sec (mean ± 1 SD); range, 53–73 m/sec
Motor across the elbow segment velocity: 62.7 ± 5.5 m/sec (mean ± 1 SD); range, 52–74 m/sec

Amplitude of the evoked muscle response:

Stimulation site	Mean ± 1 SD (mV)	Range (mV)
Wrist	6.14 ± 1.90	2.34–9.94
Below elbow	5.60 ± 1.98	1.64–9.56
Across elbow	5.77 ± 1.79	2.19–9.35

Comments: The temperature was not recorded.

Melvin JL, Harris DH, Johnson EW: Sensory and motor conduction velocities in the ulnar and median nerves. *Arch Phys Med Rehabil* 47:511–519, 1966.
Checkles NS, Russakov AD, Piero DL: Ulnar nerve conduction velocity: Effect of elbow position on measurement. *Arch Phys Med Rehabil* 52:362–365, 1971.

ULNAR NERVE MOTOR CONDUCTION LATENCY TO THE FIRST DORSAL INTEROSSEOUS MUSCLE

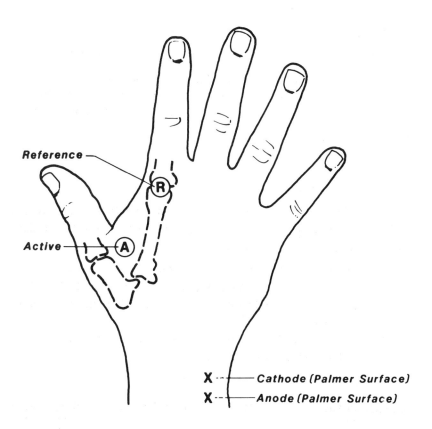

Figure 4.21. Ulnar nerve motor conduction latency to the first dorsal interosseous muscle.

Figure 4.21

Pickup:
1. The active surface electrode is placed on the abductor digit minimi (ADM) on a point midway between the distal wrist crease and the crease at the base of the fifth digit, at the junction of the dorsal palmer skin.
2. The second active surface electrode is placed on the first dorsal interosseous (FDI) at the proximal edge of the muscle, near the apposition of the first and second carpal–metacarpal joints.

Reference: The reference electrode is placed over the metacarpophalangeal joint.

Ground: The ground is placed between the stimulation and pickup sites.

Stimulation: Supramaximal stimulation of the ulnar nerve just over the flexor carpi ulnaris tendon with the cathode at the proximal wrist crease.

Electromyograph settings:
- Frequency: 8 Hz to 8 kHz
- Sweep speed: 5 msec/div
- Gain: 1,000 μV

Normal values: (N = 373 ulnar nerves in 188 persons studied)

Olney RK, Wilbourn AJ: Ulnar nerve conduction study of the first dorsal interosseous muscle. *Arch Phys Med Rehabil* 66:16–18, 1985.

Mean and Range for Distal Motor Latency by Decade:

| Age | | Latency (msec) | |
| | | ADM* | FDI* |
(years)	N	mean (range)	mean (range)
<20	14	2.5 (2.2–2.9)	3.3 (2.7–4.2)
20–29	48	2.5 (2.0–3.0)	3.4 (2.6–4.1)
30–39	103	2.4 (1.8–3.2)	3.3 (2.5–4.4)
40–49	82	2.5 (2.0–3.0)	3.2 (2.3–4.2)
50–59	84	2.6 (2.0–3.4)	3.4 (2.6–4.4)
60–69	34	2.7 (2.2–3.1)	3.6 (3.0–4.5)
>70	8	2.7 (2.3–3.1)	3.6 (3.0–4.2)

* Mean (minimum–maximum): side-to-side difference; ADM = 0.2 msec (0.0–1.0); FDI = 0.2 msec (0.0–1.3); ipsilateral difference, FDI − ADM = 0.9 msec (0.2–2.0).

Mean and Range for Amplitude by Decade:

| Age | | Amplitude (mV) | |
| | | ADM* | FDI* |
(years)	N	mean (range)	mean (range)
<20	14	13 (11–16)	15 (8–23)
20–29	48	12 (5–20)	14 (8–22)
30–39	103	12 (6–21)	15 (6–24)
40–49	82	12 (6–19)	13 (6–22)
50–59	84	11 (7–17)	13 (6–20)
60–69	34	12 (6–15)	12 (7–20)
>70	8	10 (8–13)	12 (8–15)

* Mean (minimum–maximum).

The distal motor latency to the first dorsal interosseous muscle should not exceed the distal motor latency to the contralateral first dorsal interosseous muscle by more than 1.3 msec; nor should this value exceed the distal motor latency to the ipsilateral abductor digiti minimi latency by more than 2.0 msec.

Comments:
1. Surface temperature over the first dorsal interosseous muscle was greater than 32°C.
2. The distance was not indicated.
3. The initial deflection for the CMAP recording over the first dorsal interosseous was negative. The amplitude of the CMAP was frequently increased from one to several millivolts by moving the active electrode over the center of the fleshy belly of the first dorsal interosseous muscle. This larger CMAP was usually associated with a small initial positive deflection. The initial positive deflection may be prevented when the reference is placed over the metacarpal phalangeal joint of the thumb.

ULNAR NERVE MOTOR CONDUCTION ACROSS THE ELBOW: SHORT SEGMENT STIMULATION

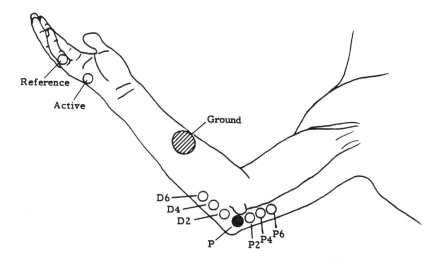

Figure 4.22. Ulnar nerve motor conduction across the elbow: short segment stimulation.

Figure 4.22

Pickup: The active surface electrode is placed over the hypothenar eminence.

Reference: The reference electrode is placed over the proximal part of the fifth finger.

Stimulation: The stimulation is applied 8 cm proximal to the active electrode at the wrist. A point "P" is located along the course of the ulnar nerve on a line passing through the medial epicondyle perpendicular to the medial border of the ulna. The distal points (D2 and D4) and the proximal points (P2, P4, and P6) are 2 and 4 cm distal or 2, 4, and 6 cm proximal, respectively, to the point "P." At 2 cm apart, each point of the ulnar nerve is supramaximally stimulated (see Fig. 4.22).

Normal values: (N = 25; 14 men and 6 women) Age, 27–58 years; mean age for men = 42; mean age for women = 35

Conduction time (msec) between points

D4–D2	D2–P	P–P2	P2–P4	P4–P6
Right (N = 12)				
0.37 ± 0.08	0.43 ± 0.10	0.38 ± 0.08	0.40 ± 0.08	0.34 ± 0.07
(0.24–0.60)	(0.29–0.48)	(0.24–0.54)	(0.24–0.48)	(0.23–0.48)
Left (N = 13)				
0.36 ± 0.07	0.44 ± 0.08	0.42 ± 0.09	0.39 ± 0.10	0.35 ± 0.05
(0.23–0.48)	(0.3–0.60)	(0.32–0.58)	(0.24–0.60)	(0.24–0.44)

Kanakamedala RV, Simons DG, Porter RW, Zucker RS: Ulnar nerve entrapment at the elbow localized by the short segment stimulation. *Arch Phys Med Rehabil* 69:959–963, 1988.

Campbell WW, Pridgeon RM, Sahni KS: Short segment incremental studies in the evaluation of ulnar neuropathy at the elbow. *Muscle Nerve* 15:1050–1054, 1992.

Stimulation site	Amplitude changes (mV)	
	Right	Left
Wrist	6.1 ± 1.3 (4.1–8.5)	7.2 ± 2.3 (4.1–11.3)
D4	5.8 ± 1.1 (3.4–7.5)	6.6 ± 2.2 (3.7–11.2)
D2	5.7 ± 1.0 (3.4–7.5)	6.5 ± 2.1 (3.4–10.7)
P	5.7 ± 1.1 (3.2–7.5)	6.4 ± 2.1 (3.7–10)
P2	5.6 ± 1.1 (3.2–7.4)	6.2 ± 2.0 (3.7–10)
P4	5.6 ± 1.1 (3.2–7.4)	6.2 ± 2.1 (3.7–10)
P6	5.6 ± 1.0 (3.2–7.2)	6.2 ± 2.1 (3.7–10)

Comments: The nerve conduction is performed with the elbow flexed to 90° and with the shoulder abducted 40°. The amplitude is measured from the baseline to the negative peak of the potential. The test is useful in localizing the exact site of the lesion of the ulnar nerve at the elbow.

Campbell et al.:
Short segment stimulation studies (1-cm interval) was used to search the discrete points of change in compound muscle action potential amplitude or configuration. A latency change over a 1-cm segment more than 0.40 msec is abnormal (mean + 2 SD).

ULNAR NERVE DISTAL SENSORY LATENCY

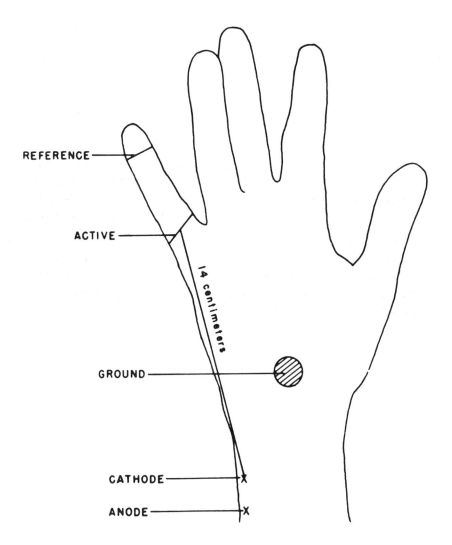

Figure 4.23. Ulnar nerve distal sensory latency (palmar surface with antidromic technique).

Figure 4.23

Antidromic:

Pickup: Ring active and reference electrodes are placed on the fifth digit with at least a 4-cm separation, if possible. The active is proximal at the base of the digit.

Ground: The ground is between the stimulating and pickup electrodes.

Stimulation: Stimulation is applied 14 cm proximally, just radial to the flexor carpi ulnaris. The cathode is distal. Stimulation also may be applied proximally at the elbow in the ulnar groove.

Orthodromic:

Pickup: The active and reference electrodes are 4 cm apart with the active placed distally 14 cm from the cathode (over the flexor carpi ulnaris tendon).

Ground: The ground is placed between the stimulating and pickup electrodes.

Stimulation: Stimulation is applied with ring electrodes around the fourth and fifth fingers, 4 cm apart, with the cathode at the base of the digits.

Electromyograph settings:
- Frequency: 8 Hz to 1.6 kHz
- Sweep speed: 5 msec/div initially; measure on 2 msec/div
- Gain: 10 μV

Normal values: (N = 120)
  Distal latency to peak: 3.2 ± 0.25 msec (mean ± 1 SD), for both orthodromic and antidromic techniques
  Forearm sensory conduction velocity: 57 ± 5.0 m/sec (mean ± 1 SD)
  Amplitude of the potential: 15–50 μV

Comments: Skin temperature was not reported. With antidromic conduction the motor artifact may appear.

Johnson EW, Melvin JL: Sensory conduction studies of median and ulnar nerves. *Arch Phys Med Rehabil* 48:25–30, 1967.

DORSAL CUTANEOUS ULNAR NERVE CONDUCTION

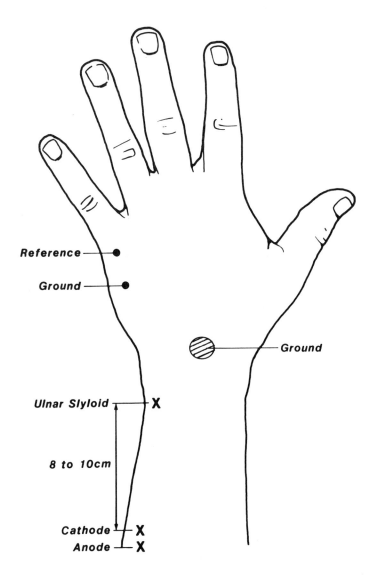

Figure 4.24. Dorsal cutaneous ulnar nerve conduction (Kim et al. antidromic technique).

Figure 4.24
Kim et al.

Pickup: The active electrode is a standard TECA type, plastic-mounted surface electrode taped along the dorsum of the fifth metacarpal bone.

Reference: The reference surface electrode is at the level of the fifth metacarpal phalangeal joint.

Ground: The ground is on the dorsum of the hand between the stimulation and pickup sites.

Stimulation: Stimulation is applied between the flexor carpi ulnaris and ulna where the nerve becomes superficial. Kim reports this as being 8–10 cm proximal to the ulnar styloid. This gave him an average distance between cathode and pickup of 11–12 cm.

Electromyograph settings:
- Frequency: 20 Hz to 2 kHz
- Sweep speed: 2 msec/div
- Gain: 20 μV

Normal values: (N = 66) Age, 21–71 years
Distal latency to peak: 2.1 $\pm$ 0.3 msec (mean $\pm$ 1 SD)
Sensory NCV: 47.8 $\pm$ 3.8 m/sec (mean $\pm$ 1 SD)
Peak-to-peak amplitude of potential: 24.2 $\pm$ 10.8 μV (mean $\pm$ 1 SD)

Comments: Kim et al.'s NCV represents distal conduction across the wrist from the site of stimulus to the pickup. The authors indicate that this technique is useful for localizing a lesion proximal or distal to the branching of the sensory dorsal branch of the ulnar nerve.

Kim DJ, Kalantri A, Guha S, Wainapel SF: Dorsal cutaneous nerve conduction: Diagnostic aid in ulnar neuropathy. *Arch Neurol* 38:321–322, 1981.

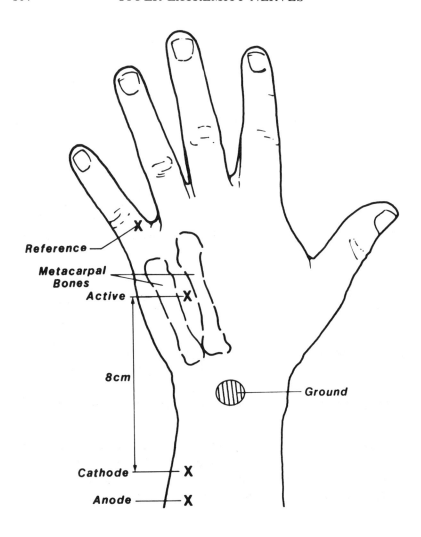

Figure 4.25. Dorsal cutaneous ulnar nerve conduction (Jabre antidromic technique).

Figure 4.25
Jabre

Pickup: Active electrode was placed on dorsum of hand at the bottom of the "V" formed between the fourth and fifth metacarpal bones (this space can be palpated).

Reference: The reference electrode is placed on the dorsum of the base of the proximal phalanx of the fifth digit.

Ground: The ground is on the dorsum of the hand between the stimulation and pickup sites.

Stimulation: Stimulation is applied 8 cm proximal to the active electrode in the space between the ulna and the flexor carpi ulnaris tendon.

Electromyograph settings:
- Frequency: 20 Hz to 2 kHz
- Sweep speed: 2 msec/div
- Gain: 20 μV

Normal values: (N = 50 limbs in 30 volunteers) Age 10–66 years
Distal latency: 2.0 ± 0.3 msec (mean ± 1 SD)
Sensory NCV (N = 16): 60 ± 4.0 m/sec (mean ± 1 SD)
Peak-to-peak amplitude: 20 ± 6.0 μV (mean ± 1 SD)

Comments: Jabre's NCV represents a segment between the wrist and the elbow. Skin temperature was not measured. He felt that this method was a simple means of localizing a lesion proximal or distal to the takeoff of the sensory dorsal branch of the ulnar nerve and for studying the ulnar nerve segment proximal to a wrist lesion when the routine sensory and motor amplitudes are depressed or absent: 11% of his normal patients have asymmetric dorsal sensory responses, with a difference of 50% or more in amplitude between the two arms.

Jabre JF: Ulnar nerve lesions at the wrist: New techniques for recording from the sensory dorsal branch of the ulnar nerve. *Neurology* 30:873–876, 1980.

MEDIAL ANTEBRACHIAL CUTANEOUS NERVE CONDUCTION AND LATENCY

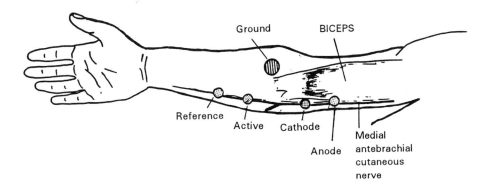

Figure 4.26.   Medial antebrachial cutaneous nerve conduction and latency.

Figure 4.26

Pickup: The active surface electrode is placed on the anteromedial surface of the forearm 9–12 cm from the cathode.

Reference: The reference is placed 3–4 cm distal to the active.

Ground: The ground is between the sites of stimulation and pickup.

Stimulation: The nerve is stimulated antidromically 2–4 cm lateral to the medial epicondyle of the humerus with the cathode located distally. This stimulation site is medial to the location of the median nerve.

Electromyograph settings:
- Frequency: 8 Hz to 2 kHz
- Sweep speed: 5 msec/div
- Gain: 50 μV

Normal values: (N = 40)
NCV: 49.3 ± 3.8 m/sec (mean ± 1 SD)
Latency to the negative peak: 1.7 to 2.6 msec (mean, 2.1 msec)
Amplitudes: 10–30 μV (mean, 20 μV)

Comments: Skin temperature of the forearm was 31–33°C.

Pribyl R, You SB, Jantra P: Sensory nerve conduction velocity of the medial antebrachial cutaneous nerve. *Electromyogr Clin Neurophysiol* 19:41–46, 1979.

CHAPTER 5

Intercostal Nerve Motor Latency

INTERCOSTAL NERVE DISTAL LATENCY AND CONDUCTION VELOCITY

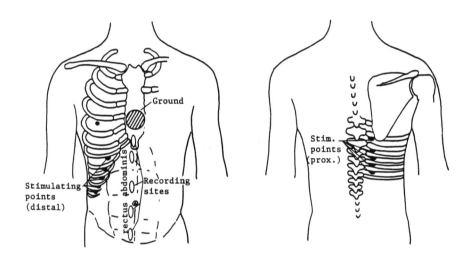

Figure 5.1. Intercostal nerve distal latency and conduction velocity.

Figure 5.1

Pickup: The active surface electrode is placed over the rectus abdominis of the same side. The most consistent recording sites for each nerve are as followed: seventh intercostal nerve (ICN) 0–1 cm above the xiphoid process; eighth ICN 1–3 cm below the xiphoid process; ninth ICN 2–5 cm above the umbilicus; 10th ICN 1–4 cm below the umbilicus; 11th ICN midway between umbilicus and pubic symphysis.

Reference: The reference electrode is placed 5 cm rostral to each active electrode except for the seventh ICN study. For the study of seventh ICN, the reference electrode is placed 3 cm above the active electrode.

Ground: The ground is placed between the stimulating and recording electrodes.

Stimulation: Two sites (distal and proximal) along the course of the same intercostal nerve are stimulated. A comma-shaped stimulator is placed 6 cm behind the costal margin and just lateral to the paraspinal muscles in the same intercostal space for the distal and proximal stimulations, respectively.

Electromyograph settings:
- Frequency: 2 Hz to 10 kHz
- Sweep speed: 5 msec/div
- Gain: 1000 μV/div
- Duration: 0.5 msec

Normal values: (N = 30 persons) Age, 14–52 years

Intercostal nerves	Distal latency (msec)	Amplitude (mV)	Conduction velocity (m/sec)
7th	3.51 ± 0.67	5.56 ± 2.42	75.07 ± 6.28
8th	3.66 ± 0.48	4.56 ± 2.19	74.87 ± 5.95
9th	3.96 ± 0.31	2.80 ± 1.54	75.52 ± 6.37
10th	4.56 ± 0.65	2.40 ± 1.48	74.78 ± 6.07
11th	4.98 ± 0.61	2.60 ± 1.37	71.67 ± 7.43

Comments: Patients lie on the opposite side of examination with the arm rested overhead to make the intercostal space wide. Holding one's breath is unnecessary. The distance between the two sites of stimulation was measured using a caliper. Supramaximal stimulation was achieved with a higher voltage (about 40%) at the proximal site than that of the distal site. All the recordings were done on the right side. For comparison, eight patients were recorded on the left.

Pradhan S, Taly A: Intercostal nerve conduction study in man. *J Neurol Neurosurg Psychiatry* 52:763–766, 1989.

CHAPTER 6

Lower Extremity Nerves

FEMORAL NERVE MOTOR LATENCY AND NERVE CONDUCTION VELOCITY

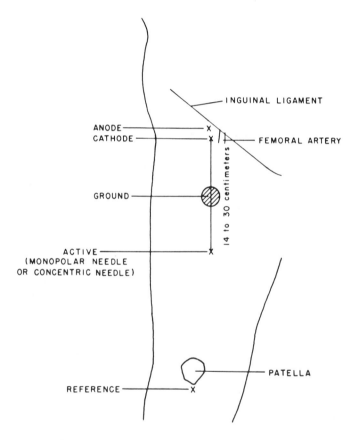

Figure 6.1. Femoral nerve motor latency and nerve conduction velocity (Gassel technique).

Figure 6.1
Gassel

Pickup: Active: concentric needles are used for pickup. (A monopolar needle and surface electrode give similar results.) No difference was noted between placement in rectus femoris, vastus medialis, or vastus lateralis muscles if distance from stimulation was kept constant. Specific values are reported for 14 and 30 cm, although the table from which Fig. 6.3 was derived can be used for other distances.

Ground: The ground is between the stimulation and pickup sites.

Stimulation: Stimulation is applied just below the inguinal ligament and lateral to the femoral artery. Usually surface electrodes are used, but occasionally a monopolar needle is needed for stimulation.

Electromyograph settings:
• Frequency: 8 Hz to 8 kHz
• Sweep speed: 5 msec/div
• Gain: 500 μV

Normal values: ($N = 42$)
Latency (14 cm): 3.7 ± 0.1 msec (SD = 0.45 msec); range, 13–15 cm
Latency (30 cm): 6.0 ± 0.15 msec (SD = 0.6 msec); range, 29–31 cm.
Mean conduction velocity calculated between 14 and 30 cm points: 70 m/sec ± 7.8%.

Gassell MM: A study of femoral nerve conduction time. *Arch Neurol* 9:607–614, 1963.
Johnson EW, Wood PK, Power JJ: Femoral nerve conduction studies. *Arch Phys Med Rehabil* 49:528–532, 1968.

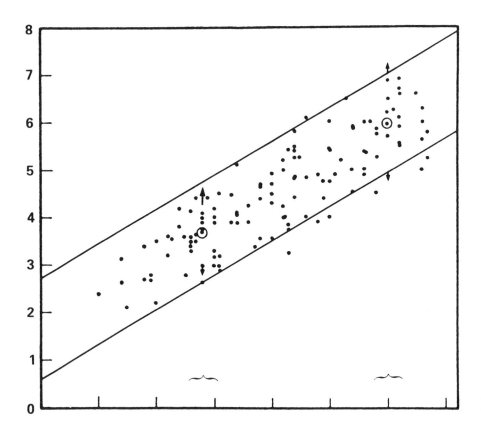

Figure 6.2. Femoral latency values by distance from the stimulating electrode. (From Gassell, 1963.)

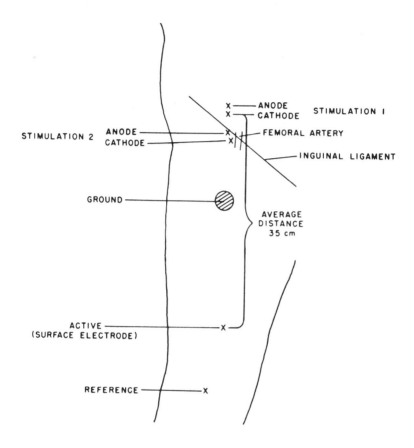

Figure 6.3. Femoral nerve motor latency and nerve conduction velocity (Johnson technique).

Figure 6.2 (see also Figure 6.3)
Johnson et al.

Pickup: Surface pickups are used, with the active surface electrode over the "center" of the vastus medialis muscle. The mean distance from above the inguinal ligament to the pickup is 35.4 ± 1.9 cm.

Reference: The reference is over the patellar ligament.

Ground: The ground is between the stimulation and pickup sites.

Stimulation: Stimulation is applied just above the inguinal ligament and lateral to the femoral artery, in addition to below the ligament. The distance across the inguinal ligament is 5.5 cm. SD = 1.6 cm. Needle electrode tends to facilitate the technique.

Normal values: (N = 100 adults)

Above the inguinal ligament latency: 7.1 ± 0.7 msec (mean ± 1 SD); range, 6.1–8.4 msec

Below the inguinal ligament latency: 6.0 ± 0.7 msec (mean ± 1 SD); range, 5.5–7.5 msec

Delay across the inguinal ligament: 1.1 ± 0.4 msec (mean ± 1 SD); range, 0.8–1.8 msec

Conduction velocity in the segment of nerve from above the inguinal ligament to the point of distal stimulation: 66.7 ± 7.4 m/sec; range, 50–96 m/sec

Conduction velocity of the segment of the nerve from below the inguinal ligament to the distal point of stimulation: 69.4 ± 9.2 m/sec; range, 50–90 m/sec

SCIATIC MOTOR NERVE CONDUCTION VELOCITY

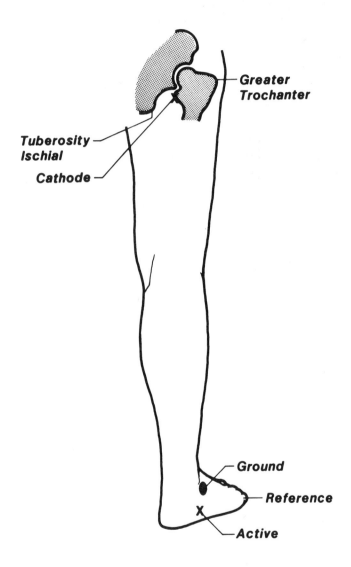

Figure 6.4. Sciatic nerve motor conduction velocity.

Figure 6.4

General: Vulnerable to entrapment as it crosses over the sciatic notch in leaving the pelvis.

Pickup:
1. The active surface electrode is placed over the abductor digiti minimi muscle.
2. The proximal active surface electrode is placed over the medial gastrocnemius muscle.

Reference: The reference is on the little toe.

Ground: The ground is on the lateral malleolus.

Stimulation:
1. Needle electrode: The cathode was placed in the gluteal skin fold equidistant from the ischial tuberosity and the greater trochanter of the femur.
2. Distal stimulation (surface) at the popliteal fossa proximal to the branching of the posterior tibial and common peroneal nerves (13–17 cm from the proximal and distal stimulation points).

Electromyograph settings:
• Frequency: 8 Hz to 8 kHz
• Sweep speed: 5 msec/div
• Gain: 1,000 μV

Normal values: ($N = 10$)
Velocity: 51.3 ± 4.4 m/sec to abductor digiti minimi
Range: 45.3–61.1 m/sec
Distance: 32.9 ± 2.4 cm (26–36.5 cm)

Comments: Electromyograph laboratory was thermostatically controlled, 72–73°F. Skin temperature was not recorded.

Yap CB, Hirota T: Sciatic nerve motor conduction velocity study. *J Neurol Neurosurg Psychiatry* 30:233–239, 1967.

PERONEAL NERVE TO EXTENSOR DIGITORUM BREVIS MOTOR NERVE CONDUCTION VELOCITY AND LATENCY

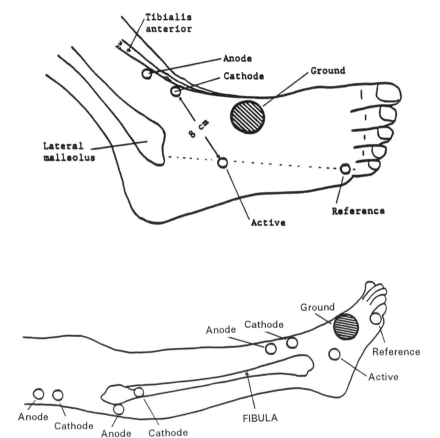

Figure 6.5. Peroneal nerve to extensor digitorum brevis motor nerve conduction velocity and latency.

Figure 6.5

Pickup: The active surface electrode is placed over the extensor digitorum brevis (EDB) muscle in the anterior lateral aspect of the proximal midtarsal area.

Reference: The reference is placed on the fifth toe.

Stimulation: Distal stimulation is applied about 8 cm proximal to the pickup, just lateral to the tibialis anterior tendon. More proximally, the nerve is stimulated just below the head of the fibula as the nerve curves around the bone. Finally, stimulation is applied in the popliteal space over the lateral third of the flexor skin crease.

Electromyograph settings:
- Frequency: 8 Hz to 8 kHz
- Sweep speed: 5 msec/div
- Gain: 1,000 μV

Normal values:
Distal latency if 8 cm used: 4.5 ± 0.8 msec (mean ± 1 SD)
Below fibula head to ankle:
Checkles et al.:
1. Tape measure (length 31.6 ± 3.4 cm) 49.9 ± 5.9 m/sec
(mean ± 1 SD); range, 41.6–64.6 m/sec (*N* = 32)
2. Calipers (length 31.3 ± 3.3 cm) 49.4 ± 5.8 m/sec (mean
± 1 SD); range, 41.2–64.0 m/sec
Jimenez et al.:
right: 51.6 ± 4.1 m/sec (mean ± 1 SD); range, 37 to 62
m/sec
left: 51.6 ± 3.5 m/sec (mean ± 1 SD); range, 42 to 63
m/sec (*N* = 39)

Checkles NS, Bailey JA, Johnson EW: Tape and caliper surface measurements in determination of peroneal nerve conduction velocity. *Arch Phys Med Rehabil* 50:214–218,
1969.
Jimenez J, Easton JK, Redford JB: Conduction studies of the anterior and posterior
tibial nerves. *Arch Phys Med Rehabil* 51:164–169, 1970.

Stimulus at:	Mean amplitude (mV)
Ankle	4.4 ± 1.2
Head of fibula	4.1 ± 1.3
Popliteal	4.0 ± 1.3

Across fibular head:
  Checkles et al.:
1. Tape measure (length 39.2 ± 3.1 cm) 51.1 ± 6.3 m/sec (mean ± 1 SD); range, 41.6–62.7 m/sec
2. Calipers (length 38 ± 3.0 cm) 49.5 ± 6.1 m/sec (mean ± 1 SD); range, 40.2–61.8 m/sec

  Jimenez et al.:
  right: 53.9 ± 4.3 m/sec (mean ± 1 SD); range, 42.3 to 63.7 m/sec
  left: 52.80 ± 4.6 m/sec (mean ± 1 SD); range, 44.1 to 65.3 m/sec

Comments: Anomalous innervation to the EDB occurs one-fifth of the time and is indicated by a different (smaller) wave shape when stimulating distally (partial anomaly) or by an absence of a wave potential (complete anomaly). The accessory peroneal nerve courses posterior and under the lateral malleolus, where stimulation is applied. The paper of Checkles et al. does not report temperatures. In the study of Jimenez et al., skin temperature in the forefoot was 29–34°C.

PERONEAL NERVE MOTOR CONDUCTION ACROSS THE KNEE: SHORT SEGMENT STIMULATION

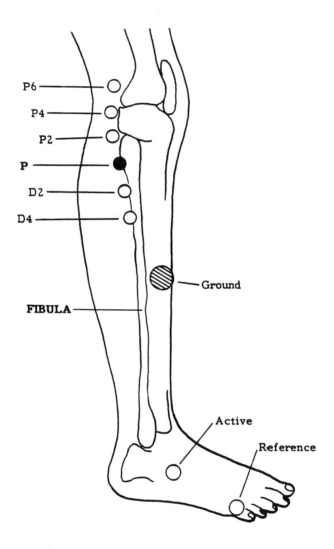

Figure 6.6. Peroneal nerve motor conduction across the knee: short segment stimulation.

Figure 6.6

Pickup: The active surface recording electrode is placed over the extensor digitorum brevis.

Reference: The reference is placed over the tendon of the extensor digitorum brevis.

Stimulation: The stimulation point "P" is identified as the tip of the fibular head. The points D2 and D4 are measured 2 and 4 cm distal to the point "P." The points P2, P4, and P6 are marked 2, 4, and 6 cm, respectively, proximal to the point "P."

Normal values:

	Conduction time (msec) between the points	
Stimulation at:	Right (N = 23)	Left (N = 21)
D4–D2	0.38 ± 0.12	0.39 ± 0.10
D2–P	0.41 ± 0.12	0.42 ± 0.13
P–P2	0.42 ± 0.09	0.43 ± 0.17
P2–P4	0.41 ± 0.10	0.41 ± 0.12
P4–P6	0.43 ± 0.08	0.44 ± 0.13

0.55 + 0.10 (mean + SD)

The amplitude changes of the proximal responses, when compared with the succeeding distal responses at 2-cm intervals: −0.2 + 0.13 mV.

Kanakamedala RV, Hong CZ: Peroneal nerve entrapment at the knee localized by short segment stimulation. *Am J Phys Med Rehabil* 68:116–122, 1989.

PERONEAL NERVE CONDUCTION VELOCITY TO TIBIALIS ANTERIOR AND PERONEUS BREVIS

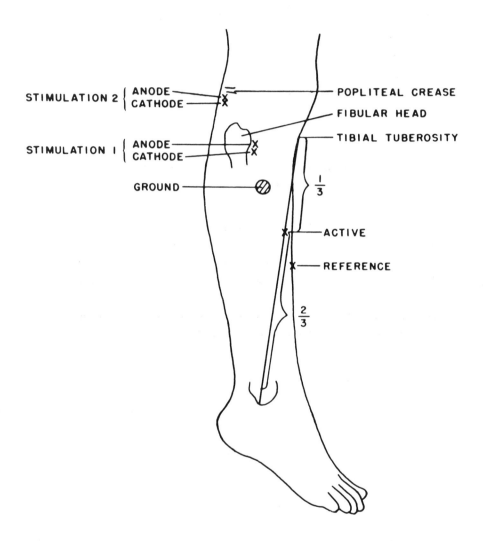

Figure 6.7. Peroneal motor nerve conduction velocity to tibialis anterior muscle.

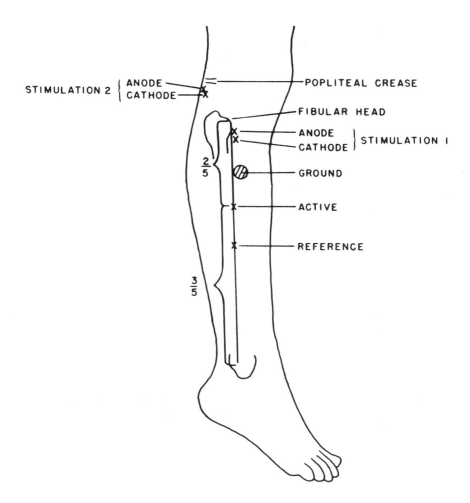

Figure 6.8. Peroneal motor nerve conduction velocity to peroneus brevis muscle.

Figures 6.7 and 6.8

Pickup: The active electrode was 32 mm (size of a TECA ground). Similar values are achieved using standard surface electrodes.

> **Tibialis Anterior:** The active surface electrode is placed at the junction of the upper third and lower two-thirds of a line between the tibial tuberosity and the tip of the lateral malleolus of the fibula.

> **Peroneus Brevis:** The active surface electrode is placed at the junction of the upper two-fifths and the lower three-fifths of a line between the head of the fibula and the tip of the lateral malleolus of the fibula.

Reference:

> **Tibialis Anterior:** The reference is placed over the medial aspect of the tibia, 4 cm distal to the active electrode.

> **Peroneus Brevis:** The reference is placed 4 cm distal to the active electrode over the muscle tendon.

Ground: The ground is between the site of stimulation and the site of pickup.

Stimulation: Stimulation is applied above the head of the fibula and below the head of the fibula with approximately 10 cm between the two points of stimulation.

Devi S, Lovelace RE, Duarte N: Proximal peroneal nerve conduction velocity: Recording from anterior tibial and peroneus brevis muscles. *Ann Neurol* 2:116–119, 1977.

Electromyograph settings:
- Frequency: 8 Hz to 8 kHz
- Sweep speed: 2 msec/div
- Gain: 250 μV

Normal values: (N = 34)

Latencies: (mean ± 1 SD)

	Above fibular head	Below fibular head
To tibialis anterior	4.7 ± 0.5 msec	3.0 ± 0.6 msec
Range	3.4–6.0 msec	2.0–4.4 msec
To peroneus brevis	5.0 ± 0.8 msec	3.0 ± 0.8 msec
Range	3.8–7.2 msec	1.7–5.4 msec

Nerve conduction velocity across fibular head:
To tibialis anterior: 66.3 ± 12.9 m/sec (mean ± 1 SD)
To peroneus brevis: 55.3 ± 10.2 m/sec (mean ± 1 SD)

Comments: Distance from point of stimulus to pickup were not specified. Skin temperature also was not specified. However, the room was kept at a constant temperature of 22.2–23.3°C.

TIBIAL MOTOR NERVE CONDUCTION VELOCITY AND MEDIAL PLANTAR AND LATERAL PLANTAR LATENCIES

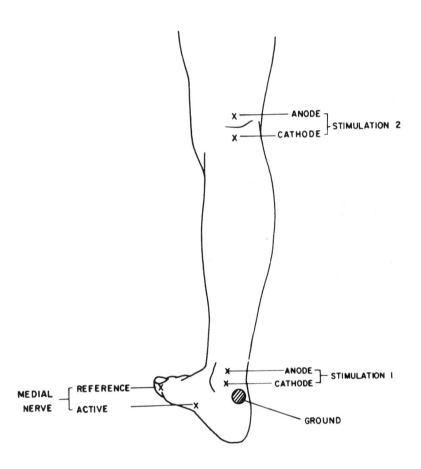

Figure 6.9. Tibial nerve motor nerve conduction velocity to the abductor hallucis muscle.

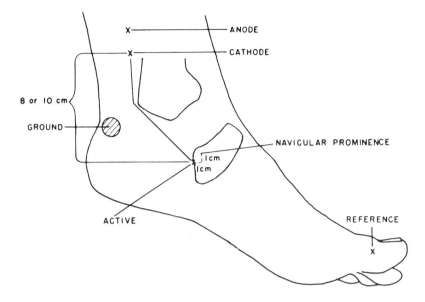

Figure 6.10. Medial plantar nerve motor latency to the abductor hallucis muscle.

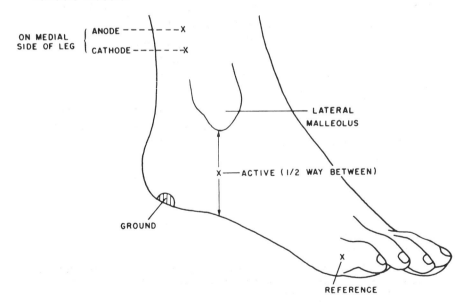

Figure 6.11. Lateral plantar nerve motor latency to the abductor digiti minimi muscle.

Figures 6.9, 6.10, and 6.11

Pickup:

Medial Plantar: The active surface electrode is 1 cm behind and 1 cm below the navicular tubercle (medial side of foot). Recording is from the abductor hallucis muscle.

Lateral Plantar: The active surface electrode is directly below the lateral malleolus, bisecting the distance from the tip of the malleolus to the sole of the foot. Recording is from the abductor digiti minimi muscle.

Reference:

Medial Plantar: The reference is on the large toe.

Lateral Plantar: The reference is on the little toe.

Ground: The ground is on the dorsum of the foot.

Stimulation: *Distal distance* is measured from the pickup of the medial plantar nerve following the course of the nerve 1 cm posterior to the medial malleolus. Distances of 8 or 10 cm can be used, with the stimulation occurring posterior to the medial malleolus and above the flexor retinaculum. The *same site of stimulation* is used for the lateral plantar nerve. Measurements are made both with calipers and with a flexible tape measure for the medial plantar nerve segments. The ankle is in the neutral position (90°).

Proximal distance is measured at the crease of the popliteal fossa, at about the junction of the lateral third and medial two-thirds. Care must be taken not to stimulate too laterally, which stimulates the peroneal nerve instead.

Fu R, DeLisa JA, Kraft GH: Motor nerve latencies through the tarsal tunnel in normal adult subjects: Standard determinations corrected for temperature and distance. *Arch Phys Med Rehabil* 61:243–248, 1980.
Jimenez J, Easton JK, Redford JB: Conduction studies of the anterior and posterior tibial nerves. *Arch Phys Med Rehabil* 51:164–169, 1970.

Electromyograph settings:
- Frequency: 8 Hz to 8 kHz
- Sweep speed: 5 msec/div
- Gain: 500 μV

Normal values: (N = 37 adults; no temperature correction, and using flexible tape measurements)

	8 cm (mean ± 1 SD)	10 cm (mean ± 1 SD)
Medial plantar latency:	3.4 ± 0.5 msec	3.8 ± 0.5 msec
Lateral plantar latency:	3.6 ± 0.5 msec	3.9 ± 0.5 msec

Motor NCV: 54.9 ± 7.6 m/sec (mean ± 1 SD): Fu et al.
51.2 ± 3.9 m/sec (mean ± 1 SD): Jimenez et al.

Amplitude (medial plantar branch of tibial nerve recording over abductor hallucis; Jimenez et al.)
Stimulus at:
Above malleolus: 11.6 ± 4.3 mV
Popliteal: 8.3 ± 1.2 mV

Comments: Skin temperature was measured below the medial malleolus, and the temperature range was 29–34°C (mean, 32.1 ± 1.4°C). The article of Fu et al. has a table of temperature corrections, as well as values obtained using calipers instead of flexible tape.

COMPOUND NERVE ACTION POTENTIALS OF THE MEDIAL AND LATERAL PLANTAR NERVE LATENCIES

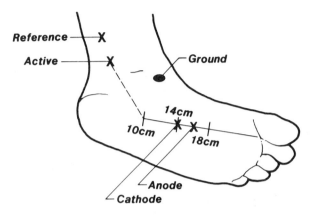

**Compound Medial Plantar Nerve
Action Potential Latency**

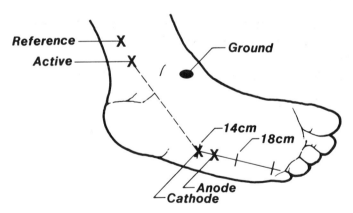

**Compound Lateral Plantar
Nerve Action Potential Latency**

Figure 6.12. Compound nerve action potentials of the medial and lateral plantar nerves.

Figure 6.12

General: These mixed nerve compound nerve action potentials are similar to pure sensory nerve potentials.

Pickup: The active electrode is placed over the tibial nerve just proximal to the flexor retinaculum, 14 cm from the stimulating cathode.

Reference electrode: The reference electrode is a bar electrode.

Ground: The ground electrode is placed over the dorsum of the foot between the cathode and the active pickup.

Stimulation: Using an orthodromic technique, the medial and lateral plantar nerves are stimulated at a site 14 cm distal to the active pickup electrode over their corresponding nerves.

Electromyograph settings:
- Frequency: 8 Hz to 1.6 kHz
- Sweep speed: 5 msec/div
- Gain: 2 µV

Normal values: (N = 41 adults)
Medial plantar nerve latency (14 cm): 3.16 ± 0.26 msec (range, 2.6–3.7 msec); amplitude greater than 10 µV (range, 10–30 µV) Lateral plantar nerve latency (14 cm): 3.15 ± 0.25 msec (range, 2.7–3.7 msec); amplitude greater than 8 µV (range, 8–20 µV). The latency is measured to the negative peak of the compound nerve action potential.

Comments: The mean temperature of the feet in the tarsal tunnel was 30.7°C, the medial sole was 29.8°C, and the lateral sole was 39.2°C. The distance is measured with a flexible metal tape.

Saeed MA, Gatens PF: Compound nerve action potentials in the medial and lateral plantar nerves through tarsal tunnel. *Arch Phys Med Rehabil* 63:304–307, 1982.

TIBIAL SENSORY NERVE CONDUCTION VELOCITY—MEDIAL PLANTAR AND LATERAL PLANTAR

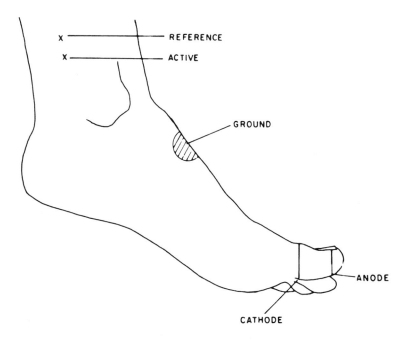

Figure 6.13.   Medial plantar sensory nerve conduction velocity (orthodromic technique).

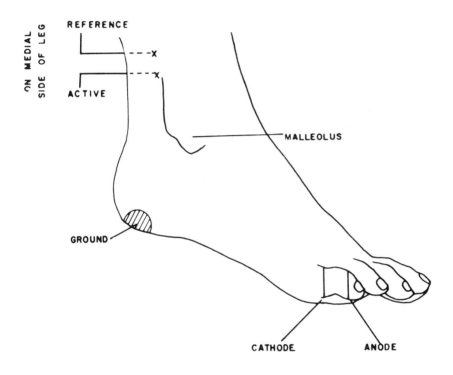

Figure 6.14. Lateral plantar sensory nerve conduction velocity (orthodromic technique).

Figures 6.13 and 6.14

Pickup: The active electrode is placed above the flexor retinaculum and medial to the medial malleolus for both medial and lateral plantar nerves.

Ground: The ground is placed on the dorsum of the foot.

Stimulation: The stimulus intensity needed to obtain the maximal amplitudes is usually three times the sensory threshold.

Orthodromically:

Medial Plantar: Stimulation is applied by means of a ring electrode on the great toe.

Lateral Plantar: Stimulation is applied by means of a ring electrode on the fifth toe.

Electromyograph settings:
• Frequency: 8 Hz or 1.6 kHz
• Sweep speed: 2 or 5 msec/div
• Gain: 5–10 µV

Distance: For the medial plantar nerve, the distance is measured with a tape from the first digit ring electrode to the ankle pickup. For the lateral plantar nerve, calipers are used to measure the distance from the fifth digit ring electrode to the ankle pickup. No specific standard distance was noted.

Normal values: (N = 20 adults)

	Terminal SNCV	Mean amplitude
Medial plantar	35.22 ± 3.63 m/sec (mean ± 1 SD)	3.61 µV (range, 2–6)
Lateral plantar	31.68 ± 4.39 m/sec (mean ± 1 SD)	1.89 µV (range, 1–5)

Oh SJ, Sarala PK, Kuba T, Elmore RS: Tarsal tunnel syndrome: Electrophysiological study. *Ann Neurol* 5:327–330, 1979.

Interval from the stimulus artifact to the negative peak of the compound sensory nerve action potential.

Comments: An averager must be used (the averager used 32–256 stimulations). Skin temperature was taken on the sole of the foot and measured 29.5–33.5°C.

SAPHENOUS SENSORY NERVE LATENCY AND CONDUCTION VELOCITY

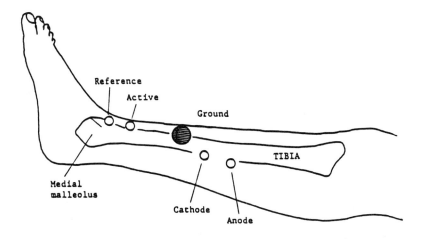

Figure 6.15. Saphenous sensory nerve latency and conduction velocity.

Figure 6.15

Pickup: The distal (reference) electrode is placed anterior to the highest prominence of the medial malleolus of the tibia, in the space between the malleolus and the medial border of the tibialis anterior tendon. The proximal active electrode is located 3 cm above the reference and just medial to the aforementioned tendon, whose direction is parallel to a line drawn between recording electrodes.

Ground: The ground is placed between the stimulation and pickup sites.

Stimulation: Antidromic stimulation is applied 14 cm above the proximal recording electrode and deep to the medial border of the tibia. Firm pressure is exerted, pushing the electrodes between the medial gastrocnemius muscle and the tibia. The cathode is distal. The gastrocnemius muscle can be relaxed by positioning it in plantarflexion.

Electromyograph settings:
- Frequency: 8 Hz to 1.6 kHz
- Sweep speed: 5 msec/div
- Gain: 10 µV

Normal values: (N = 40 adults)

$$\text{Velocity} = \frac{\text{interelectrode distance}}{\text{sensory latency}}$$

$$= 41.7 \pm 3.4 \text{ m/sec (mean} \pm 1 \text{ SD)}$$

Latency to negative peak of the evoked compound sensory nerve action potential: 3.6 ± 0.4 msec (mean ± 1 SD)
Amplitude: 9.0 ± 3.4 µV (mean ± 1 SD).

Comments: The main problem is that the gain often is 5 µV or less, which requires averaging. Since the sural nerve gives higher amplitudes, it is often the preferred nerve to study. Room temperature was maintained at 22.8°C during the study. The limbs were covered during the procedure.

Wainapel SF, Kim DJ, Ebel A: Conduction studies of the saphenous nerve in healthy subjects. *Arch Phys Med Rehabil* 59:316–319, 1978.

SUPERFICIAL PERONEAL SENSORY NERVE CONDUCTION VELOCITY AND LATENCY

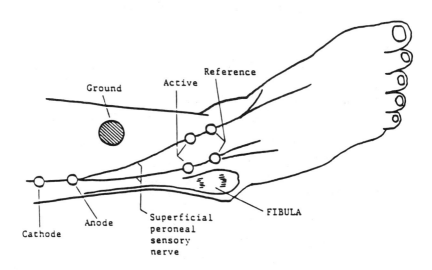

Figure 6.16. Superficial peroneal sensory nerve conduction velocity and latency.

Figure 6.16

Pickup: The active and reference electrodes are placed over *each* of the medial and intermediate dorsal cutaneous branches, with the active being 3 cm proximal.

Ground: The ground is placed between the stimulating and pickup electrodes.

Stimulation: Using antidromic techniques, the site of stimulation was 14 cm from the proximal recording electrodes on the anterolateral aspect of the calf.

Electromyograph settings:
* Frequency: 8 Hz to 16 khz
* Sweep speed: 2 msec/div
* Gain: 20 μV

Normal values: (N = 80 adults)

Medial Dorsal Cutaneous:
Latency to peak: 3.4 ± 0.4 msec; range, 2.7–4.7 msec (mean ± 1 SD)
Sensory conduction velocity: 51.2 ± 5.7 m/sec; range, 38.2–63.6 m/sec
Amplitude: 18.3 ± 8.0 μV; range, 5–44 μV

Intermediate Dorsal Cutaneous:
Latency to peak: 3.4 ± 0.4 msec; range, 2.8–4.6 msec (mean ± 1 SD)
Sensory conduction velocity: 51.3 ± 5.4 m/sec; range, 38.8–63.6 m/sec
Amplitude: 15.1 ± 8.2 μV; range, 4–40 μV

Comment: Medial and intermediate dorsal cutaneous branches were located by inspection and palpation during plantar flexion and inversion of the foot. Room temperature maintained at 23°C. Patients with skin temperatures below 28°C were excluded.

Izzo KL, Sridhara CR, Lemont H, Rosenholtz H: Sensory conduction studies of branches of the superficial peroneal nerve. *Arch Phys Med Rehabil* 62:24–27, 1981.

DEEP PERONEAL NERVE SENSORY CONDUCTION VELOCITY AND LATENCY

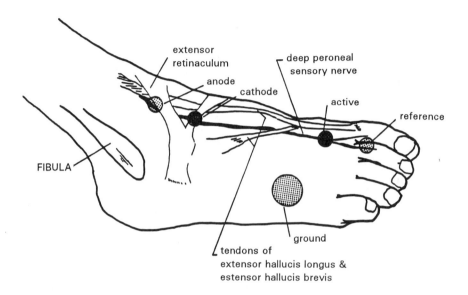

Figure 6.17. Deep peroneal nerve sensory conduction velocity and latency.

Figure 6.17

Pickup: The active surface electrode is placed at the interspace between the first and second metatarsal heads.

Reference: The reference surface electrode is placed 3 cm distally on the second toe.

Ground: The ground is between the sites of stimulation and pickup.

Stimulation: The nerve is stimulated antidromically at the ankle, 12 cm proximal from the active electrode and just lateral to the extensor hallucis longus tendon.

Electromyograph settings:
- Frequency: 20 Hz to 2 khz
- Sweep speed: 1 msec/div
- Gain: 2–5 μV/div

Normal values: (N = 40) Age, 21–50 years; mean age, 35
NCV: 42 ± 5 m/sec (range, 33–53)
Latency to the onset: 2.9 ± 0.4 (2.1–3.6)
Latency to the negative peak: 3.6 ± 0.4 (2.7–4.2)
Amplitude (baseline to the negative peak): 3.4 ± 1.2 μV

Comment: Skin temperature of the foot was 29°C or above.

Posas et al.

Pickup: The recording electrode is placed over the first dorsal web space 10 cm distal to the stimulating electrode.

Stimulation: The nerve is stimulated antidromically at the ankle 2 cm distal to extensor retinaculum.

Normal values: (N = 36)
Latency at the peak: 3.24 ± 0.5 msec
Amplitude (peak to peak): 5.16 ± 0.474 μV

Lee HJ, Bach JR, DeLisa JA: Deep peroneal sensory nerve: Standardization in nerve conduction study. *Am J Phys Med Rehabil* 69:202–204, 1990.
Posas HN, Rivner MH: Nerve conduction studies of the medial branch of the deep peroneal nerve. *Muscle Nerve* 13:862, 1990.

SURAL SENSORY NERVE LATENCY

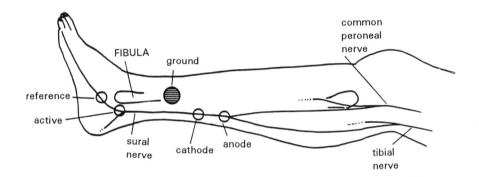

Figure 6.18.   Sural sensory nerve latency.

Figure 6.18

Pickup: The active is posterior and below the distal lateral malleolus of the fibula.

Reference: The reference is placed 3 cm distally.

Ground: The ground is placed between the cathode and the active pickup.

Stimulation: Stimulation is applied slightly lateral to the midline in the lower third of the posterior aspect of the leg with the cathode distally. The patient feels shocks radiate to the heel and foot. Sites 10, 14, or 17 cm from the active electrode are stimulated antidromically.

Electromyograph settings:
- Frequency: 8 Hz to 1.6 kHz
- Sweep speed: 5 msec/div
- Gain: 10 μV

Normal values:

Latency to peak:

Distance measured	Mean latency
10 cm	2.84 ± 0.27 msec (mean ± 1 SD; $N = 37$); range, 2.3–3.38 msec
14 cm	3.50 ± 0.25 msec (mean ± 1 SD; $N = 56$); range, 3.0–4.0 msec
17 cm	4.02 ± 0.30 msec (mean ± 1 SD; $N = 56$); range, 3.42–4.62 msec
20 cm	4.58 ± 0.36 msec (mean ± 1 SD; $N = 54$); range, 3.86–5.3 msec

Amplitude of evoked sensory potential: 5–30 μV.

Comments: Tests at 14 and 17 cm were most easily evoked. An averager was not necessary. Limb temperatures were not recorded, but any limbs that were cool to palpation were warmed or excluded from the study.

Schuchmann JA: Sural nerve conduction: A standardized technique. *Arch Phys Med Rehabil* 58:166–168, 1977.

LATERAL DORSAL CUTANEOUS BRANCH OF THE SURAL NERVE CONDUCTION

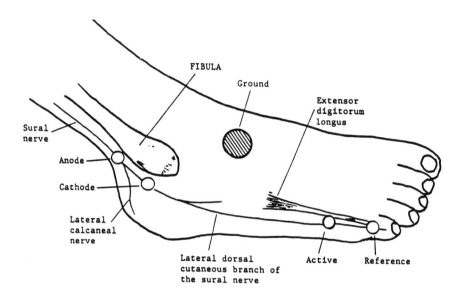

Figure 6.19. Lateral dorsal cutaneous branch of the sural nerve conduction.

Figure 6.19

Pickup: The active surface electrode is placed at the midportion of the fifth metatarsal bone and just lateral to the extensor digitorum longus tendon for the fifth toe.

Reference: The reference is placed about 4 cm distal to the active electrode.

Ground: The ground is placed on the dorsum of the foot.

Electromyograph settings:
- Frequency: 20 Hz to 2 kHz
- Sweep speed: 1 msec/div
- Gain: 5 μV/div

Normal values: (N = 40; 25 men, 15 women) age, 23–52 years; mean age, 33
   NCV: 37.6 ± 4.8 m/sec (with onset)
       30.7 ± 3.7 m/sec (with peak)
   Latency: 3.2 ± 0.4 msec (to the onset)
       3.9 ± 0.5 msec (to the peak)
   Amplitude: 5.8 ± 2.1 μV (baseline to peak)

Comments: Antidromic study. The surface skin temperature at the center of the dorsal foot was maintained at or above 31°C. The distance between the cathode and the active electrode was 12 cm.

Lee HJ, Bach JR, DeLisa JA: Lateral dorsal cutaneous branch of the sural nerve: Standardization in nerve conduction study. *Am J Phys Med Rehabil* 71:318–320, 1992.

MEDIAL CALCANEAL NERVE LATENCY

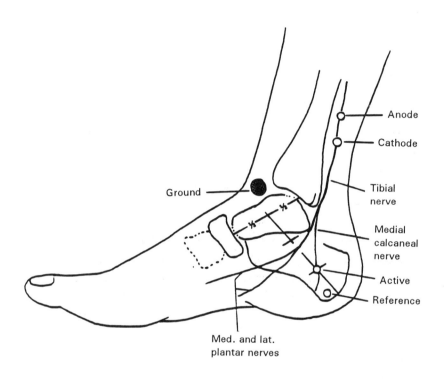

Figure 6.20.   Medial calcaneal nerve latency.

Figure 6.20

Pickup: The active surface electrode is placed one-third of the distance from the apex of the heel to the midpoint between the navicular and tip of the medial malleolus.

Reference: The reference is placed at the apex of the heel.

Ground: The ground electrode is placed over the dorsum of the foot.

Stimulation: The tibial nerve is stimulated antidromically 10 cm proximal to the active recording electrode.

Electromyograph settings:
  • Frequency: 20 Hz to 2 kHz
  • Sweep speed: 1–2 msec/div
  • Gain: 10–20 μV/div

Normal values: (N = 20 patients, 40 feet)

Latency (msec)	Mean ± SD	Range	Side-to-side difference
Onset	1.7 ± 0.3	1.4–2.0	0.1
Peak	2.5 ± 0.3	2.2–2.8	0.1
Amplitude (μV) (baseline to peak)	18 ± 13	8–34	4

Comments: The optimal site for the placement of recording electrode was determined by cadaveric dissection. Skin temperature was not controlled.

Del Toro DR, Park TA, Mandel JD, Wertsch JJ: Development of a nerve conduction study technique for the medial calcaneal nerve. *Muscle Nerve* 15:1194, 1992.

DORSAL NERVE OF THE PENIS NERVE CONDUCTION VELOCITY AND LATENCY

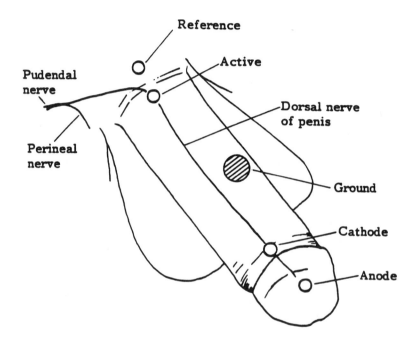

Figure 6.21.   Dorsal nerve of the penis nerve velocity and latency.

Figure 6.21

Pickup: The active surface recording electrode is placed at the most proximal base of the penis.

Reference: The reference electrode is placed 4 cm proximal to the active electrode above symphysis pubis.

Ground: The ground is placed on the medial thigh.

Stimulation: The cathode is placed just proximal to the dorsal glans, and the anode on the dorsal glans.

Electromyograph settings:
- Frequency: 30 Hz to 2 kHz
- Gain: 5 μV

Normal values: (N = 20)
NCV: 36.2 ± 3.2 m/sec
Latency: 2.34 ± 0.35 msec
Amplitude: 2.29 ± 1.08 μV

Comments: Orthodromic study. Skin temperature was measured from the midshaft of the penis. The mean temperature was 31.8°C (range, 30–33.5°C). The interelectrode distance ranged from 5.4 to 11.5 cm (mean, 8.6 ± 1.5 cm). A penile traction device was used. The test may be valuable to evaluate the penile sensory component of erectile dysfunction.

Clawson DR, Cardenas DD: Dorsal nerve of the penis nerve conduction velocity: A new technique. *Muscle Nerve* 14:845–849, 1991.

LATERAL FEMORAL CUTANEOUS NERVE LATENCY
AND CONDUCTION VELOCITY

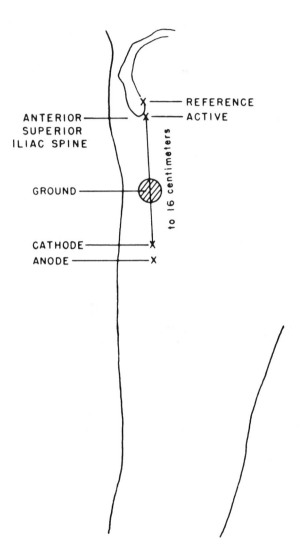

Figure 6.22. Lateral femoral cutaneous latency and nerve conduction velocity (Sarala orthodromic technique).

Figure 6.22
Sarala et al.

Orthodromic:

Pickup: The active surface disc electrode is placed 1 cm medial to the anterior superior iliac spine.

Reference: The reference is placed about 4 cm more cephalad.

Stimulation: Stimulation is applied using percutaneous bipolar stimulating electrodes placed 11–16 cm directly inferior to the anterior iliac spine on the anterior aspect of the thigh.

Electromyograph settings:
- Frequency: 8 Hz to 1.6 kHz
- Sweep speed: 5 msec/div
- Gain: 10 μV

Butler ET, Johnson EW, Kaye ZA: Normal conduction velocity in the lateral femoral cutaneous nerve. *Arch Phys Med Rehabil* 55:31–32, 1974.

Sarala PK, Nishihara T, Oh SJ: Meralgia paresthetica—Electrophysiologic study. *Arch Phys Med Rehabil* 60:30–31, 1979.

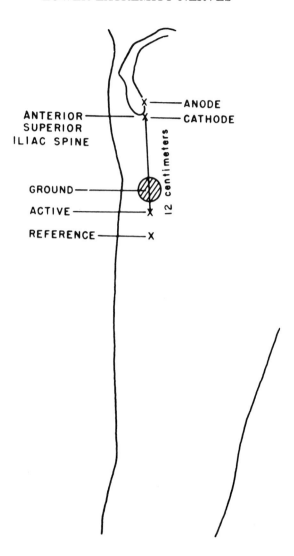

Figure 6.23. Lateral femoral cutaneous latency and nerve conduction velocity (Butler antidromic technique).

Figure 6.23
Butler et al.

Antidromic:

Pickup: Two strips of lead (1.2 × 1.9 cm) fixed in a plastic bar are placed 4 cm apart and 12 cm directly inferior to the anterior superior iliac spine on the anterior aspect of the thigh.

Stimulation: A 3-inch monopolar needle with a disc anode or a bipolar needle can be used. The needle is inserted above the inguinal ligament about 1 cm medial to the anterior superior iliac spine. The nerve is fairly superficial, and the depth of insertion is influenced by the degree of subcutaneous tissue.

Normal values:

$$\text{Velocity} = \frac{\text{distance}}{\text{latency to negative peak}}$$

$$= 57.5 \pm 8.61 \text{ m/sec (mean } \pm \text{ 2 SD);}$$

range, 45.0–68.2 m/sec

(Sarala et al.: $N = 20$ normal adults)

$$= 47.9 \pm 3.7 \text{ m/sec (mean } \pm \text{ 2 SD);}$$

range, 43–55 m/sec

(Butler et al.: $N = 24$ normal adults)

Latency: 1.8–3.1 msec over 12–16 cm (Sarala et al.); for 12 cm, 2.6 ± 0.2 msec (mean ± 1 SD) (Butler et al.); range, 2.3–3.1 msec.
Amplitude of the nerve potential: 10–25 μV (Butler et al.)

Comments: Skin temperature of the thigh ranged from 31.0 to 34.7°C in the study of Sarala et al. An averager (using 32–64 stimuli) was necessary in that study, as the amplitude of the nerve potential was 2–10 μV.

POSTERIOR FEMORAL CUTANEOUS NERVE CONDUCTION

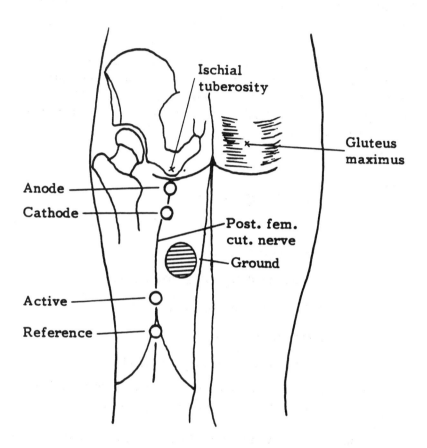

Figure 6.24.   Posterior femoral cutaneous nerve conduction.

Figure 6.24

Pickup: The active electrode is placed in the midline of the posterior thigh 6 cm proximal to the midpopliteal region.

Reference: The reference electrode is placed 3 cm distally from the active electrode.

Ground: The ground is placed just proximal to the active electrode.

Stimulation: Stimulation is applied 12 cm proximal to the active recording electrode on a line connecting the active electrode with the ischial tuberosity.

Electromyograph settings:
- Frequency: 20 Hz to 2 kHz
- Sweep speed: 1 or 2 msec/div
- Gains: 5 μV/div

Normal values: (N = 80) Age, 20–78 years; mean age, 34
Latency to the negative peak: 2.8 ± 0.2 msec (2.3–3.4)
Amplitude (peak to peak): 6.5 ± 1.5 μV (4.1–12.0)

Comments: The cathode of the stimulating electrode is placed in the groove between the medial and lateral hamstrings. The skin temperature in the posterior thigh was maintained between 32 and 33°C.

Dumitru D, Nelson MR: Posterior femoral cutaneous nerve conduction. *Arch Phys Med Rehabil* 71:979–982, 1990.

L-5 AND S-1 SPINAL ROOT STIMULATION

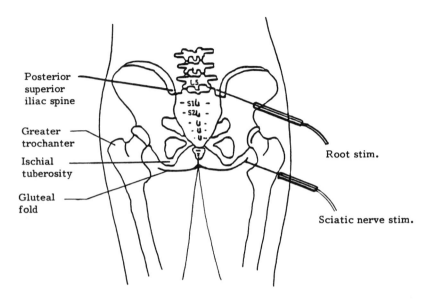

Figure 6.25. L-5 and S-1 spinal root stimulation.

Figure 6.25

Pickup: Recording (active and reference) electrodes are placed over the appropriate muscle. The common recording sites are as follows: soleus, gastrocnemius, abductor hallucis, flexor hallucis brevis, abductor digiti quinti, semimembranosus, etc.

Ground: The ground electrode is placed between the stimulating and recording electrodes.

Stimulation: A monopolar needle (Teflon coated) cathode is inserted about 1 cm medial and slightly caudal to the posterior superior iliac spine and the same type of needle inserted on the opposite side in an identical manner. A 50- to 75-mm needle is required. The anode (surface electrode) is placed on the anterior abdomen just opposite the needle electrode or placed over the spinous process.

Normal values:

Kraft and Johnson:
Conduction latency to soleus: 15.4 ± 1.3 msec
Side to side difference: 0.2 msec (0–0.8 msec)

Macdonell, Cros, and Shahani:
Needle electrode stimulation was compared with magnetic coil stimulation in the lumbosacral nerve root. With both techniques the latency obtained did not differ significantly.
Conduction latency to tibialis anterior: 13.5 ± 1.2 msec (11.4–15.9)
Conduction latency to flexor hallucis brevis: 25.1 ± 2.0 msec (21.7–29.7)

MacLean:
To measure conduction across the sacral plexus, the sciatic nerve also was stimulated with the needle electrode, inserting it at the gluteal skin fold midway between the greater trochanter of the femur and the ischial tuberosity. The recording electrodes are placed over the abductor hallucis. The test is performed with the patient prone, using two pillows under the belly and one under the ankle.
Latency across the sacral plexus: 3.9 ± 0.7 msec (2.5–4.9)
Right-to-left difference: 0–1.0 msec

Kraft GH, Johnson EW: Proximal nerve conduction and late responses. American Association of Electromyography and Electrodiagnosis Workshop, September 1986.
Macdonell RA, Cros D, Shahani BT: Lumbosacral nerve root stimulation comparing electrical with surface magnetic coil techniques. *Muscle Nerve* 15:885–890, 1992.
MacLean IC: Spinal nerve stimulation. American Association of Electromyography and Electrodiagnosis Course B, October 1988.

CHAPTER 7

Reflex, Wave, and Long Latency

BLINK RESPONSES LATENCY

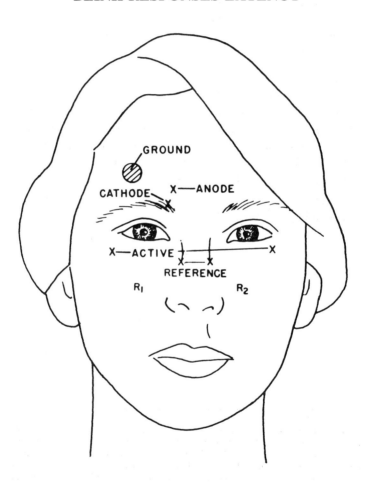

Figure 7.1. Blink responses latency.

Figure 7.1

General: Electrical stimulation of the supraorbital nerve elicits the blink reflex response, which consists of two separate components: an early R1 and a late R2. Visual and auditory stimuli give a response with only one component. Whereas R1 is evoked only on the side of electrical stimulation, R2 is recorded bilaterally with unilateral electrical stimulation. The patient is either positioned in an armchair, relaxed and with the eyes half-closed, or placed in a warm room, supine, with the eyes gently closed.

Pickup: The active surface electrode is placed on the belly of the orbicularis oculi below the canthus. To pick up consensual R2 on a second channel, a second pickup is attached to the opposite orbicularis oculi muscle. A second ground is not needed.

Reference: The reference is placed on the side of the nose.

Ground: The ground is placed on the forehead or cheek.

Stimulation: Electrical stimulation is applied over the supraorbital nerve, which is in the groove that is palpable at the medial third of the superior orbit, with the cathode placed over the supraorbital foramen. The infraorbital or mental nerve can be used instead of the supraorbital. Stimulation intensity is usually approximately 3–8 mA (up to 16–20 mA), with duration of stimulus between 0.1 and 1 msec. Stimulus of low intensity causes the second response of the blink reflex to have a prolonged latency. Thus, it is necessary to determine the stimulus intensity that will evoke the maximum R2 amplitude. With better stimulus control, there is less variability and more reproducibility of responses.

Kimura J, Powers JM, Van Allen MW: Reflex response of orbicularis oculi muscle to supraorbital nerve stimulation: Study in normal subjects and in peripheral facial paresis. *Arch Neurol* 21:193–199, 1969.

Kimura J, Giron LT, Young SM: Electrophysiological study of Bell's palsy. Electrically elicited blink reflex in assessment of prognosis. *Arch Otolaryngol* 102:140–143, 1976.

Kimura J, Bodensteiner J, Yamada T: Electrically elicited blink reflex in normal neonates. *Arch Neurol* 34:246–249, 1977.

Electromyograph settings:
- Frequency: 8 Hz to 8 kHz
- Sweep speed: 5 msec/div (may need 10 msec/div if R2 latency is prolonged)
- Gain: 50–100 μV/div
- Rate: not to be more than 1/sec (a faster rate may produce habituation)

Normal values: (N = 83 normal adults, supraorbital nerve stimulation)

R1 usually is a biphasic or triphasic wave (occasionally polyphasic). It tends to habituate slowly and is a brief, relatively synchronous reflex. It is more stable with repeated trials and better suited for assessing nerve conduction of the trigeminal and facial nerves.

R2 is polyphasic and habituates quickly with a decrease in amplitude and duration with repetitive stimulation. R2 correlates with clinically observed blink of the eyelids.

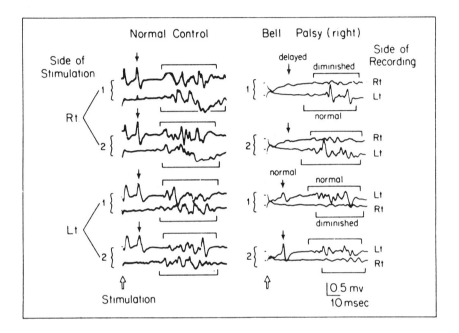

Figure 7.2. Two right-sided and two left-sided stimulations were delivered in each case to show consistency. In the patient, R_1 *(arrows)* and R_2 *(single brackets)* were delayed and small on the right side and normal on the left side regardless of the side stimulated. This finding indicates a lesion involving the efferent arc of reflex (facial nerve) on the right side. (From Kimura et al., 1976.)

R1 Component Latency: 10.6 ± 2.5 msec (mean ± 3 SD). It is delayed if it exceeds 13.0 msec. In normal patients, the difference between values for R1 on each side is less than 1.2 msec. Since R1 appears only ipsilaterally, to compare right with left, both sides must be stimulated. Reflex latency is measured from the stimulus artifact to the initial deflection of the evoked potential.

R2 Component Latency: Direct R2 (ipsilateral to the side of stimulus) is 31 ± 10 msec (mean ± 3 SD). It is delayed if it exceeds 40 msec. The reflex latency is measured from the stimulus artifact to the initial deflection of the potential. Consensual R2 latency (contralateral to the side of stimulus) is 32 ± 11 msec (mean ± 3 SD). It is delayed if it exceeds 41 msec. The difference between values for R2 consensual and R2 direct is normally less than 5 msec (mean ± 3 SD). This measurement requires only "one" stimulus, since R2 appears ipsilaterally and contralaterally to the side stimulated.

Amplitude: R1: 0.38 ± 0.23 mV
R2: 0.53 ± 0.24 mV

Neonates: (*N* = 30)

R1 Component latency: 12.1 ± 0.96 msec (mean ± 1 SD)

R2 Direct Component Latency: 35.85 ± 2.45 msec (mean ± 1 SD). The contralateral R2 often is absent. It was bilaterally absent in one-third and usually only ipsilateral in the other two-thirds.

Amplitude: R1: 0.51 ± 0.18 mV
R2: 0.39 ± 0.19 mV

Comments:
1. Latency is measured from the stimulus artifact to the initial deflection of the evoked potential (R1 or R2). Dr. Kimura suggests using the shortest latency of eight stimulations.
2. Both R1 and R2 waves probably are due to a polysynaptic brain stem reflex, the blink reflex, with the afferent arc provided by the sensory branches of the trigeminal nerve and the efferent arc provided by the facial nerve motor fibers.
   R1 is affected by lesions in:
   trigeminal nerve (afferent arc)
   pons (central arc)
   facial nerve (efferent arc)
   R2 is affected by:
   level of consciousness
   habituation
   lateral medullary lesion
   contralateral hemispheric lesion
   parkinsonism
   medications [diazepam (Valium)]
3. When the supraorbital nerve is stimulated, both R1 and R2 are regularly elicited in normals.
4. When the infraorbital nerve is stimulated, R2 is always present, but R1 is inconsistent in normals.
5. When the mental nerve is stimulated, R2 is inconsistent, and R1 is present only rarely in normals.

BULBOCAVERNOSUS REFLEX LATENCY

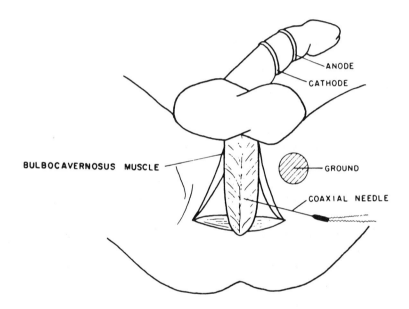

Figure 7.3. Bulbocavernosus reflex latency.

Figure 7.3

Pickup: The active electrode is a coaxial needle inserted into the bulbo-cavernosus muscle. This muscle is superficial and is located under the scrotum on either side of the midline. Needle placement can be confirmed by squeezing the glans penis and observing the bulbocavernosus reflex. A monopolar needle can be inserted into the bulbocavernosus muscle.

Reference: The reference·skin electrode is near the placement of the monopolar needle described above.

Ground: The ground is placed in a convenient location near the perineum.

Stimulation: Stimulation is on the dorsal side of the penile shaft and can be done using ring electrodes of a surface stimulator. The voltage required in this case usually is 50–200 V, or 5–20 mA, and the duration is 0.1 msec. Siroky et al. report using a 0.5-msec duration.

Electromyograph settings:
- Frequency: 8 Hz to 8 kHz
- Sweep speed: 10 msec/div
- Gain: 250 μV

Normal values:
Values were measured to the onset of the negative peak, which is often somewhat diffuse.

Siroky et al.: 35 ± 2 msec (mean ± 1 SD); range, 28–42 msec (N = 52 adult men).

Dick et al.: 31 msec: average; range, 24–40 msec (N = 10 adult men).

Comments: This study also can be done on women. Either the clitoris can be stimulated or a special stimulator can be attached to a Foley catheter and placed intraurethrally. Several other investigators also have reported values. It appears that under 42 msec is normal with most techniques. However, Siroky's study defined abnormal as greater than 45 msec. Skin temperature was not reported.

Siroky MB, Sax DS, Krane RJ: Sacral signal tracing: The electrophysiology of the bulbo-cavernosus reflex. *J Urol* 122:661–664, 1979.
Dick HC, Bradley WE, Scott FB, Timm GW: Pudendal sexual reflexes. Electrophysiologic investigations. *Urology* 3:376–379, 1974.

H REFLEX OF THE FLEXOR CARPI RADIALIS

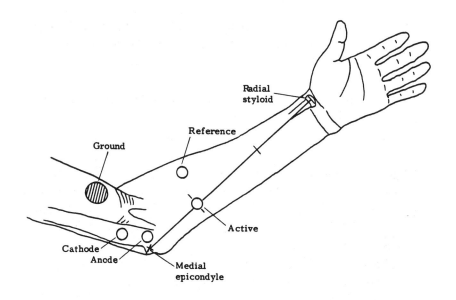

Figure 7.4.   H reflex of the flexor carpi radialis.

Figure 7.4
Jabre

Pickup: The active recording surface electrode is placed over the belly of the flexor carpi radialis, which is at about one-third of the line between the medial epicondyle and the radial styloid.

Reference: The reference is placed over the bracheoradialis.

Ground: The ground is placed between the stimulator and the active electrode.

Stimulation: The median nerve is stimulated using bipolar surface electrodes with the cathode proximal. A 0.5- to 1.0-msec rectangular pulse is used. The frequency of stimuli is not more than 0.5 Hz.

Electromyograph settings:
- Frequency: 20 Hz to 10 khz
- Sweep speed: 5 msec/div
- Gains: 200 μV/div

Normal values: (N = 50, S = 30; 12 men and 27 women) Age, 15–56 years.
Latency (msec): 15.9 ± 1.5
Amplitude (mV): 1.6 ± 0.4.

Comments: Room temperature was maintained at 70°F. Amplitudes were measured from the baseline to the negative peak. No identifiable H reflex was obtained in about 10% of an otherwise healthy volunteer population. The difference in latency between the right and the left is not more than 1 msec.

de Visser et al.

Pickup: A coaxial electrode was inserted into the flexor carpi radialis.

Stimulation: The median nerve at the elbow was stimulated using bipolar surface electrodes.

Electromyograph settings:
- Stimulation duration: 0.5 msec of a rectangular pulse
- Frequency of stimuli: 0.2 Hz

Normal values: (S = 52; 28 women and 24 men) Age, 20–85 years (mean age 50.8 years)
Latency (msec): 16.8 ± 1.1 (right and left difference, 0.38 ± 2.4)

Comments: The room temperature was maintained between 23 and 25°C. The skin temperature in the upper extremity ranged from 32 to 34°C. The test may be valuable in studying proximal lesions, such as the C6 or C7 radiculopathies and brachial plexopathies.

Jabre JF: Surface recording of the H-reflex of the flexor carpi radialis. *Muscle Nerve* 4: 435–438, 1981.
de Visser O, Schimsheimer RJ, Hart AAM: The H-reflex of the flexor carpi radialis muscle: A study in controls and radiation-induced brachial plexus lesions. *J Neurol Neurosurg Psychiatry* 47:1098–1101, 1984.

H-WAVE LATENCY TO THE GASTROCNEMIUS

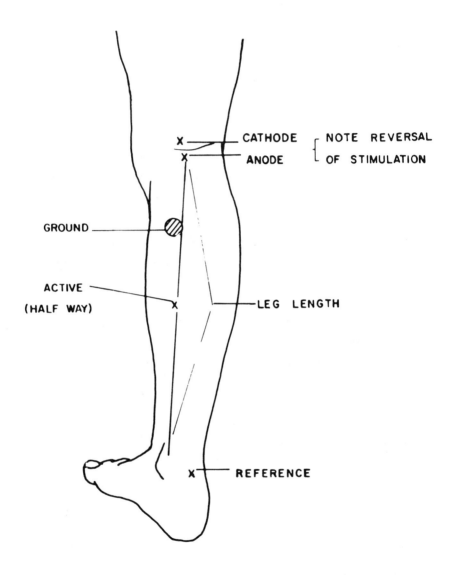

Figure 7.5.   H-wave latency to the gastrocnemius.

Figure 7.5

Pickup: The patient is prone with the feet suspended over the edge of the table or with a pillow placed under the ankles. The active surface electrode is placed on a point of bisection on the line connecting the popliteal crease and the proximal flare of the medial malleolus.

Reference: The reference is placed over the Achilles tendon.

Ground: The ground is placed between the sites of stimulation and pickup. This is especially important in H reflexes and minimizes artifacts.

Stimulation: Low-intensity current (submaximal stimulus) is used. The cathode is proximal (reverse of normal) and is placed over the tibial nerve in the popliteal fossa at the level of the popliteal crease. The nerve is just lateral to the popliteal artery or at the midpopliteal crease. (*Note:* A common error is to stimulate the peroneal nerve, which gives a wave that can be mistaken for the H reflex. Check for gastrocnemius contraction and the absence of peroneal contraction.)

Distance: Leg length is measured from the site of stimulation in the midpopliteal crease to the medial malleolus. (*Note:* This is not the tip of the medial malleolus, but represents a point over the tibial nerve just before it passes behind the most proximal part of the medial malleolus.)

Electromyograph settings:
- Frequency: 8 Hz to 8 kHz
- Sweep speed: 10 msec/div
- Gain: 200 or 500 μV
- Intensity of stimulus: approximately 25–30 V
- Frequency of stimulus: 0.5 pulses/sec
- Duration of stimulus: 1.0 msec

Normal values: ($N = 100$)
Predicted H latency (msec): $9.14 + 0.46 \times$ leg length (cm) $+ 0.1 \times$ age (years); measured value should be within 5.5 msec (250's) of the theoretical value
A difference between two legs of 1.2 msec (3 SEs) may be considered significant, assuming equal leg lengths.

Braddom RL, Johnson EW: Standardization of H reflex and diagnostic use in S1 radiculopathy. *Arch Phys Med Rehabil* 55:161–166, 1974.

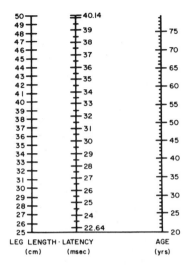

Figure 7.6. Nomogram of the simultaneous regression of H wave latency on leg length and age. (From Braddom and Johnson, 1970.)

Figure 7.6

Comments:

1. The H wave is thought to be due to the H reflex, a monosynaptic reflex evoked by direct electrical stimulation of large group Ia afferent fibers.

2. The H wave is recognized as an unchanging muscle evoked–action potential, which occurs at a latency of 28–35 msec in normals when measured from the gastrocnemius–soleus muscle in adults. It appears at submaximal stimulus either before or shortly after the appearance of the M response. With increase in stimulus intensity, the maximal H wave can be seen when the M response is submaximal. Further increases in the stimulus intensity increase the amplitude of the M response and reduce the amplitude of the H wave. At supramaximal stimulus, the H wave disappears and sometimes is replaced by an F wave.

3. Dr. Johnson suggests measuring latency and comparing it with predicted value. If latency is prolonged, or history and physical are highly suggestive of radiculopathy, then contralateral latency should be determined. A 1.2-msec or greater difference may be significant. In addition, an abnormal H-reflex latency requires evaluation of sensory conduction (e.g., sural nerve) and motor conduction (e.g., tibial or peroneal nerve) to rule out neuropathy.

4. The H wave normally is present at birth, but after the age of 6 months it is present only in the gastrocnemius–soleus and flexor carpi radialis muscles and occasionally can be recorded from the hamstrings and quadriceps muscles.

5. The H wave is triphasic, with an initial positive deflection and a large negative deflection in the gastrocnemius–soleus muscle. The highest amplitude of the H-reflex is up to 50–100% of the maximum M wave.

6. Active contraction of the antagonist muscle can inhibit the H reflex.

7. Marked shortening or lengthening of the muscle from which the H wave is being recorded can inhibit the reflex.

8. Sleep also may inhibit the reflex.

9. The H-wave latency shows high sensitivity to S-1 radiculopathy.

10. The H-wave latency is abnormal in a strictly sensory S-1 radiculopathy.

11. The H-wave latency becomes abnormal immediately or shortly after injury to S-1 nerve root.

12. The H-wave latency allows better differentiation between L-5 and S-1 radiculopathy.

13. Amplitude and duration of the H wave are too variable to be used clinically.

14. The H wave may not be present bilaterally in persons over the age of 60 years.

H-WAVE LATENCY TO THE SOLEUS

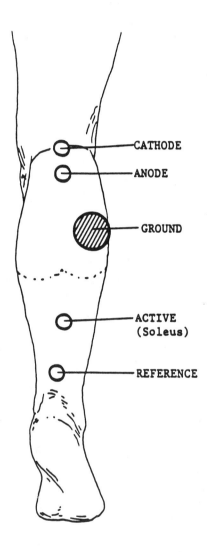

Figure 7.7. H-wave latency to the soleus.

Figure 7.7

Pickup: The active surface electrode is placed over the soleus muscle.

Reference: The reference is placed over the Achilles tendon distal to the active electrode.

Ground: The ground is placed between the stimulating and the active electrodes.

Stimulation: Stimulation is delivered to the tibial nerve over the popliteal fossa with the cathode proximal.

Normal values: H-reflex latency according to height (msec)
Short (147–160 cm): 28.46 ± 1.8
Medium (163–175 cm): 29.9 ± 2.12
Tall (178–193 cm): 31.5 ± 1.2

Comments: Latencies more than 2 SDs or absent responses were considered abnormal.

Tonzola RF, Ackil AA, Shahani BT, Young RR: Usefulness of electrophysiological studies in the diagnosis of lumbosacral root disease. *Ann Neurol* 9:305–308, 1981.

F WAVE IN THE UPPER EXTREMITY

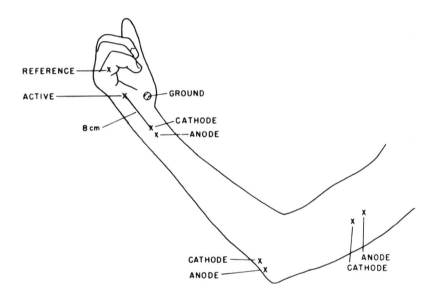

Figure 7.8.   F wave in the upper extremity, testing the ulnar side.

Figure 7.8

General: The F wave is not a reflex because the afferent and efferent arc of this response consist of the same alpha motor axon.

Pickup: The active surface electrode for the median nerve is over the abductor pollicis brevis. The active surface for the ulnar nerve is over the abductor digiti quinti. (This placement is the same as standard median or ulnar motor surface nerve placement.)

Reference: For the median nerve, the reference is on the distal phalanx of the thumb; for the ulnar nerve, it is on the fifth digit.

Ground: The ground is between the stimulation and pickup sites.

Stimulation: Stimulation can be applied at the wrist, elbow, or in the axilla; however, axillary stimulation is difficult unless the collision technique is used. Exact sites of stimulation are not described. The stimulating electrode is distal and not proximal. Supramaximal stimulation is used.

Electromyograph settings:
- Frequency: 8 Hz to 8 kHz
- Sweep speed: 5 msec/div
- Gain: 250 μV

Distance: The distance from the point of stimulus to the seventh cervical spine is measured as follows: Surface measurements are made with the patient in the upright position and the arm abducted 90°. The hand is supinated for the median nerve and pronated for the ulnar nerve. Measurements are made along the course of the nerve to the axilla, then around the back of the shoulder (posteriorly) to the seventh cervical spinous process (T-1 is most prominent; seventh cervical is second most prominent).

Kimura J: F-wave velocity in the central segment of the median and ulnar nerves. A study in normal subjects and in patients with Charcot–Marie–Tooth disease. *Neurology (Minn)* 24:539–546, 1974.

Normal values: (N = 33)

Latency is measured to onset of the F wave and is the minimal latency after several trials (8–10 F waves).

Latency values (mean ± 1 SD msec)

Site	Median nerve	Ulnar nerve
Wrist	29.1 ± 2.3	30.5 ± 3.0
Elbow	24.8 ± 2.0	26.0 ± 1.8
Axilla	21.7 ± 2.8	21.9 ± 1.9

Latency difference between two stimulus points (mean ± 1 SD msec)

Site	Median nerve	Ulnar nerve
Elbow–wrist	4.3 ± 0.8	4.1 ± 0.8
Axilla–elbow	3.5 ± 0.5	4.1 ± 0.9

$$\text{F wave velocity (m/sec)} = \frac{\text{(distance from stimulus point to C-7 spine)(2 mm)}}{\text{(F latency} - \text{M latency)} - 1 \text{ msec}}$$

F-wave velocity

Median nerve	m/sec (mean ± 1 SD)
Wrist–spinal cord	59.2 ± 3.9
Elbow–spinal cord	62.2 ± 5.2
Axilla–spinal cord	64.3 ± 6.4

Ulnar nerve	m/sec (mean ± 1 SD)
Wrist–spinal cord	56.7 ± 2.9
Elbow–spinal cord	59.4 ± 4.7
Axilla–spinal cord	63.1 ± 5.9

Characteristics of F wave versus H wave and M wave:

1. In contrast with the H wave, the F wave can be recorded from almost every skeletal muscle in the adult. The latency of the F wave is longer, with more distal sites of stimulation.
2. The amplitude of the F wave usually is less than that of the H wave. The F wave often is not present with each stimulus.

3. Supramaximal stimulus, which abolishes the H wave, is used for recording F waves.
4. The F wave has a smaller amplitude than the M wave and is variable in latency and configuration when recorded with surface electrodes.

Comments:
1. Latency values are not useful until the exact sites of stimulation are indicated and standards are established.
2. It becomes abnormal immediately after an injury.
3. One cannot distinguish between acute and chronic radiculopathy.
4. It receives innervation from multiple nerve roots; hence, it may be normal when only one root is destroyed.
5. F waves do provide a means to measure conduction along the most proximal segment of a nerve.

F WAVE IN THE LOWER EXTREMITY

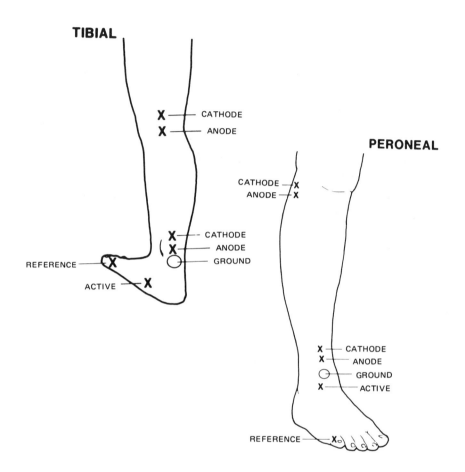

Figure 7.9. F wave in the lower extremity.

Figure 7.9

General: The F wave is not a reflex because the afferent and efferent arc of this response consist of the same alpha motor axon.

Peroneal Nerve (Patient Prone):

Pickup: The active surface electrode is placed over the extensor digitorum brevis muscle in the anterior lateral aspect of the proximal midtarsal level.

Reference: The reference is placed on the fifth digit.

Ground: The ground is placed between the stimulation and pickup sites.

Stimulation: Stimulation can be applied at the ankle, just lateral to the tibialis anterior tendon, or in the popliteal space over the lateral third of the flexor skin crease. The cathode is proximal, and supramaximal stimulation is used.

Electromyograph settings:
- Frequency: 8 Hz to 8 kHz
- Sweep speed: 5 msec/div
- Gain: 200–500 μV

Distance: The distance is measured from the stimulation site to the lower border of the thoracic-12 spinous process by way of the greater trochanter of the femur.

Normal values: (N = 66) The shortest of 10 latencies is taken.
Peroneal nerve F-wave latency from ankle: 51.3 ± 4.7 msec (mean ± 1 SD)
Peroneal nerve F-wave latency from knee: 42.7 ± 4.0 msec (mean ± 1 SD)
Peroneal nerve F-wave NCV (ankle to spinal cord): 53.5 ± 3.7 msec (mean ± 1 SD)
Peroneal nerve F-wave NCV (knee to spinal cord): 56.3 ± 4.9 mscc (mean ± 1 SD)

Kimura J, Bosch P, Linday GM: F-wave conduction velocity in the central segment of the peroneal and tibial nerves. *Arch Phys Med Rehab* 56:492–497, 1975.

$$\text{F-wave velocity (m/sec)} = \frac{\begin{array}{c}\text{(distance from stimulus to T-12)} \\ \times\ 2\ \text{(mm)}\end{array}}{\text{(F latency} - \text{M latency)} - 1\ \text{(msec)}}$$

Tibial Nerve (Patient Prone):

Pickup: The active surface pickup is placed over the abductor hallucis muscle, 1 cm behind and 1 cm below the navicular tubercle.

Reference: The reference is placed on the first digit.

Ground: The ground is placed between the stimulation and pickup sites.

Stimulation: Stimulation can be applied at the ankle, 1 cm posterior to the medial malleolus, or at the knee in the popliteal fossa. The cathode is proximal, and supramaximal stimulation is used.

Distance: Distance is measured from the stimulation sites to the lower border of the thoracic-12 spinous process by way of the greater trochanter of the femur.

Electromyograph settings:
- Frequency: 8 Hz to 8 kHz
- Sweep speed: 5 msec/div
- Gain: 200–500 μV

Normal values: ($N = 66$) The shortest of 10 latencies is taken.
> Tibial nerve F-wave latency from ankle: 52.3 ± 4.3 msec (mean ± 1 SD)
> Tibial nerve F-wave latency from knee: 43.5 ± 3.4 msec (mean ± 1 SD)
> Tibial nerve F-wave NCV (ankle to spinal cord): 51.3 ± 2.9 msec (mean ± 1 SD)
> Tibial nerve F-wave NCV (knee to spinal cord): 54.4 ± 3.6 msec (mean ± 1 SD)

Comment: Stimulation at the knee usually is tolerated better than at the ankle. Also see comments, page 179.

SYMPATHETIC SKIN RESPONSE

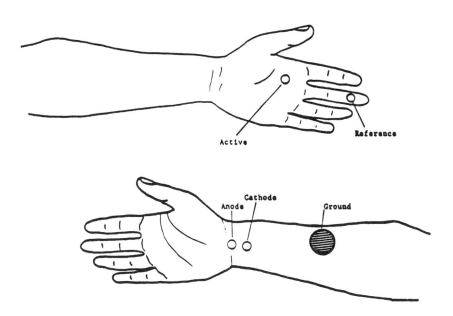

Figure 7.10. Sympathetic skin response.

Figures 7.10 and 7.11

Recording: The recording surface electrodes are placed on the hand and foot contralateral to the stimulus.
1. *Hand:* The active electrode is placed on palm, 3 cm proximal to the second web space and the reference on the distal phalanx of the third digit.
2. *Foot:* The active electrode is placed on plantar surface, 3 cm proximal to the first web space and the reference over the second toe.

Ground: The ground is placed at the wrist or ankle proximal to the recording electrodes.

Stimulation:
1. *Hand:* The stimulation is applied over the contralateral median nerve at the wrist; the cathode is placed proximally.
2. *Foot:* The stimulating cathode is placed over the second plantar interspace in the midfoot and the anode is attached to the second toe.

Electromyograph settings:
• Frequency: 2 Hz (0.5) to 5 kHz (500–2,000 Hz)
• Sweep: 300–500 msec/div
• Gain: 50–500 μV/div
• Duration: 0.2 msec

Sympathetic Skin Response

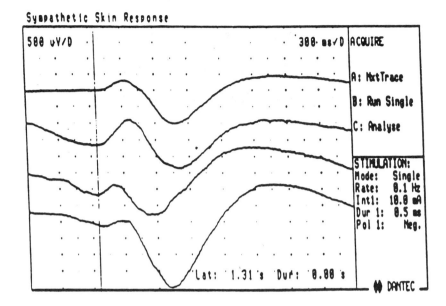

Figure 7.11. Sympathetic skin responses recorded from hand (palmar surface).

Normal Values: ($N = 30$)

	Latency (sec)	Amplitude (μV)
Palmar PASP	1.52 ± 0.13	479 ± 105
Plantar PASP	2.07 ± 0.16	101 ± 40

Sympathetic conduction velocity: 1.28 ± 0.18 m/sec

Comments: Ambient room temperature remained 20–23°C and limb temperature 34°C. The lights were dimmed and the room was quiet. The patients were relaxed. The stimulus intensities are 15–20 mA, with a duration of 0.2 msec. The interval of stimuli is more than 15 sec.

Knezevic W, Bajada S: Peripheral autonomic surface potential: A quantitative technique for recording sympathetic conduction in man. *J Neurol Sci* 67:239–251, 1985.

CHAPTER 8

Motor Nerve Conduction Velocity Studies in Premature Infants, Infants, and Children

Figures 8.1, 8.2, and 8.3

1. The motor nerve conduction velocity (MNCV) values of newborns are about half those of adults.
2. By age 3 years, the MNCV values are in the lower adult range.
3. By the age of 5 years, the MNCV values are essentially the same as those for adults.
4. Premature infant values (Cerra and Johnson):
   a. Premature ulnar MNCV (N = 19): 20.2 ± 2.6 m/sec (mean ± 1 SD); range, 16.5–24.6 m/sec.
   b. Premature peroneal MNCV (N = 17): 19.1 ± 4.2 m/sec (mean ± 1 SD); range, 13.7–28.3 m/sec.
5. The MNCV for the median, peroneal, and ulnar nerves for term infants, children, and adolescents are graphed in Figures 8.1, 8.2, and 8.3. These figures, which express the mean ± 2 SD, are derived from the work of Ingrid Gamstorp.
6. In children, the medial and posterior tibial nerves are the most readily accessible for study.

Cerra D, Johnson EW: Motor conduction velocity in premature infants. *Arch Phys Med Rehabil* 43:160–164, 1962.

Gamstorp I: Normal conduction velocity of ulnar, median and peroneal nerves in infancy, childhood and adolescence. *Acta Paediatr Scand* 146(Suppl):68–76, 1963.

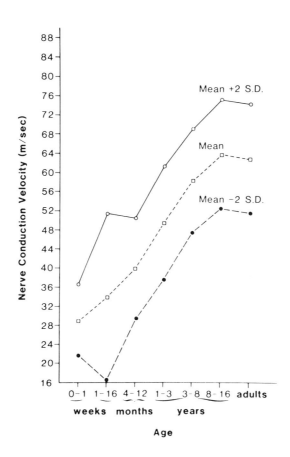

Figure 8.1. Median motor nerve conduction velocity (mean ± 2 SD) for term infants, children, and adolescents.

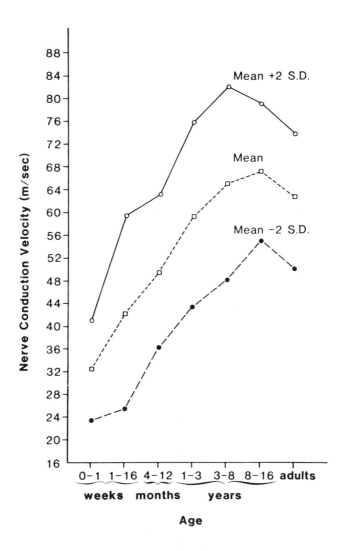

Figure 8.2. Ulnar motor nerve conduction velocity (mean ± 2 SD) for term infants, children, and adolescents.

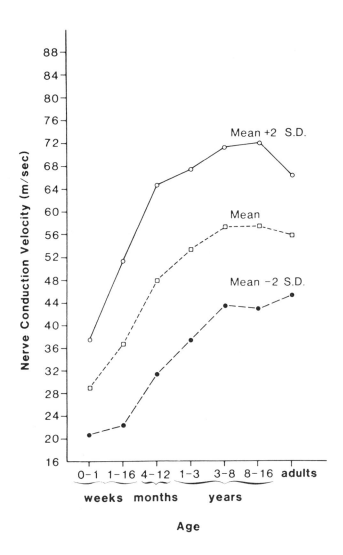

Figure 8.3.   Peroneal motor nerve conduction velocity (mean ± 2 SD) for term infants, children, and adolescents.

CHAPTER 9

Repetitive Stimulation (Neuromuscular Junction)

Figure 9.1

Repetitive stimulation techniques can be useful in diagnosing diseases of the neuromuscular junction; however, technical errors can give erroneous results, and careful attention to technique is essential.

1. For 24 hours before testing, the patient must receive no medication that affects the neuromuscular junction.
2. The results must be printed on light-sensitive paper or stored and photographed for accurate measurement.
3. The muscle and joint(s) it crosses are immobilized to minimize movement artifact, and the stimulating and recording electrodes are secured to avoid any movement. Immobilization is best with the muscles stretched and joint(s) extended.
4. The skin temperature is 34°C (94°F) to avoid false negative results.
5. All stimuli must be supramaximal.
6. In myasthenic syndrome (Lambert–Eaton syndrome), the deficit is present in any muscle tested.
7. If the patient is suspected of having botulism, any clinically weak muscle is tested.
8. In myasthenia gravis, muscle weakness increases with exertion but improves with rest and with anticholinesterase drugs. Proximal muscle testing is much more sensitive than distal; however, testing proximal is technically more difficult.

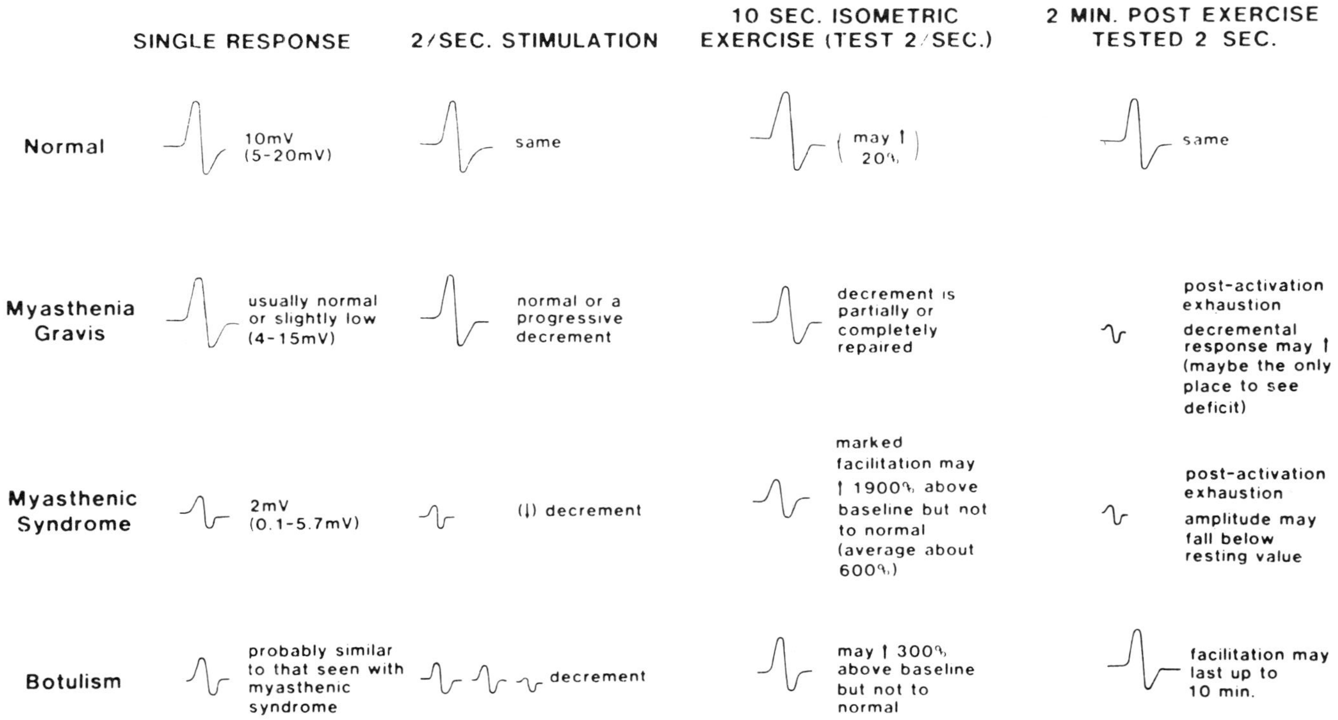

	SINGLE RESPONSE	2/SEC. STIMULATION	10 SEC. ISOMETRIC EXERCISE (TEST 2/SEC.)	2 MIN. POST EXERCISE TESTED 2 SEC.
Normal	10mV (5-20mV)	same	(may ↑ 20%)	same
Myasthenia Gravis	usually normal or slightly low (4-15mV)	normal or a progressive decrement	decrement is partially or completely repaired	post-activation exhaustion decremental response may ↑ (maybe the only place to see deficit)
Myasthenic Syndrome	2mV (0.1-5.7mV)	(↓) decrement	marked facilitation may ↑ 1900% above baseline but not to normal (average about 600%)	post-activation exhaustion amplitude may fall below resting value
Botulism	probably similar to that seen with myasthenic syndrome	decrement	may ↑ 300% above baseline but not to normal	facilitation may last up to 10 min.

Figure 9.1. Repetitive stimulation (a decrement must be reproducible on a number of trials).

Proximal stimulation:

a. *Facial nerve:* Stimulate at the angle of the jaw with the active electrode over the nasalis muscle. Use a 2 × 2 gauze to act as a compression dressing filling the void at the side of the nose.

b. *Upper trunk brachial plexus:* Stimulate at Erb's point with the active electrode over the deltoid muscle. This technique is painful, and movement artifact can be a problem.

c. *Musculocutaneous nerve:* Stimulate in the axilla with the active electrode over the biceps brachii muscle. With this technique, the stimulus can be unstable.

d. *Femoral nerve:* Stimulate in the inguinal region with the active electrode over the vastus medialis muscle. This technique can be painful.

e. *Spinal accessory nerve:* Stimulate the nerve as it descends along the posterior border of the sternocleidomastoid muscle with the active electrode over the upper trapezius at the angle of the neck and shoulder. The patient is upright in a chair; the arms are adducted and extended with the hand holding on to the bottom of the chair. Exercise is obtained by having the patient shrug the shoulders against his/her own resistance.

Distal stimulation:

a. *Ulnar nerve:* Most investigators test the ulnar nerve distally. Stimulate the ulnar nerve at the wrist with the active electrode over the abductor digiti minimi muscle.

b. *Median nerve:* Stimulate the median nerve at the wrist with the active electrode over the abductor pollicis brevis muscle. The disadvantage of this technique is that the thumb is difficult to immobilize.

9. During each portion of the test (the single response, the 2/sec stimulation, the 10-sec postexercise), the potential amplitude often decreases during the first four responses. Thus, most investigators measure the fifth response, compare its amplitude to that of the first response of the train, and calculate the percentage of change.

10. In a rigidly controlled system, a decrement by the fifth successive potential (compared to the first) of 10% is definitely abnormal in distal muscles. In proximal muscles, where rigid control is more difficult to obtain, only decrements of more than 20% are considered abnormal.
11. The following are important to observe during testing:
    a. Amplitude of the initial response to a single nerve supramaximal stimulation
    b. Presence or absence of a decrement during repetitive stimulation at a slow rate
    c. Presence or absence of a decrement or increment after isometric exercise and then stimulation at a slow rate
    d. Postactivation facilitation
    e. Postactivation exhaustion
    f. Change in response after anticholinesterase drugs.
12. Actual technique:
    a. To obtain the single response: In an unexercised muscle, initially use a high voltage to obtain a supramaximal response; then look at the peak-to-peak amplitude of the initial muscle action potential.
    b. Wait 1 min before stimulating at a frequency of 2 or 3/sec for 3 sec, looking for a decrement. For screening purposes, a train of three to five stimuli is adequate. To test reproducibility of the decrement, a muscle must be rested 1 min between tests.
    c. Wait at least 1 min (until the amplitude is back to the initial amplitude and use it as the baseline before exercise) before having the patient perform isometric exercises for 10 sec (30 sec if the muscle is not clinically weak).
    d. Ten seconds after the exercise facilitation is completed, start to stimulate at 2 or 3/sec for 3 sec. Repeat this at 30 sec and at 1, 2, 3, and 5 min to check for postactivation exhaustion or facilitation. (According to the literature, 2 min appears to be the most sensitive time.)
13. Figure 9.1 indicates results seen with repetitive stimulation in normals and in patients with myasthenia gravis, myasthenic syndrome, and botulism.

14. A more sensitive method for evaluating the status of the neuro-muscular junction is jitter study of a motor fiber pair by single fiber electromyography.

15. Each laboratory should establish its approach and technique for evaluating possible dysfunction of the neuromuscular junction. Technique is perfected by performing a number of tests on normal persons.

REFERENCES

Botelho SY, Deaterly DF, Austin S, Comroe JH Jr: Evaluation of the electromyogram of patients with myasthenia gravis. *AMA Arch Neurol Psychiatry* 67:441–450, 1952.

Harvey AM, Masland RL: A method for the study of neuromuscular transmission in human subjects. *Bull Johns Hopkins Hosp* 68:81–93, 1941.

Lambert EH: Diagnostic value of electrical stimulation of motor nerves. *Electroencephalogr Clin Neurophysiol* 14(Suppl 22):9–16, 1962.

Oh SJ: *Electromyography: Neuromuscular Transmission Studies.* Baltimore: Williams & Wilkins, 1988.

Schumm F, Stohr M: Accessory nerve stimulation in the assessment of myasthenia gravis. *Muscle Nerve* 7:147–151, 1984.

Slomic A, Rosenfalck A, Buchthal F: Electrical and mechanical response of normal and myasthenic muscle with particular reference to the staircase phenomenon. *Brain Res* 10:1–78, 1968.

CHAPTER 10

Somatosensory Evoked Potentials

GENERAL GUIDELINES FOR SOMATOSENSORY EVOKED POTENTIAL TESTING

Surface electrical excitation of large myelinated fibers in peripheral nerves produces afferent volleys that ascend in the posterior columns–medial lemnisus–thalmocortical projections to the primary somatosensory cortex. These afferent volleys can be recorded over the peripheral nerve, spinal cord, and scalp with various surface recording montages (electrode locations) in humans. Appropriate selection of stimulation/recording techniques, meticulous preparation of the patient and testing environment, and adequate recording instrumentation are necessary for optimal acquisition of somatosensory evoked potentials (SEPs). The following sections cover the fundamentals of an approach to the patient for SEP testing, stimulation/recording techniques, designation/nomenclature, and clinical applications.

Patient Preparation

When scheduling a patient for SEP testing, a short description of the study should be provided to acquaint the patient with the testing procedure and to reduce anxiety. A history and physical examination should be performed to decide which nerves are to be tested. Other peripheral and central nervous system lesions also should be identified so that the test results reflect assessment of the clinical problem being addressed. Medications and prior surgical procedures of peripheral nerves, plexi, spinal cord, or brain should be recorded.

Myogenic silence is mandatory to prevent contamination of the evoked potential by electromyographic (EMG) activity and to eliminate somatomotor evoked potentials (time/event-related evoked motor potentials recorded over the paraspinal muscles).[1] These latter potentials are facilitated by muscle contraction; therefore, myogenic silence is necessary. Silence in the testing room also should be promoted with low-intensity lighting, and short periods of nerve stimulation without averaging should be performed to acquaint the patient with the procedure and the testing environment before data are taken. Patients either can lie in a supine or prone position for either lower or upper extremity nerve stimulation or may sit in a chair for upper extremity SEP testing. Patients with low-back pain may have to have a pillow placed under their pelvis or lie on their side to have the study performed. If a sedative has to be used to achieve relaxation, chloral hydrate is recommended, for it has no observable effects on presynaptic or postsynaptic potentials. Valium can modify the amplitude and configuration of midlatency potentials from upper extremity nerve stimulation.[2]

Stimulation Techniques

Mixed sensory/motor or sensory nerves can be stimulated with surface stimulation techniques. Motor threshold can be used as an indicator of adequate stimulus intensity; however, 1.5 times motor threshold activates more myelinated fibers, thus producing larger spinal and scalp responses. This stimulus intensity usually is tolerated satisfactorily by most patients. Two to three times sensory threshold is used for sensory nerve stimulation; however, stimulus intensity depends on the patient's tolerance. When doing bilateral studies, it is important to use identical stimulus intensities for valid comparison of data. Stimulation rates of 3 Hz are tolerated comfortably by the patient; however, in certain disease states, lower rates of 0.5 or 1 Hz may have to be used. A stimulus rate that is not an integral of 60 Hz (i.e., 4.7 Hz) may have to be used if 60 Hz interference is present. A 0.1- or 0.2-msec duration stimulus is satisfactorily tolerated. In certain clinical conditions in which nerve excitability and conduction are impaired, stimulus rates of 0.5 Hz and stimulus durations as long as 1 msec may have to be used. H-response thresholds or stimulus intensities to obliterate the H response also can be employed if the tibial nerve is used for stimulation.[3,4]

When stimulating a peripheral nerve, the cathode should be proximal to the anode. The ground electrode is placed between the stimulator and recording electrodes, preferably closer to the recording electrodes to minimize stimulus artifact.

Bilateral (simultaneous) peripheral nerve stimulation can be used and bilateral short, medium, and long latency components of the scalp responses can be analyzed. For analysis of unilateral lesions, unilateral stimulation is accepted as the most appropriate form of stimulation.

Dermatomal stimulation can be performed by stimulating the skin in a specific dermatome at sensory or two or three times the sensory threshold and the response is recorded over the scalp. Peripheral nerve or spinal potentials are unable to be recorded by conventional recording techniques with this form of stimulation. Clinical application of this methodology is currently being explored.

Recording Techniques

Conventional 0.5-cm gold or silver-silver cup electroencephalogram (EEG) electrodes can be used to record the SEPs over the peripheral nerve, spine, or scalp; 1-cm stainless steel subdermal EEG electrodes can be used for recording over the scalp. In using surface electrodes, the skin under the electrode should be prepared with a pumice paste (this also applies to the ground electrode) to minimize skin–electrode impedance. Impedance measurements should be kept under 1,200 Ω. Because SEPs are low in amplitude (0.1–3 µV), an averager is required to increase the signal-to-noise ratio to produce a measurable response. A total of 128 to 1,000 sweeps may have to be averaged to obtain a measurable and reproducible response. The number of sweeps averaged to obtain a measurable response depends on the age, electrical contamination from the environment, EMG, activity, weight, recording electrode montage, and impedance–amplifier–averager characteristics. At least two recordings should be obtained to confirm the presence of a response.[5] A 50-msec analysis time usually is used for upper extremity SEPs and a 100-msec analysis time for lower extremity SEPs. This can be altered according to the clinical condition being investigated. Amplifier gains of 100,000 (10 µV/div) usually are adequate for signal acquisition. Amplitude bandwidth of 10 to 5,000 Hz is adequate for peripheral and spinal recordings. A 0- to 2,000-Hz bandpass is satisfactory for scalp responses; however, if far-field potentials are to be accentuated, the lower bandpass should be increased to 300 to 500 Hz.[6]

Four-channel evoked potential systems are recommended for accurate clinical interpretation of data. If two-channel evoked potential systems are used, repeat studies may be needed to delineate focal or diffuse lesions.

Bipolar (differential) or monopolar (referential) recording montages (electrode locations) can be used for SEPs. In general, monopolar recordings are larger in amplitude, frequently contain volume-conducted electrical events (nonneural and neural), and reflect increased contamination from EMG, electrocardiogram (ECG), movement artifact, and unwanted electromagnetic interference from the environment. Because of the summation characteristics of bipolar recordings, the peaks and the generated waveforms may not represent valid anatomic–physiologic correlates; however, peak latency measurements reflect propagated sensory nerve action potentials.

Extremity skin temperature should be kept between 30° and 35°C when clinical judgments are being made only from absolute latency measurements. Central conduction is not appreciably affected by cool extremities. Allowing patients to adjust to ambient room temperature (23–26°C) is acceptable; however, reduced peripheral conduction measurements may have to be adjusted according to peripheral limb temperature.[7–9]

Far-field potentials (potentials where the biologic origin is located at a considerable distance from the recording electrodes) can be recorded with an active cephalic electrode and noncephalic (leg, arm) electrode by stimulating a mixed peripheral nerve. The electrical generators of these potentials are not uniformly agreed upon, and clinical applications have not been perfected.

Figure 10.1
The international 10–20 system (Figure 10.1) is a system of electrode placement on the scalp in which electrodes are placed either 10% or 20% of the total distance between the nasion and inion in the sagittal plane and between right and left preauricular points in the coronal plane. Placement of electrodes over the scalp is delineated in the text under each section dealing with specific nerve stimulation. Peripheral nerve and spinal electrode placements also are designated.

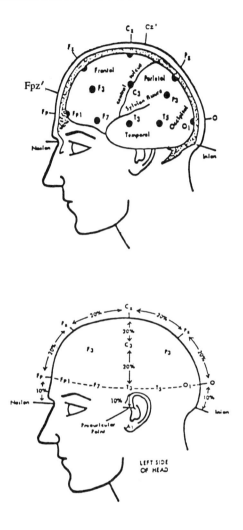

Figure 10.1. Location of scalp electrodes in the 10–20 system. *Top:* Relationship among central sulcus, sylvian fissure, lobes of the brain, and electrode positions. *Bottom:* In the 10–20 system, electrodes are placed either 10% or 20% of the total distance between.

Designated abbreviations for the 10–20 system:

Brain area	Left hemisphere	Midline	Right hemisphere
Frontal pole	F_{p1}		F_{p2}
Frontal	F_3		F_4
Inferior frontal	F_7		F_8
Midfrontal		F_z	
Midtemporal	T_3		T_4
Posterior temporal	T_5		T_6
Central	C_3		C_4
Vertex or midcentral		C_z	
Parietal	P_3		P_4
Midparietal		P_z	
Occipital	O_1		O_2

	Nonscalp leads		
Auricular	A_1		A_2

Designation of SEP Components, Nomenclature, and Measurement Parameters

Short-latency SEPs refer to that portion of a waveform of the SEP normally occurring within 25 msec after stimulation of a nerve in the upper extremity at the wrist, 40 msec after stimulation of a nerve in the lower extremity at the knee, and 50 msec after stimulation of the nerve in the lower extremity at the ankle. A midlatency SEP refers to that portion of a waveform of an SEP occurring within 25 to 100 msec after stimulation of a nerve in the upper extremity at the wrist; within 40 to 100 msec after stimulation of the nerve in the lower extremity at the knee; and within 50 to 100 msec after stimulation of a nerve in the lower extremity at the ankle. A long-latency SEP refers to that portion of an SEP occurring at a time greater than 100 msec after stimulation of a nerve in the upper extremity at the wrist or in the lower extremity at the knee or ankle.

Accepted nomenclature for identifying an SEP obtained by stimulating a specific nerve is the appropriate way to identify the SEP (i.e., median nerve SEP, peroneal nerve SEP). Peaks of SEPs are identified by polarity [(N) negative, upward on recordings in example; (P) positive, downward on recordings in examples] and average peak latency in the normal patient to the nearest millisecond. For example, N9 indicates a brachial plexus response occurring 9 msec (latency measured to the first major negative peak) after stimulation of the median nerve at the wrist in a normal person.

Ipsilateral latencies and side-to-side latency differences, amplitude, and duration measurements also are performed; however, the most reliable measurement is the peak latency. Interpeak latencies also are valuable in interpretation of clinical data. Amplitude measurements of SEP components are variable and, in general, amplitude differences (side-to-side comparison) greater than 50% are considered abnormal. Duration measurements also are highly variable and usually not clinically relevant at this time. Waveform morphology, particularly of the scalp SEPs, also is an important parameter; however, objective and analytical techniques have to be developed for accurate analysis of waveform morphology. These measurements are not considered here; however, several references are provided for the reader's interest.[10,11]

Clinical Applications of SEPs

Four channels usually are recommended to record upper or lower extremity SEPs. The first channel monitors the peripheral sensory nerve action potential and the other recordings are made over the shoulder (brachial plexus), cervical spine, and scalp.

Segmental sensory upper extremity SEP testing consists of stimulating the following cutaneous nerves:

lateral antebrachial cutaneous nerve (musculocutaneous nerve, lateral cord, upper trunk, C5 dorsal root)

superficial sensory radial nerve (radial nerve, posterior cord, upper trunk, C5 and C6 dorsal roots)

third digit (median nerve, lateral cord, middle trunk, C7 dorsal root)

fifth digit (ulnar nerve, medial cord, lower trunk, C8 and T1 dorsal roots).

Median nerve stimulation at the wrist (mixed motor/sensory nerve) activates C5, C6, C7, and C8 sensory fibers; therefore, this nerve is not adequate for localizing proximal brachial plexus or cervical root lesions. Median nerve SEPs are used to detect diffuse or multifocal central nervous system (CNS) disease or to detect localization of disease processes peripherally. Ulnar nerve stimulation at the wrist retains its segmental (C8, T1) input and is preferable to fifth digit stimulation because it produces larger peripheral and central responses. Dermatomal SEPs can be performed; however, peripheral sensory nerve action potentials, brachial plexus, or cervical responses are unable to be recorded using this technique. Also, muscle and joint afferents are not stimulated by performing dermatomal stimulation. Localizing peripheral or central lesions using this technique currently is being investigated.

Absolute latency measurements vary with arm length; therefore, arm length (measured from the stimulus site to the C7 spinous process) must be recorded and the latency modified by the algorithm of 0.2 × arm length + 2.7 cm.[12] Interpeak latencies (elbow–shoulder, shoulder–cervical spine, cervical spine–scalp) are calculated to determine peripheral versus central conduction times. Abnormal peripheral sensory conduction can produce CNS abnormalities; therefore, by eliminating the peripheral conduction measurement, a more accurate assessment of central transmission could be attained.

Segmental sensory testing of the lower extremities consists of stimulating the following cutaneous nerves:

lateral femoral cutaneous nerve (L2–L3)
saphenous nerve (L3, L4)
superficial peroneal nerve (ankle, L5)
sural nerve (ankle, L5, S1).

The tibial nerve (mixed motor/sensory; L4, L5, S1) can be stimulated at both the knee and ankle. Peroneal nerve stimulation (mixed motor/ sensory nerve) usually is performed at the knee (L4, L5, S1). When stimulating the tibial and peroneal nerves (mixed nerve), sensory fibers from multiple segmental spinal levels are activated; therefore, localization of lumbosacral plexus and spinal nerve lesions using this particular technique may be of limited value. Because of the difficulty in recording over the spinal cord from the lower extremity nerve stimulation in the adult, an accurate assessment of the conduction properties of ascending volleys in spinal pathways is difficult. Frequently, assessment of somatosensory transmission depends on scalp recordings, making difficult precise localization of one or more lesions of the somatosensory system at the spinal or subcortical levels. Spine-to-scalp propagation velocities are helpful in assessing central transmission time as well as interpeak latencies. Absolute latencies are a function of limb length and body height. By using interpeak latencies, the variable of height can be eliminated; however, if absolute latencies are used, a regression curve relating body height to latency must be employed.[13]

In humans, lesions of the peripheral or CNS can be classified topographically as focal, multifocal, or diffuse. In the peripheral nervous system, SEPs are useful in following peripheral nerve injury and in the diagnosis of entrapment syndromes. Proximal sensory neuropathies (i.e., traumatic, infectious, idiopathic) and radiculopathies also can be assessed by SEPs and complement the conventional electrophysiologic procedures of the peripheral nervous system in establishing the extent and severity of sensory system involvement. Diffuse lesions of the peripheral nervous system and spinal cord can produce SEP abnormalities and include the following entities: metabolic disorders (diabetes, uremia),[1a,1b,14] multiple sclerosis,[15,16] nutritional deficiencies,[17] CNS degenerative diseases,[18] and distal axonopathies.[19,20] This latter group consists of distal axonal degeneration occurring in the peripheral nervous system and in the central projections of the primary sensory neuron. The distal axonopathies include the spinocerebellar degenerations, nutritional disorders, diabetic and uremic polyneuropathies, paraneoplastic neuropathies, and toxic neuropathies (acrylamide, N-hexane).

The use of SEPs in assessing patients with multiple sclerosis has gained wide acceptance. Almost consistent abnormal SEPs have been noted in the patients with definite multiple sclerosis when there is clinical involvement of the system being tested.[15] SEPs are useful in identifying probable and possible multiple sclerosis and in uncovering silent lesions in these persons. Multimodal testing [SEPs, visual evoked potentials (VEPs), brain stem auditory evoked potentials (BAEPs)] is useful in evaluating multiple sclerosis, and SEPs and VEPs reportedly have a higher diagnostic yield than BAEPs. Trojaborg and Peterson[16] believe that the best yield in multiple sclerosis is given by SEPs from lower extremity nerve stimulation because a larger segment of the central

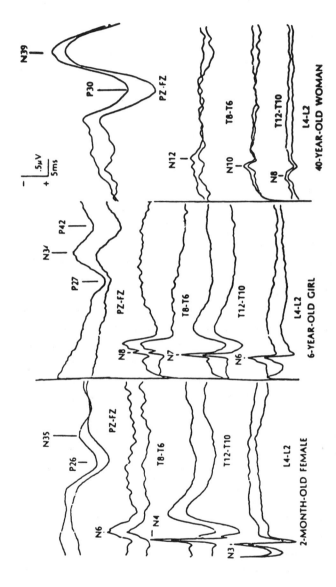

Figure 10.2. Spinal and scalp somatosensory responses to unilateral peroneal nerve stimulation (knee). Comparison of bipolar surface-recorded spinal and scalp SEPs from unilateral peroneal nerve stimulation (knee) in a 2-month-old infant, 6-year-old girl, and 40-year-old woman.

neuraxis is surveyed, which enhances the detection of any conduction defecit.

Spinal trauma, tumor, and myelodysplasia[21-25] are focal lesions of the spinal cord that SEPs can assess. The use of SEPs in intraoperative monitoring has gained wide acceptance and is useful in assessing ascending spinal pathways when patients are under general anesthesia.[26] SEPs also have been useful in detecting lesions in the brain stem and hemispheres. Abnormalities in scalp SEPs have been recorded in brain stem tumors, infarctions, and hemorrhages[27-30] when large-fiber proprioceptive and somesthetic pathways are involved. SEPs also have been used in monitoring patients in coma and in assessing brain-dead patients.[28,31]

Pediatric applications of SEPs have been described in focal and diffuse neurologic deficits.[18,24,32,33] Maturational considerations must be employed when making measurements in both the peripheral and central segments of the somatosensory pathway before interpreting SEPs. It is not until approximately 8 years of age that the central afferent pathways reach adult conduction ranges. Figure 10.2 shows the comparison of bipolar (differential) surface-recorded spinal and scalp SEPs from unilateral peroneal nerve stimulation in a 2-month-old infant, 6-year-old girl, and 40-year-old woman. These responses show a progressive diminution of the amplitudes of the spinal responses as one ages, whereas the scalp responses become larger.

REFERENCES

1a. Cracco RQ, Anziska BJ, Cracco JB, Vas GA, Rossini PM, Maccabee PJ: Short-latency somatosensory evoked potentials to median and peroneal nerve stimulation: Studies in normal subjects and patients with neurologic disease. *Ann NY Acad Sci* 388:412–425, 1982.
1b. Cracco JB, Cracco RQ: Spinal somatosensory evoked potentials: Maturational and clinical studies. *Ann NY Acad Sci* 388:526–537, 1982.
2. Prevec TS: Effect of Valium on the somatosensory evoked potential. In: Desmedt JH (ed): *Progress in Clinical Neurophysiology. Vol 7: Clinical Uses of Cerebral Brainstem and Spinal Somatosensory Evoked Potentials.* Basel: Karger, 1980;311–318.
3. Baran EM, Grover W, Brown L: Stimulus-response characteristics of spinal evoked potentials. *Electroencephalogr Clin Neurophysiol* 52:108P, 1981. (Abstract)
4. Dimitrijevic MR, Larsson LE, Lehmkuhl D, Sherwood A: Evoked spinal cord and nerve root potentials in humans using a non-invasive recording technique. *Electroencephalogr Clin Neurophysiol* 45:331–340, 1978.

5. Donchin E, Calloway E, Cooper R, et al.: Publication criteria for studies of evoked potentials (EP) in man. Report of a committee. In: Desmedt JH (ed): *Process in Clinical Neurophysiology. Vol 1: Attention, Voluntary Contraction, and Event-Related Cerebral Potentials.* Basel: Karger, 1977;1–11.
6. Rossini PM, Cracco RQ, Cracco JB, House WJ: Short latency somatosensory evoked potentials to peroneal nerve stimulation: Scalp topography and the effect of different frequency filters. *Electroencephalogr Clin Neurophysiol* 52:540–552, 1981.
7. Halar EM, DeLisa JA, Brozovich FV: Nerve conduction velocity: Relationship of skin, subcutaneous, and intramuscular temperatures. *Arch Phys Med Rehabil* 61: 199–203, 1980.
8. Abramson DI, Hlavova A, Rickert B, et al.: Effect of ischemia on median and ulnar motor nerve conduction velocities at various temperatures. *Arch Phys Med Rehabil* 51:463–470, 1970.
9. Abramson DI, Hlavova A, Rickert B, et al.: Effect of ischemia on latencies of the median nerve in the hand at various temperatures. *Arch Phys Med Rehabil* 51: 471–480, 1970.
10. Baran EM, Jacobs M, Kresch E, Odland J: Correlation coefficient analysis of somatosensory evoked potential waveforms. *Muscle Nerve* 7:571, 1984.
11. Jaeger S, Baran E, Mandel S, Whitenack S, Kresch E, Bess H, Odland JD: Mid-latency somatosensory evoked potential abnormalities in proximal sensory neuropathies. *Muscle Nerve* 8:618, 1985. (Abstract)
12. Eisen A, Stevens JC: *Upper Limb Somatosensory Evoked Potentials.* An American Association of Electromyography and Electrodiagnosis Workshop, September 1984.
13. Baran EM, Daube J: *Lower Extremity Somatosensory Evoked Potentials.* An American Association of Electromyography and Electrodiagnosis Workshop, September 1984.
14. Gupta PR, Dorfman LJ: Spinal somatosensory conduction in diabetes. *Neurology* 31:841–845, 1981.
15. Chiappa KH: Pattern shift visual, brainstem auditory, and short-latency somatosensory evoked potentials in multiple sclerosis. *Neurology* 30(7PT2):110–123, 1980.
16. Trojaborg W, Petersen E: Visual and somatosensory evoked cortical potentials in multiple sclerosis. *J Neurol Neurosurg Psychiatry* 42:323–330, 1979.
17. Krumholtz A, Weiss HD, Goldstein PJ, Harris KC: Evoked responses in vitamin B12 deficiency. *Ann Neurol* 9:407–409, 1981.
18. Cracco JB, Bosch VV, Cracco RQ: Cerebral and spinal somatosensory evoked potentials in children with CNS degenerative disease. *Electroencephalogr Clin Neurophysiol* 49:437–445, 1980.
19. Arezzo JC, Schaumburg HH, Vaughan HG Jr, Spencer PS, Barna JA: Hind limb somatosensory evoked potentials in the monkey: The effects of distal axonopathy. *Ann Neurol* 12:24–32, 1982.
20. Pedersen L, Trojaborg W: Visual, auditory, and somatosensory pathway involvement in hereditary cerebellar ataxia, Friedreich's ataxia, and familial spastic paraplegia. *Electroencephalogr Clin Neurophysiol* 52:283–297, 1981.
21. Cracco RQ: Spinal evoked response: Peripheral nerve stimulation in man. *Electroencephalogr Clin Neurophysiol* 35:379–386, 1973.
22. Baran EM: Lumbar and thoracic spinal evoked potentials in man: Frontiers in engineering and health care. In: Proceedings of the Fourth Annual Conference of IEEE Engineering in Medicine and Biology Society, New York: IEEE, 44–49, 1982.
23. Baran EM: Spinal and scalp somatosensory evoked potentials in spinal disorders. In: Course C (ed): *Somatosensory Evoked Potentials.* Rochester, MN: American Association of Electromyography and Electrodiagnosis, 1983;57–66.
24. Cracco JB, Cracco RQ: Somatosensory spinal and cerebral evoked potentials in children with occult spinal dysraphism. *Neurology* 29:543, 1979. (Abstract)

25. Rowed DW, McLean JAG, Tator CH: Somatosensory evoked potentials in acute spinal cord injury: Prognostic value. *Surg Neurol* 9:203–210, 1978.

26. Brown RH, Nash CL: Current status of spinal cord monitoring. *Spine* 4:466–470, 1979.

27. Anziska B, Cracco RQ: Short latency somatosensory evoked potentials: Studies in patients with focal neurological disease. *Electroencephalogr Clin Neurophysiol* 49: 227–239, 1980.

28. Hume AL, Cant BR, Shaw NA: Central somatosensory conduction time in comatose patients. *Ann Neurol* 5:379–384, 1979.

29. Noel P, Desmedt JE: Somatosensory cerebral evoked potentials after vascular lesions of the brainstem and diencephalon. *Brain* 98:113–128, 1975.

30. Pavot AP, Ignacio DR, Lightfoote WF II: Diagnostic value of multimodality evoked potentials in stroke. *Arch Phys Med Rehabil* 64:492–493, 1983. (Abstract)

31. Goldie WD, Chiappa KH, Young RR, Brooks EB: Brainstem auditory and short-latency somatosensory evoked responses in brain death. *Neurology* 31:248–256, 1981.

32. Hrbek A, Karlberg P, Kjellmer I, Olsson T, Riha M: Clinical application of evoked electroencephalographic responses in newborn infants: I. Perinatal asphyxia. *Dev Med Child Neurol* 19:34–44, 1977.

33. Desmedt JE, Brunko E, Debecker J: Maturation of the somatosensory evoked potentials in normal infants and children, with special reference to the early N1 component. *Electroencephalogr Clin Neurophysiol* 40:43–58, 1976.

MEDIAN NERVE SOMATOSENSORY EVOKED POTENTIALS

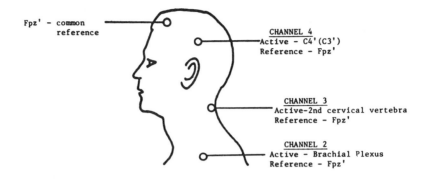

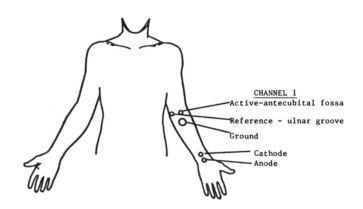

Figure 10.3. Median nerve SEPs. *Top:* Brachial plexus, second cervical vertebra, and C4′ (C3′) recording sites with Fpz′ as common reference. *Bottom:* Wrist stimulation and elbow recording sites.

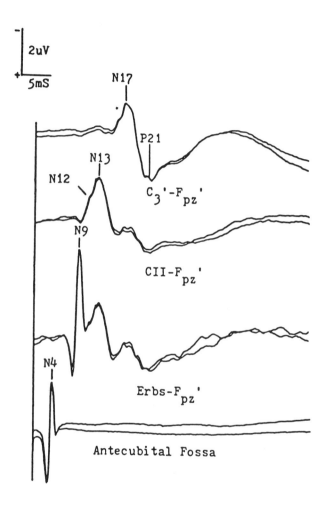

Figure 10.4. Left median nerve stimulation (wrist).

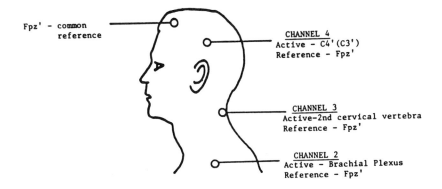

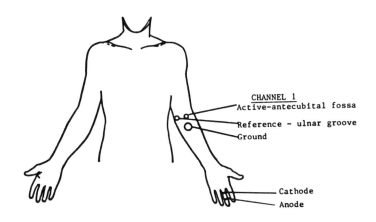

Figure 10.5. Median nerve SEPs. *Top:* Brachial plexus, second cervical vertebra, and C4' (C3') recording sites with Fpz' as common reference. *Bottom:* Third digit stimulation and elbow recording sites.

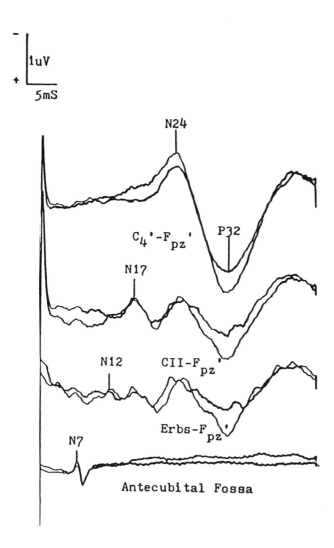

Figure 10.6. Left median nerve stimulation (third digit).

Figures 10.3 to 10.6
Stimulation/Recording Technique

Pickup (four sites):

Elbow (first channel): Surface electrodes are placed over the elbow; one over the antecubital fossa (active electrode) at a point bisecting a line drawn from the lateral to the medial humeral epicondyle; the other over the ulnar nerve in the ulnar groove (reference electrode).

Shoulder (second channel): The active electrode is placed over the brachial plexus at a point 2–3 cm bisecting an angle formed by the posterior border of the clavicular head of the sternocleidomastoid muscle and the clavicle. Resisted flexion of the head accentuates the clavicular head of the sternocleidomastoid muscle. The reference electrode can be either a common cephalic site (Fpz′) or the contralateral brachial plexus recording electrode.

Cervical spine (third channel): The active electrode is placed over the second cervical spinous process and referenced to the cephalic common reference (Fpz′).

Anziska B, Cracco RQ: Short latency SEP's to median nerve stimulation: Comparison of recording methods and origin of components. *Electroencephalogr Clin Neurophysiol* 52:531–539, 1981.

Chiappa KH: *Evoked Potentials in Clinical Medicine.* Raven Press, New York, 1983.

Chiappa KH, Choi S, Young RR: Short latency somatosensory evoked potentials following median nerve stimulation in patients with neurological lesions. In Desmedt JE (ed): *Progress in Clinical Neurophysiology, Vol 7: Clinical Uses of Cerebral, Brainstem, and Spinal Somatosensory Evoked Potentials.* Basel: Karger, 1980;264–281.

Eisen A: *The Somatosensory Evoked Potential.* (Minimonograph No. 19.) American Association of Electromyography and Electrodiagnosis. Rochester, Minnesota, 1982, pp. 1–19.

Eisen A, Stevens JC: *Upper Limb Somatosensory Evoked Potentials.* An American Association of Electromyography and Electrodiagnosis Workshop, September 1984.

Jones SJ: Short latency potentials recorded from the neck and scalp following median nerve stimulation in man. *Electroencephalogr Clin Neurophysiol* 43:853–863, 1977.

Scalp (fourth channel): The active electrode is placed at C3' (C4'), which is located 2 cm behind C3 (C4). These scalp locations are identified in Figures 10.3 and 10.6. The reference electrode is Fpz'.

Options: The above four-channel recording system (montage) can be changed. Instead of an elbow recording on channel 1, an active scalp recording (C3' or C4') can be referenced to the contralateral shoulder. In this recording, far-field potentials are recorded and designated as P9, P11, P13–14. These recordings frequently are sensitive to EMG artefact and environmental electrical contamination; therefore, meticulous stimulus/recording techniques must be followed.

Ground: The ground electrode is placed as close as possible to the first pair of recording electrodes, avoiding contact either with the recording electrodes or the electrode paste under the electrodes.

Stimulation:

Wrist: The median nerve is stimulated at the wrist with surface electrodes. It is located between the palmaris longus and flexor carpi radialis tendons. The anode of the stimulating electroding pair should be distally at the level of the proximal wrist crease.

Digit: The third digit is stimulated with ring electrodes 4 cm apart and the anode is placed distal to the cathode.

Equipment settings:
- Analysis time: 40–60 msec
- Gain: 10 μV
- Frequency bandwidth: (a) elbow, shoulder, cervical recordings, 10–3,000 Hz; (b) scalp recordings, 0–2,000 Hz
- Averager (sweeps averaged): 200–1,000 sweeps

Normal values: ($N = 20$) Adult values, 18–37 years

Wrist stimulation:

	Peak latency (msec) (mean ± 1 SD)	Side-to-side latency difference (range, msec)
Elbow	4.3 ± 0.3	0.24–0.99
Shoulder	9.9 ± 0.6	0.44–1.74
Cervical		
1st peak	12.1 ± 0.2	0.47–1.89
2nd peak	13.4 ± 0.3	0.43–1.52
Scalp		
N1	19.2 ± 1.1	0.72–3.10
P1	25.2 ± 2.1	1.08–4.05

	Peak amplitude (μV) (mean ± 1 SD)	Side-to-side amplitude difference (range, μV)
Elbow	3.4 ± 0.7	0.11–2.54
Shoulder	2.1 ± 0.6	0.17–0.94
Cervical		
1st peak	1.5 ± 0.4	0.14–1.31
2nd peak	1.9 ± 0.3	0.16–1.28
Scalp		
N1	0.6 ± 0.2	0.19–1.81
N1–P1	2.1 ± 0.9	0.21–2.31

	Interpeak latencies (msec)
Elbow to shoulder	4.9 ± 0.2
Shoulder to cervical spine (2nd peak)	3.8 ± 0.3
Cervical spine to scalp (N1)	5.6 ± 0.5
Shoulder to scalp (N1)	9.3 ± 0.4

Comments: Amplitude measurements for N1 (first negative peak) of the scalp response are taken from the onset of the negative deflection to the peak of the negative deflection. Amplitude measurements for N1–P1 segment are taken from the peak of N1 to the peak of P1 (first positive peak). (The above values are from E. Baran et al., *unpublished data.*)

Third digit stimulation:

	Peak latency (msec) (mean ± 1 SD)	Side-to-side latency difference (range, msec)
Elbow	˙7.9 ± 0.9	0.43–1.32
Shoulder	13.1 ± 0.8	0.31–1.42
Cervical	16.9 ± 1.3	0.28–1.84
Scalp		
N1	22.6 ± 1.3	0.68–2.47
P1	28.8 ± 4.1	0.97–3.41

	Peak amplitude (μV) (mean ± 1 SD)	Side-to-side amplitude difference (range, μV)
Elbow	Too variable	Too variable
Shoulder	Too variable	Too variable
Cervical	Too variable	Too variable
Scalp		
N1	0.5 ± 0.1	0.14–0.41
N1–P1	1.4 ± 0.7	0.16–1.72

	Interpeak latencies (msec)
Elbow to shoulder	5.4 ± 0.4
Shoulder to cervical spine	3.6 ± 0.6
Cervical spine to scalp (N1)	5.9 ± 0.7
Shoulder to scalp (N1)	9.9 ± 1.2

Comments: The amplitude of the responses at the elbow, shoulder, and cervical levels were highly variable, making a normal database not possible. The scalp responses were the most reliable for amplitude measurements but are also highly variable. (The above values are from E. Baran et al., *unpublished data.*)

ULNAR NERVE SOMATOSENSORY EVOKED POTENTIALS

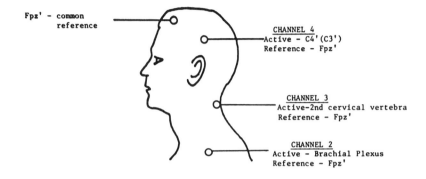

Fpz' - common
reference

CHANNEL 4
Active - C4'(C3')
Reference - Fpz'

CHANNEL 3
Active-2nd cervical vertebra
Reference - Fpz'

CHANNEL 2
Active - Brachial Plexus
Reference - Fpz'

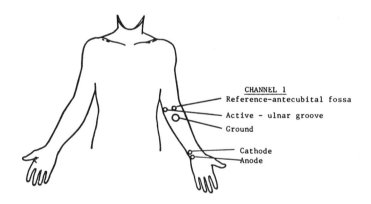

CHANNEL 1
Reference-antecubital fossa

Active - ulnar groove

Ground

Cathode
Anode

Figure 10.7.   Ulnar nerve SEPs. *Top:* Brachial plexus, second cervical vertebra, and C4' (C3') recording sites with Fpz' as common reference. *Bottom:* Wrist stimulation and elbow recording sites.

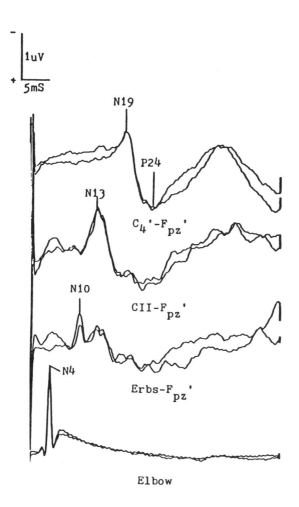

Figure 10.8. Left ulnar nerve stimulation (wrist).

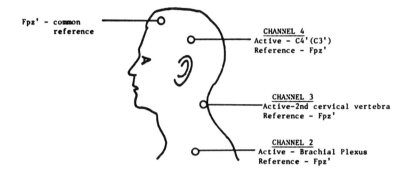

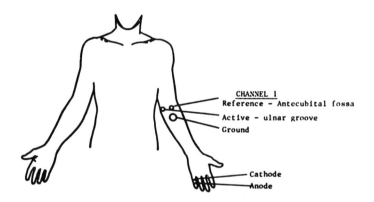

Figure 10.9. Ulnar nerve SEPs. *Top:* Brachial plexus, second cervical vertebra, and C4′ (C3′) recording sites with Fpz′ as common reference. *Bottom:* Fifth digit stimulation and elbow recording sites.

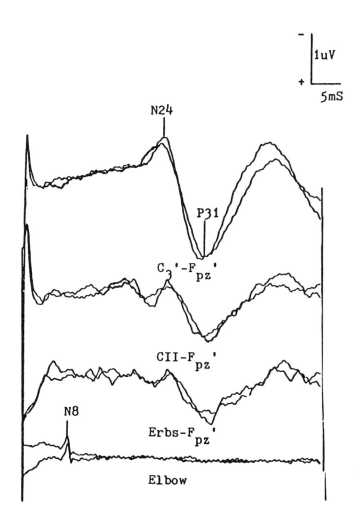

Figure 10.10. Right ulnar nerve stimulation (fifth digit).

Figures 10.7 to 10.10

Stimulation/Recording Technique

Pickup (four sites):

Elbow (first channel): Surface electrodes are placed over the elbow; one over the ulnar groove (active electrode) on a line drawn from the lateral to the medial humeral epicondyle and the other over the antecubital fossa (reference electrode) bisecting the line drawn between the two humeral epicondyles. The active and reference electrode positions are the reverse of those used for median nerve SEPs; therefore, by reversing the input polarities of the leads in the amplifier from the median nerve SEPs, the correct recording montage is achieved without altering the electrode positions on the arm.

Shoulder (second channel): Same as for median nerve SEPs.

Cervical spine (third channel): Same as for median nerve SEPs, page 208.

Scalp (fourth channel): Same as for median nerve SEPs.

Options: Same as for median nerve SEPs, page 208.

Ground: The ground electrode is the same as for the median nerve.

Stimulation:

Wrist: The ulnar nerve is stimulated at the wrist medial (ulnar side) to the tendon of the flexor carpi ulnaris. The anode of the stimulating electrode pair should be placed distally at the level of the proximal wrist crease.

Digit: The fifth digit is stimulated with ring electrodes 4 cm apart, and the anode is placed distal to the cathode.

Equipment settings: Equipment settings are the same as for the median nerve.

Chiappa KH: *Evoked Potentials in Clinical Medicine.* Raven Press, New York, 1983.
Eisen A, Stevens JC: *Upper Limb Somatosensory Evoked Potentials.* An American Association of Electromyography and Electrodiagnosis Workshop, September 1984.

Normal values: (N = 20) Adult values, 18–37 years

Wrist stimulation:

	Peak latency (msec) (mean ± 1 SD)	Side-to-side latency difference (range, msec)
Elbow	4.3 ± 0.5	0.31–1.18
Shoulder	9.9 ± 0.8	0.39–1.80
Cervical	14.0 ± 1.1	0.38–1.44
Scalp		
N1	19.5 ± 1.1	0.45–1.77
P1	24.1 ± 2.6	0.95–4.22

	Peak amplitude (μV) (mean ± 1 SD)	Side-to-side amplitude difference (range, μV)
Elbow	2.1 ± 0.6	0.01–1.51
Shoulder	1.5 ± 0.4	0.17–1.83
Cervical	0.9 ± 0.31	0.13–0.92
Scalp		
N1	1.1 ± 0.6	0.19–1.62
N1–P1	1.9 ± 0.8	0.10–2.88

	Interpeak latencies (msec)
Elbow to shoulder	5.7 ± 0.5
Shoulder to cervical spine	4.3 ± 0.8
Cervical spine to scalp (N1)	6.0 ± 0.8
Shoulder to scalp (N1)	9.6 ± 1.4

Comments: Amplitude measurements are performed as described in the median nerve SEP section. All ulnar responses are lower in amplitude and more variable than the median nerve SEPs, making measurements difficult. (The above values are from E. Baran et al., *unpublished data*.)

Fifth digit stimulation:

	Peak latency (msec) (mean ± 1 SD)	Side-to-side latency difference (range, msec)
Elbow	8.0 ± 0.6	0.38–1.46
Scalp		
N1	24.0 ± 1.8	0.71–2.34
P1	31.0 ± 3.4	0.95–3.67

	Peak amplitude (μV) (mean ± 1 SD)	Side-to-side amplitude difference (range, μV)
Elbow	0.6 ± 0.1	0.09–0.83
Scalp		
N1	0.7 ± 0.3	0.05–0.78
N1–P1	1.1 ± 0.6	0.01–1.89

Interpeak latency (msec): Elbow–scalp (N1) 14.0 ± 1.7.

Comments: The responses recorded over the shoulder and cervical spine frequently were small and difficult to measure; therefore, they are not included in the normal database. (The above values are from E. Baran et al., *unpublished data.*)

SUPERFICIAL SENSORY RADIAL NERVE
SOMATOSENSORY EVOKED POTENTIALS

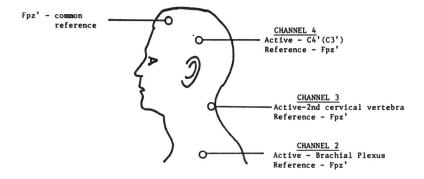

Fpz' - common
      reference

CHANNEL 4
Active - C4'(C3')
Reference - Fpz'

CHANNEL 3
Active-2nd cervical vertebra
Reference - Fpz'

CHANNEL 2
Active - Brachial Plexus
Reference - Fpz'

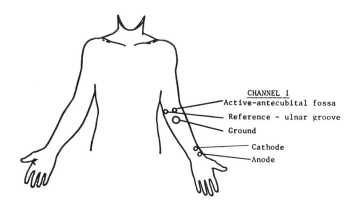

CHANNEL 1
Active-antecubital fossa

Reference - ulnar groove

Ground

Cathode

Anode

Figure 10.11. Superficial sensory radial nerve SEPs. *Top:* Brachial plexus, second cervical vertebra, and C4' (C3') recording sites with Fpz' as common reference. *Bottom:* Wrist stimulation and elbow recording sites.

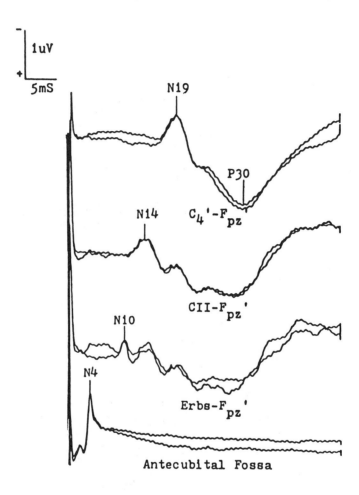

Figure 10.12. Left superficial sensory radial nerve stimulation (wrist).

Figures 10.11 and 10.12
Stimulation/Recording Technique

Pickup (four sites):

Elbow (first channel): The recording electrode positions are the same as for the median nerve SEPs, page 208.

Shoulder (second channel): Same as for median nerve SEPs.

Cervical spine (third channel): Same as for median nerve SEPs.

Scalp (fourth channel): Same as for median nerve SEPs, page 208.

Options: None.

Ground: The ground electrode is the same as for the median nerve SEPs.

Stimulation:

Wrist: The superficial sensory radial nerve is stimulated over the dorsolateral aspect of the wrist approximately 2 cm proximal to the radial styloid process. The anode of the stimulator should be placed distally.

Equipment settings: Equipment settings are the same as for the median nerve.

Normal values: ($N = 20$) Adult values, 18–37 years

Kritchevsky M, Wiederholt WC: Short-latency somatosensory evoked potentials. *Arch Neurol* 35:706–711, 1978.

	Peak latency (msec) (mean ± 1 SD)	Side-to-side latency difference (range, msec)
Elbow	3.7 ± 0.5	0.23–0.86
Shoulder	9.5 ± 0.6	0.24–0.97
Cervical	13.3 ± 1.1	0.47–1.86
Scalp		
N1	18.8 ± 1.2	0.49–1.84
P1	25.4 ± 4.3	1.03–3.49

	Peak amplitude (μV) (mean ± 1 SD)	Side-to-side amplitude difference (range, μV)
Elbow	1.1 ± 0.4	0.12–1.06
Shoulder	0.8 ± 0.2	0.08–0.68
Cervical	0.5 ± 0.2	0.04–0.69
Scalp (N1)	0.8 ± 0.3	0.03–0.87

	Interpeak latencies (msec)
Elbow–shoulder	5.6 ± 0.7
Shoulder–scalp (N1)	9.1 ± 1.3

Comments: Amplitude measurements are performed as described in the median nerve SEP section. Amplitudes of all sensory radial responses are small and variable. (The above values are from E. Baran et al., *unpublished data.*)

TRANSBRACHIAL PLEXUS MEDIAN NERVE SOMATOSENSORY EVOKED POTENTIALS

See Figures 10.3 to 10.6 and Figure 10.13

Stimulation/Recording Technique

Recordings (four sites):

Elbow (first channel): Same as for median nerve SEPs.

Axilla (second channel): Active electrode is placed in the apex of the axilla that lies between the first rib clavicle and the upper edge of the subscapularis muscle. The reference electrode is the contralateral shoulder or Fpz'.

Suprascapular (third channel): Same as for shoulder median nerve SEPs.

Cervical spine (fourth channel): Same as for median nerve SEPs.

Ground: The ground electrode is the same as for the median nerve SEP.

Stimulation:

Wrist: Same as for median nerve SEPs.

Equipment settings: Same as for median nerve SEPs.

Normal values: (N = 30) Adult values, 18–40 years

Baran E, Stagliano N, Whitenack S, Jaeger S, Kresch E: Sensory conduction abnormalities and brachial plexus lesions. *Muscle Nerve* 15:1186–1187, 1992.

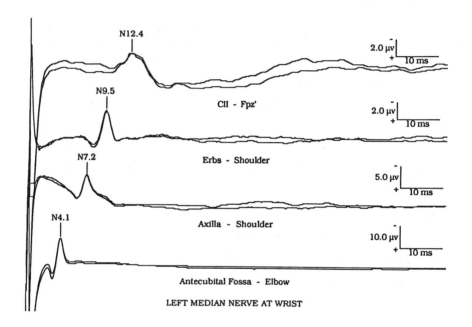

Figure 10.13. Left median nerve at wrist.

Wrist stimulation:

	Peak latency (msec) (mean ± 1 SD)	Side-to-side latency difference (range, msec)
Elbow	4.4 ± 0.4	0.32–1.19
Axilla	8.1 ± 0.6	0.33–1.72
Supraclavicular	9.9 ± 0.7	0.39–1.82
Cervical	13.1 ± 1.1	0.38–1.46

	Peak amplitude (μV) (mean ± 1 SD)	Side-to-side amplitude difference (range, μV)
Elbow	4.6 ± 0.5	0.01–1.52
Axilla	4.0 ± 0.5	0.18–1.76
Supraclavicular	3.9 ± 0.3	0.17–1.86
Cervical	1.8 ± 0.3	0.13–0.96

	Interpeak latencies (msec)
Elbow to axilla	3.3 ± 0.1
Axilla to supraclavicular	2.1 ± 0.2
Supraclavicular to cervical spine	2.5 ± 0.3

TRANSBRACHIAL PLEXUS ULNAR NERVE SOMATOSENSORY EVOKED POTENTIALS

See Figures 10.7 to 10.10 and Figure 10.14

Stimulation/Recording Technique:

Recordings (four sites):

Elbow (first channel): Same as for ulnar nerve SEPs

Axilla (second channel): Same as for median transbrachial plexus SEPs.

Suprascapular (third channel): Same as for median nerve SEPs.

Cervical spine (fourth channel): Same as for median nerve SEPs.

Ground: The ground electrode is the same as for the median nerve SEPs.

Stimulation: Same as for ulnar nerve SEPs.

Equipment settings: Same as for median nerve SEPs.

Normal values: (N = 30) Adult values, 18–40 years

Baran E, Stagliano N, Whitenack S, Jaeger S, Kresch E: Sensory conduction abnormalities and brachial plexus lesions. *Muscle Nerve* 15:1186–1187, 1992.

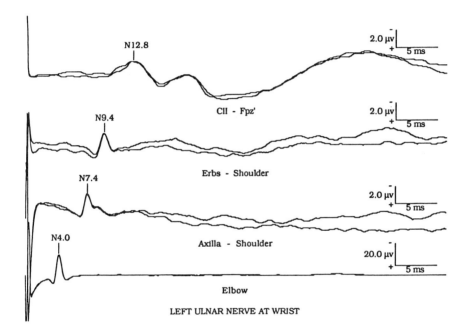

Figure 10.14. Left ulnar nerve at wrist.

Wrist stimulation:

	Peak latency msec (mean ± 1 SD)	Side-to-side latency difference (range, msec)
Elbow	4.4 ± 0.4	0.31–1.19
Axilla	8.2 ± 0.5	0.34–1.74
Supraclavicular	9.9 ± 0.7	0.38–1.44
Cervical	13.4 ± 0.6	0.37–1.46

	Peak amplitude (μV) (mean ± 1 SD)	Side-to-side amplitude difference (range, msec)
Elbow	4.5 ± 0.5	0.01–1.52
Axilla	3.8 ± 0.2	0.16–1.85
Supraclavicular	2.5 ± 0.4	0.17–1.80
Cervical	1.8 ± 0.2	0.12–0.98

	Interpeak latencies (msec)
Elbow to axilla	3.2 ± 0.2
Axilla to supraclavicular	2.1 ± 0.3
Supraclavicular to cervical spine	2.5 ± 0.4

TRANSBRACHIAL PLEXUS SUPERFICIAL SENSORY RADIAL NERVE SOMATOSENSORY EVOKED POTENTIALS

See Figures 10.11 and 10.12, and 10.15

Stimulation/Recording Technique

Recordings (four sites):

Elbow (first channel): Same as for median nerve SEPs.

Axilla (second channel): Same as for transbrachial median nerve SEPs.

Suprascapular (third channel): Same as for median nerve SEPs.

Cervical Spine (fourth channel): Same as for median nerve SEPs.

Ground: The ground electrode is the same as for the median nerve SEPs.

Stimulation: Same as for superficial radial sensory nerve SEPs.

Equipment settings: Same as for median nerve SEPs.

Normal values: (N = 30) Adult values, 18–40 years

Baran E, Stagliano N, Whitenack S, Jaeger S, Kresch E: Sensory conduction abnormalities and brachial plexus lesions. *Muscle Nerve* 15:1186–1187, 1992.

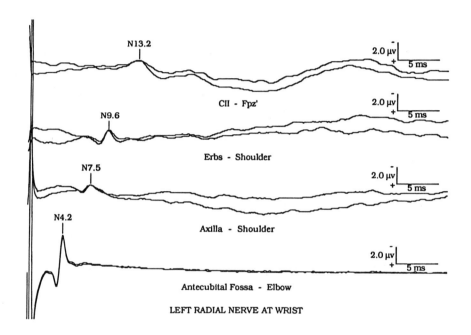

Figure 10.15. Left radial nerve at wrist.

Wrist stimulation:

	Peak latency msec (mean ± 1 SD)	Side-to-side latency difference (range, msec)
Elbow	3.8 ± 0.4	0.23–0.87
Axilla	8.2 ± 0.4	0.34–1.78
Supraclavicular	9.4 ± 0.5	0.24–1.42
Cervical	13.4 ± 1.2	0.47–1.89

	Peak amplitude (μV) (mean ± 1 SD)	Side-to-side amplitude difference (range, μV)
Elbow	2.7 ± 0.4	0.12–1.08
Axilla	2.3 ± 0.3	0.11–1.12
Supraclavicular	1.6 ± 0.4	0.08–0.72
Cervical	1.0 ± 0.3	0.04–0.91

	Interpeak latencies (msec)
Elbow to axilla	3.3 ± 0.2
Axilla to supraclavicular	2.2 ± 0.3
Supraclavicular to cervical spine	2.5 ± 0.4

LATERAL ANTEBRACHIAL CUTANEOUS NERVE
SOMATOSENSORY EVOKED POTENTIALS

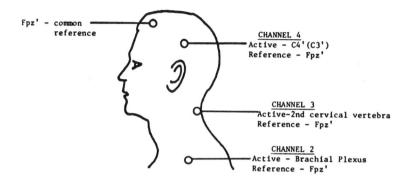

Fpz' - common
reference

CHANNEL 4
Active - C4'(C3')
Reference - Fpz'

CHANNEL 3
Active-2nd cervical vertebra
Reference - Fpz'

CHANNEL 2
Active - Brachial Plexus
Reference - Fpz'

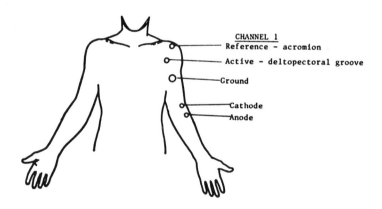

CHANNEL 1
Reference - acromion

Active - deltopectoral groove

Ground

Cathode

Anode

Figure 10.16.   Lateral antebrachial cutaneous nerve SEPs. *Top:* Brachial plexus, second cervical vertebra, and C4' (C3') recording sites with Fpz' as common reference. *Bottom:* Lateral elbow stimulation.

Figures 10.16 and 10.17

Stimulation/Recording Technique

Pickup (four sites):

Anterior shoulder (first channel): The active surface electrode is placed in the deltopectoral groove of the shoulder at the greater tubercle level of the humerus. The reference electrode is placed over the tip of the acromion.

Supraclavicular position (second channel): Same as for median nerve SEPs, page 208.

Cervical spine (third channel): Same as for median nerve SEPs.

Scalp (fourth channel): Same as for median nerve SEPs, page 208.

Options: None.

Ground: The ground electrode is placed over the middle of the biceps brachii muscle.

Stimulation: The lateral antebrachial cutaneous nerve is stimulated at the elbow 2 cm lateral to the biceps brachii tendon with the anode of the stimulator placed distal to the cathode.

Equipment settings: Same as for median nerve SEPs.

Normal values: (N = 20) Adult values, 18–37 years

Eisen A, Stevens JC: *Upper Limb Somatosensory Evoked Potentials.* An American Association of Electromyography and Electrodiagnosis Workshop, September 1984.

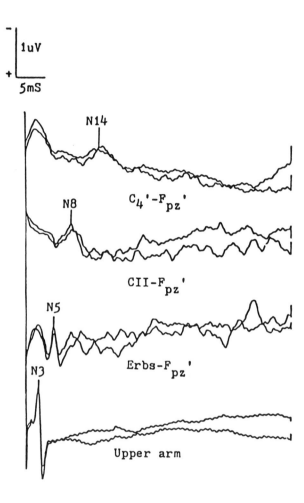

Figure 10.17. Left lateral antebrachial cutaneous nerve stimulation (elbow).

	Peak latency (msec) (mean ± 1 SD)	Side-to-side latency difference (range, msec)
Anterior shoulder	3.1 ± 0.4	0.22–0.82
Supraclavicular	4.9 ± 0.5	0.28–1.02
Cervical spine	7.8 ± 0.3	0.37–1.91
Scalp (N1)	14.1 ± 0.7	0.51–2.1

	Peak amplitude (μV) (mean ± 1 SD)	Side-to-side amplitude difference (range, μV)
Anterior shoulder	0.8 ± 0.3	0.05–0.86
Supraclavicular	0.7 ± 0.2	0.07–0.64
Cervical spine	0.5 ± 0.2	0.04–0.56
Scalp (N1)	Variable	Variable

	Interpeak latencies (msec)
Anterior shoulder–supraclavicular	1.6 ± 0.4
Supraclavicular–cervical spine	2.7 ± 0.3
Cervical spine–scalp (N1)	6.5 ± 0.7
Supraclavicular–scalp (N1)	10.0 ± 1.6

Comments: Amplitude measurements are performed as described in the median nerve SEP section. The scalp responses were so variable that a mean could not be statistically generated. (The above values are from E. Baran et al., *unpublished data*.)

TIBIAL NERVE SOMATOSENSORY EVOKED POTENTIALS

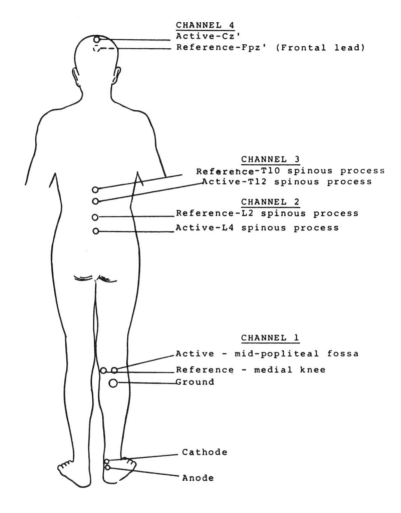

Figure 10.18. Tibial nerve SEPs. Ankle stimulation with popliteal, spinal, and scalp recording sites.

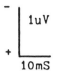

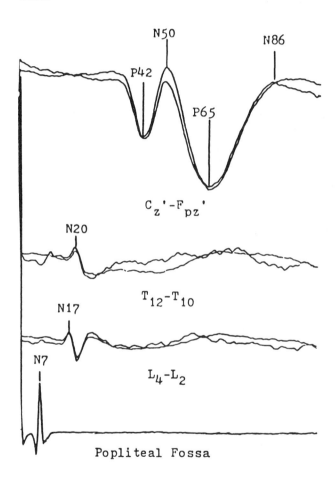

Figure 10.19. Right tibial nerve stimulation (ankle).

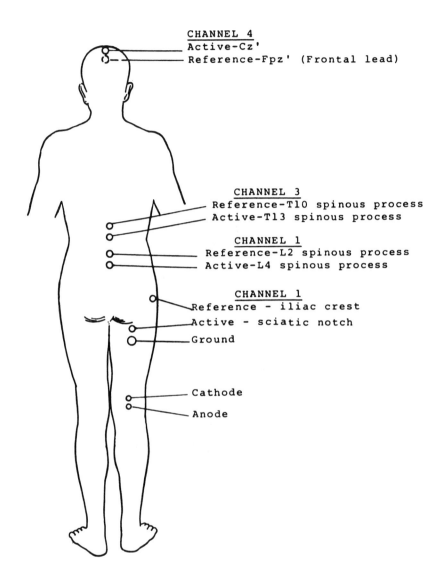

Figure 10.20. Tibial nerve SEPs. Knee stimulation with sciatic notch, spinal, and scalp recording sites.

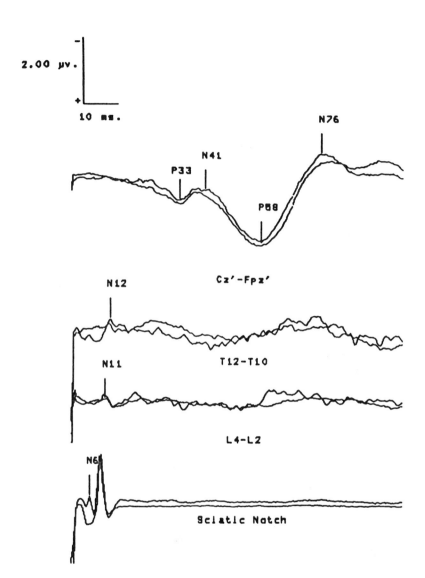

Figure 10.21.   Right tibial nerve at knee.

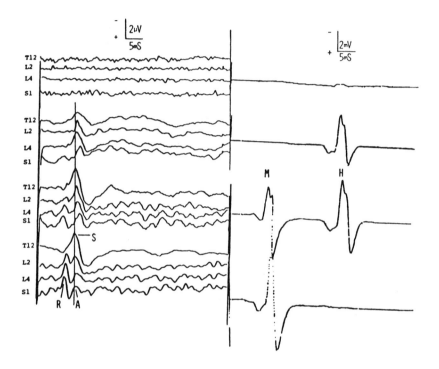

Figure 10.22. Surface spinal recordings via unilateral tibial nerve stimulation at popliteal fossa with increasing stimulus strength in a normal 6-year-old girl. The increasing stimulus strength is monitored by the H reflex and M responses on the right. Monopolar recordings with C7 spinous process reference.

Figures 10.18 to 10.22

Stimulation/Recording Technique

Pickup (four sites):

Popliteal fossa (first channel): The active surface electrode is placed over the tibial nerve approximately 2 cm above the popliteal fossa midway between a line drawn between the combined tendons of the semimembranous and semitendinosis muscles medially and the tendon of the biceps femoris muscle laterally. These landmarks are prominent if the patient slightly flexes the knee when lying in the supine position. The reference electrode is placed over the medial joint line (tibial–femoral articulation).

Lumbar spine (L4–L2) (second channel): The active electrode is placed over the L4 spinous process that is identified by bisecting a line drawn between the superior aspects of the left and right iliac crest. The reference electrode should be placed approximately 3 cm cephalad to the L4 recording electrode. This approximates the spinous process of L2.

Thoracic spine (T12–T10) (third channel): The active electrode should be placed over the T12 spinous process, which is identified by counting four spinous processes above the L4 spinous process. The reference electrode is placed approximately 3 cm cephalad to the T12 electrode. The position of the reference electrode approximates the T10 spinous process.

Baran E, Daube J: *Lower Extremity Somatosensory Evoked Potentials.* An American Association of Electromyography and Electrodiagnosis Workshop, September 1984.

Chiappa KH: *Evoked Potentials in Clinical Medicine.* New York: Raven Press. 1983.

Delbeke J, McComas AJ, Kopec SJ: Analysis of evoked lumbosacral potentials in man. *J Neurol Neurosurg Psychiatry* 41:293–302, 1978.

Dimitrijevic MR, Larson LE, Lehmkuhl D, et al.: Evoked spinal cord and nerve root potentials in humans using noninvasive recording technique. *Electroencephalogr Clin Neurophysiol* 45:331–340, 1978.

Phillips LH, Daube JR: Lumbosacral spinal evoked potentials in humans. *Neurology* 30: 1175–1183, 1980.

Scalp (fourth channel): The active electrode is placed at the Cz' (2 cm posterior to Cz). The reference electrode is placed at Fpz' (2 cm behind Fp).

Options: The above four-channel recording system is for stimulation of the tibial nerve at the ankle. When stimulating the tibial nerve at the knee, the peripheral sensory nerve action potential is recorded over the sciatic notch. The active electrode is placed over the sciatic notch, and the reference electrode is placed over the greater trochanter. The spinal recordings (L4–L2, T12–T10) are bipolar recordings. If the spinal responses at the spinal level are small or absent using the bipolar montage, the reference electrode (L2 or T10) can be placed in other locations (contralateral iliac crest, contralateral ear lobe, or T6 spinous process). This will result in a monopolar (differential) recording that is usually larger but may contain more noise.

　　Bipolar recording montages are used for the spinal and scalp recordings. Because these electrodes are near the generator sources, both electrodes are hence "active." For purposes of convention, the recordings for both the spinal and scalp recordings are labeled "active" and "reference." The tibial nerve also can be stimulated at the popliteal fossa with stimulus intensities to produce H and M responses recorded over the triceps surae. The spinal recordings reveal responses that may represent dorsal and ventral root activity. Figure 10.22 shows spinal responses with stimulus intensities to produce an H response without an M response, an M response that is equal to the H response, and an M response with no H response. In this latter recording, R represents volleys from the group I, group II fibers, and the electrical origin of A is less well understood; S represents the spinal cord response.

　　A cervical recording (C7) referenced to the scalp also may be used when stimulating the tibial nerve in the lower extremity; however, these cervical recordings may be small and may contain considerable EMG artifact.

Ground: The ground electrode is placed as close to the first pair of recording electrodes, avoiding contact with either the recording electrodes or the electrode paste under the electrodes.

Stimulation:

Ankle: With the patient in the supine or prone position, surface-stimulating electrodes are placed behind the medial malleolus. The exact point of stimulation is identified by measuring 1 cm behind and 1 cm below the navicular tubercle (medial side of the foot). This point approximates the middle of the belly of the abductor hallucis muscle. Next, measure 8 cm proximal to this point, following the course of the tibial nerve 1 cm posterior to the medial malleolus. The electrode at this point is the anode. Place the cathode 4 cm proximal to the anode.

Popliteal fossa: The tibial nerve at the popliteal fossa is stimulated approximately 2 cm above the popliteal crease at a point that is midway between a line drawn between the tendons of the lateral and medial hamstring muscles. These landmarks are prominent if the patient flexes the knee slightly when lying in the supine position. The anode should be placed 4 cm distal to the cathode.

Equipment settings:
- Analysis time: 50–100 msec
- Gain: 10 μV
- Frequency bandwidth: (a) the peripheral sensory nerve action potential and the spinal responses, 10–3,000 Hz; (b) scalp recordings, 0–2,000 Hz
- Averager (sweeps averaged): 200–1,000 sweeps

Normal values: ($N = 38$) Adult values, 19–45 years; height, 140–188 cm

Ankle stimulation (Baran and Daube; Phillips and Daube; Chiappa):

	Peak latency (msec) (mean ± 1 SD)	Side-to-side latency difference (range, msec)
Popliteal fossa	8.4 ± 0.9	0.18–0.88
L4–L2	17.9 ± 1.4	0.14–1.48
T12–T10	21.6 ± 1.6	0.12–1.29
Scalp		
P1	38.5 ± 2.8	0.45–3.05
N1	48.1 ± 4.1	0.67–5.92
P2	61.2 ± 6.5	1.59–12.18
N2	79.7 ± 9.4	3.42–15.47

	Peak amplitude (μV) (mean ± 1 SD)	Side-to-side amplitude difference (range, μV)
Popliteal fossa	2.3 ± 0.6	0.12–1.92
L4–L2	0.7 ± 0.2	0.16–0.65
T12–T10	0.8 ± 0.3	0.14–0.72
Scalp		
P1	1.1 ± 0.3	0.13–0.97
P1–N1	1.4 ± 0.5	0.19–1.42
N1–P2	1.8 ± 0.4	0.35–1.58
P2–N2	21.0 ± 0.6	0.42–1.94

	Interpeak latencies (msec)
Popliteal fossa/L4–L2	9.3 ± 0.8
L4–L2/T12–T10	3.5 ± 0.2
T12–T10/scalp (P1)	15.5 ± 1.7
T12–T10/scalp (P1)	Conduction velocity, 35.4 ± 1.6 m/sec

Comments: Amplitude measurements for P1 (first positive peak) of the scalp response are taken from the onset of P1 to the peak of P1. Amplitude measurements for the P1–N1 segment are taken from the peak of P1 to the peak of N1, for the N1–P2 segment from the peak of N1 to the peak of P2, and for the P2–N2 segment from the peak of P2 to the peak of N2. (Part of the above values are from E. Baran et al., *unpublished data.*)

Popliteal fossa stimulation (Delbeke et al.; Dimitrijevic et al.):

	Peak latency (msec) (mean ± 1 SD)	Side-to-side latency difference (range, msec)
Sciatic notch	5.4 ± 0.3	0.21–0.82
L4–L2	10.9 ± 0.8	0.19–1.51
T12–T10	12.8 ± 1.1	0.15–1.32
Scalp		
P1	31.2 ± 2.6	0.52–3.24
N1	39.4 ± 4.6	0.74–6.14
P2	53.7 ± 5.9	1.62–12.91
N2	72.4 ± 9.8	3.76–14.31

	Peak amplitude (µV) (mean ± 1 SD)	Side-to-side amplitude difference (range, µV)
Sciatic notch	1.1 ± 0.5	0.14–1.28
L4–L2	0.8 ± 0.3	0.19–0.84
T12–T10	0.9 ± 0.3	0.15–0.88
Scalp		
P1	1.6 ± 0.4	0.12–1.42
P1–N1	1.9 ± 0.7	0.18–1.51
N1–P2	2.1 ± 0.5	0.27–1.76
P2–N2	2.8 ± 0.8	0.47–2.52

	Interpeak latencies (msec)
Sciatic notch/L4–L2	5.3 ± 0.6
L4–L2/T12–T10	1.7 ± 0.3
T12–T10/scalp (P1)	18.4 ± 2.1
T12–T10/scalp (P1)	Conduction velocity, 34.6 ± 1.9 m/sec

Comments: Same as under ankle stimulation. (The above values are from E. Baran et al., *unpublished data.*)

PERONEAL NERVE SOMATOSENSORY EVOKED POTENTIALS

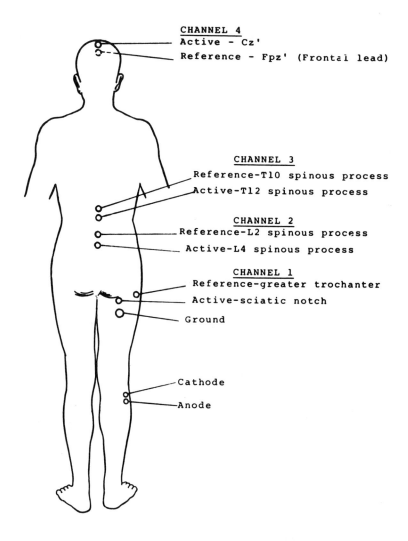

CHANNEL 4
Active - Cz'
Reference - Fpz' (Frontal lead)

CHANNEL 3
Reference-T10 spinous process
Active-T12 spinous process

CHANNEL 2
Reference-L2 spinous process
Active-L4 spinous process

CHANNEL 1
Reference-greater trochanter
Active-sciatic notch
Ground

Cathode
Anode

Figure 10.23.   Peroneal nerve SEPs. Stimulation at fibular neck with sciatic notch, spinal, and scalp recording sites.

Figures 10.23 and 10.24

Stimulation/Recording Technique

Pickup (four sites):

Sciatic notch (first channel): The active electrode is placed over the sciatic notch, identified by bisecting a line drawn between the greater trochanter and the ischial tuberosity. The reference electrode is placed over the greater trochanter.

Lumbar spine (L4–L2) (second channel): The active electrode is placed over the L4 spinous process that is identified by bisecting a line drawn between the superior aspects of the left and right iliac crest. The reference electrode should be placed approximately 3 cm cephalad to the L4 recording electrode. This approximates the spinous process of L2.

Thoracic spine (T12–T10) (third channel): The active electrode should be placed over the T12 spinous process, which is identified by counting four spinous processes above the L4 spinous process. The reference electrode is placed approximately 3 cm cephalad to the T12 electrode. The position of the reference electrode approximates the T10 spinous process.

Scalp (fourth channel): The active electrode is placed at the Cz' (2 cm posterior to Cz). The reference electrode is placed at Fpz' (2 cm behind FP).

Options: None.

Ground: The ground electrode is placed as close to the first pair of recording electrodes at the level of the sciatic notch, avoiding contact with either the recording electrodes or the electrode paste under the electrodes.

Baran E: Spinal cord responses to peripheral nerve stimulation in man. *Arch Phys Med Rehabil* 61:10–17, 1980.

Baran E: Lumbar and thoracic spinal evoked potentials in man: Frontiers in engineering and health care. *Proceedings of the Fourth Annual Conference of IEEE Engineering in Medicine and Biology Society.* New York: IEEE, 1982;44–49.

Cracco RQ, Anziska BJ, Cracco JB, et al.: Short latency somatosensory evoked potentials to median and peroneal nerve stimulation: Studies in normal subjects and patients with neurologic disease. *Ann NY Acad Sci* 388:412–425, 1982.

Chiappa KH: *Evoked Potentials in Clinical Medicine.* New York: Raven Press. 1983.

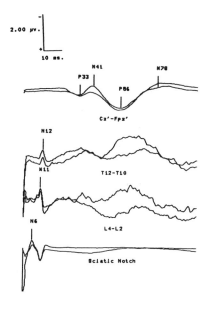

Figure 10.24.   Right peroneal nerve at knee.

Stimulation:

> *Knee:* The peroneal nerve is identified as it passes lateral to the fibular neck. The cathode is placed 4 cm proximal to the anode, lateral to the fibular neck.

Equipment settings:
- Analysis time: 50–100 msec
- Gain: 10 μV
- Frequency bandwidth: (a) The sciatic notch potential and spinal recordings; 10–3,000 Hz; (b) scalp recordings, 0–2,000 Hz
- Averager (sweeps averaged): 200–1,000

Normal values: (N = 38) Adult values, 19–45 years; height, 140–188 cm

Knee stimulation:

	Peak latency (msec) (mean ± 1 SD)	Side-to-side latency difference (range, msec)
Sciatic notch	5.7 ± 0.4	0.29–0.91
L4–L2	10.4 ± 0.6	0.08–0.71
T12–T10	11.1 ± 0.9	0.07–0.82
Scalp		
N1	27.1 ± 1.4	0.42–3.18
P1	32.5 ± 2.4	0.59–5.87
N2	41.3 ± 3.9	1.92–11.72
P2	55.8 ± 5.1	4.21–18.46
	Peak amplitude (μV) (mean ± 1 SD)	Side-to-side amplitude difference (range, μV)
Sciatic notch	0.8 ± 0.3	0.18–0.83
L4–L2	0.7 ± 0.3	0.36–1.29
T12–T10	0.8 ± 0.4	0.41–1.32
Scalp		
N1	0.4 ± 0.2	0.08–0.34
N1–P1	1.1 ± 0.4	0.14–0.75
P1–N2	1.7 ± 0.7	0.17–1.72
N2–P2	1.9 ± 0.5	0.43–1.59
		Interpeak latencies (msec)
Sciatic notch/L4–L2		4.4 ± 0.7
L4–L2/T12–T10		1.5 ± 0.3
T12–T10/scalp (P1)		15.4 ± 0.8
		Conduction velocity, 37.4 ± 2.1 m/sec

Comments: The amplitude measurement of N1 of the scalp response is taken from the baseline to the peak of N1. The amplitude of segments (N1–P1, P1–N2, N2–P2) is measured in the same manner as the tibial scalp SEP segments. (Part of above values are from E. Baran et al., *unpublished data.*)

SURAL NERVE SOMATOSENSORY EVOKED POTENTIALS

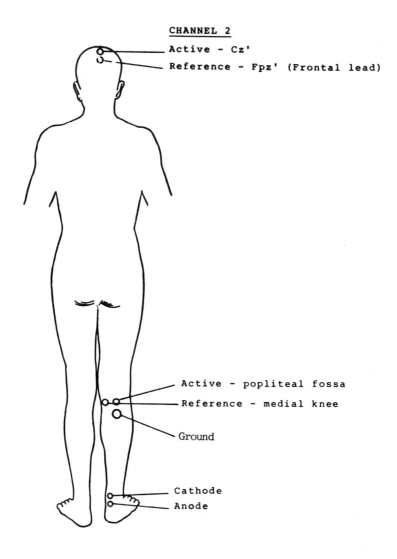

Figure 10.25. Sural nerve SEPs. Lateral ankle stimulation with popliteal and scalp recordings.

Figures 10.25 and 10.26

Stimulation/Recording Technique

Pickup (two sites):

Popliteal fossa (first channel): Same as for tibial nerve SEPs, page 240.

Scalp (fourth channel): Same as for tibial nerve SEPs, page 240.

Options: None.

Ground: The ground electrode is placed close to the first pair of recording electrodes in the popliteal fossa, avoiding contact with either the recording electrodes or the electrode paste under the electrodes.

Stimulation:

Ankle: With the patient in a supine or prone position, surface-stimulating electrodes are placed approximately 2 cm behind the lateral malleolus. The anode is placed at the level of the lateral malleolus, and the cathode is placed 4 cm proximal to the anode.

Equipment settings:
- Analysis time: 100 msec
- Gain: 10 μV
- Frequency bandwidth: (a) The peripheral sensory nerve action potential, 10–3,000 Hz; (b) scalp recordings, 0–2,000 Hz
- Averager (sweeps averaged): 200–1,000 sweeps

Normal values: (N = 22) Adult values, 19–45 years; height, 140–188 cm

Eisen A: *The Somatosensory Evoked Potential.* (Minimonograph #19.) An American Association of Electromyography and Electrodiagnosis Workshop, September 1982.
Eisen A, Stevens JC: *Upper Limb Somatosensory Evoked Potentials.* An American Association of Electromyography and Electrodiagnosis Workshop, September 1984.

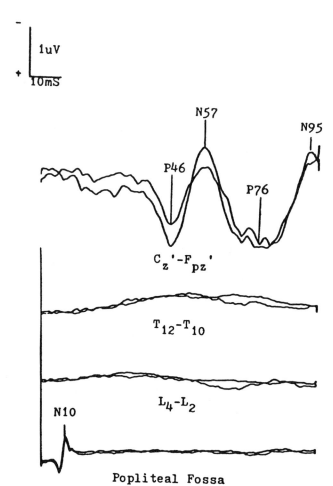

Figure 10.26.   Left sural nerve stimulation (ankle).

Ankle stimulation:

	Peak latency (msec) (mean ± 1 SD)	Side-to-side latency difference (range, msec)
Popliteal fossa	8.7 ± 0.5	0.17–0.84
Scalp		
N1	33.4 ± 2.2	0.48–3.10
P1	44.3 ± 3.7	0.59–5.71
N2	51.7 ± 5.9	1.42–10.84
P2	64.8 ± 7.3	2.91–14.88

	Peak amplitude (μV) (mean ± 1 SD)	Side-to-side amplitude difference (range, μV)
Popliteal fossa	1.8 ± 0.5	0.16–1.62
Scalp		
N1	0.3 ± 0.2	0.05–0.48
N1–P1	1.1 ± 0.5	0.11–1.24
P1–N2	1.4 ± 0.7	0.11–1.24
N2–P2	1.6 ± 0.9	0.37–1.58

Interpeak latency (msec): popliteal fossa/scalp (N1), 22.4 ± 3.1.

Comments: Spinal responses are unable to be recorded satisfactorily in adults; however, they are recordable in children. (Part of the above values are from E. Baran et al., *unpublished data.*)

LATERAL FEMORAL CUTANEOUS NERVE
SOMATOSENSORY EVOKED POTENTIALS

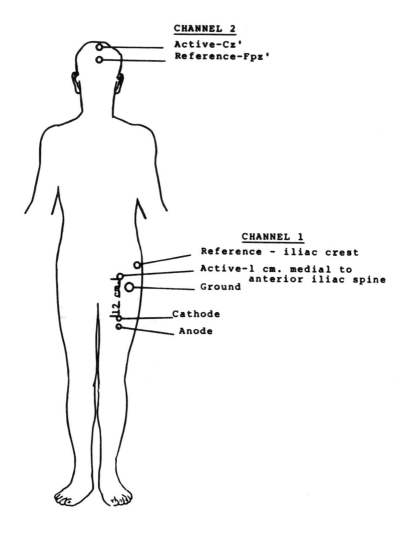

Figure 10.27. Lateral femoral cutaneous nerve SEPs. Anterior thigh stimulation with anterior superior iliac spine and scalp recordings.

Figures 10.27 and 10.28

Stimulation/Recording Technique

Pickup (two sites):

Anterior iliac spine (first channel): The active surface electrode is placed 1 cm medial to the anterior superior iliac spine. The reference electrode is placed over the ipsilateral greater trochanter.

Scalp (fourth channel): The same as for tibial nerve SEPs.

Options: None.

Ground: The ground electrode is placed close to the first pair of recording electrodes over the groin, avoiding contact with either the recording electrodes or the electrode paste under the electrodes.

Stimulation:

Anterior thigh: The cathode of the stimulator electrode is placed over a point 12 cm directly below the anterior superior iliac spine, and the anode is placed 4 cm distal to the cathode.

Equipment settings:
- Analysis time: 50–100 msec
- Gain: 10 μV
- Frequency bandwidth: (a) The peripheral sensory nerve action potential, 10–3,000 Hz; (b) scalp recordings, 0–2,000 Hz
- Averager (sweeps averaged): 500–1,000 sweeps

Normal values: (N = 12) Adult values, 19–45 years; height, 140–188 cm

---

Eisen A: *The Somatosensory Evoked Potential*, pp 1–19. (Minimonograph #19.) American Association of Electromyography and Electrodiagnosis, Rochester, Minnesota, 1982.

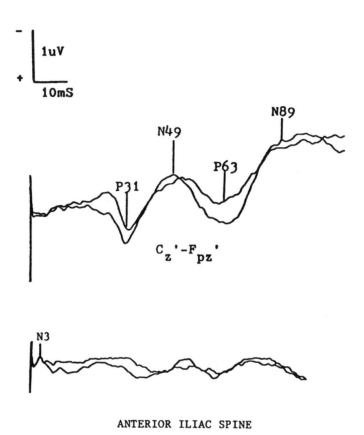

ANTERIOR ILIAC SPINE

Figure 10.28. Left lateral femoral cutaneous nerve stimulation (thigh).

Anterior thigh stimulation:

	Peak latency (msec) (mean ± 1 SD)	Side-to-side latency difference (range, msec)
Iliac spine	2.9 ± 0.5	0.31–0.75
Scalp		
P1	30.2 ± 2.4	0.41–2.89
N1	42.5 ± 4.5	0.61–6.72
P2	52.5 ± 8.8	1.58–9.46

	Peak amplitude (μV) (mean ± 1 SD)	Side-to-side amplitude difference (range, μV)
Iliac spine	0.42 ± 0.21	0.08–0.41
Scalp		
P1	0.32 ± 0.12	0.09–0.28
P1–N1	0.41 ± 0.19	0.15–0.41
N1–P2	0.56 ± 0.23	0.17–0.44

Interpeak latency (msec): iliac spine/scalp P1, 25.2 ± 2.8.

Comments: Spinal responses are unable to be recorded in adults or children. (The above values are from E. Baran et al., *unpublished data.*)

SUPERFICIAL SENSORY PERONEAL NERVE
SOMATOSENSORY EVOKED POTENTIALS

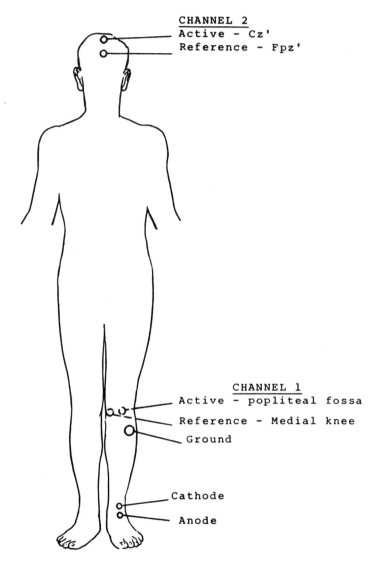

CHANNEL 2
Active - Cz'
Reference - Fpz'

CHANNEL 1
Active - popliteal fossa

Reference - Medial knee

Ground

Cathode

Anode

Figure 10.29. Superficial sensory peroneal nerve SEPs. Anterior ankle stimulation with popliteal fossa and scalp recordings.

Figures 10.29 and 10.30

Stimulation/Recording Technique

Pickup (two sites):

Popliteal fossa (first channel): Same as for tibial nerve SEPs, page 240.

Scalp (fourth channel): Same as for tibial nerve SEPs, page 240.

Options: None.

Ground: Same as for tibial nerve SEPs.

Stimulation:

Anterior ankle: The cathode of the stimulating electrode is placed at the junction of the lateral and middle thirds of a line drawn between the lateral and median malleoli. The anode is placed 4 cm distal to the cathode.

Equipment settings:
- Analysis time: 50–100 msec
- Gain: 10 μV
- Frequency bandwidth: (a) The peripheral sensory nerve action potential, 10–3,000 Hz; (b) scalp recordings, 0–2,000 Hz
- Averager (sweeps averaged): 500–1,000 sweeps

Normal values: (N = 15) Adult values, 19–45 years; height, 140–188 cm

Eisen A: *The Somatosensory Evoked Potential,* pp 1–19. (Minimonograph #19.) American Association of Electromyography and Electrodiagnosis, Rochester, Minnesota, 1982.

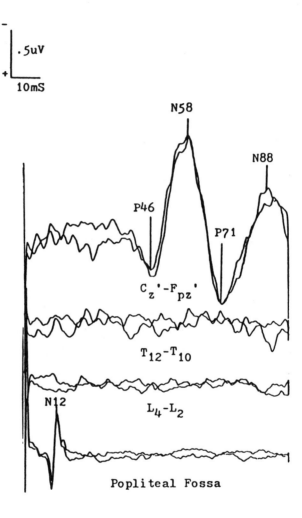

Figure 10.30.   Superficial sensory peroneal nerve (ankle).

Anterior ankle stimulation:

	Peak latency (msec) (mean ± 1 SD)	Side-to-side latency difference (range msec)
Popliteal fossa	11.6 ± 0.8	0.16–0.73
Scalp		
P1	45.2 ± 2.4	0.39–2.
N1	58.5 ± 4.2	0.52–5.84
P2	70.8 ± 6.2	1.8 –8.73
N2	89.4 ± 8.7	2.75–10.82

	Peak amplitude (μV) (mean ± 1 SD)	Side-to-side amplitude difference (range, μV)
Popliteal fossa	0.43 ± 0.19	0.07–0.41
Scalp		
P1	0.28 ± 0.13	0.12–0.28
P1–N1	1.12 ± 0.35	0.15–1.19
N1–P2	1.48 ± 0.39	0.18–1.22
P2–N2	0.94 ± 0.25	0.16–0.72

Interpeak latency (msec): popliteal fossa/scalp P1, 31.4 ± 1.7 m/sec.

Comments: Spinal responses are unable to be recorded in adults or children. (The above values are from E. Baran et al., *unpublished data.*)

SAPHENOUS NERVE SOMATOSENSORY EVOKED POTENTIALS

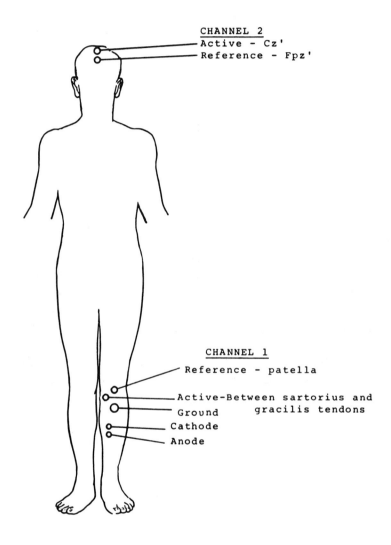

Figure 10.31.   Saphenous nerve SEPs. Lower leg stimulation with medial knee and scalp recordings.

Figures 10.31 and 10.32

Stimulation/Recording Technique

Pickup (two sites):

Medial knee (first channel): The active electrode is placed between the tendons of the sartorius and the gracilis muscles on a line 1 cm above the inferior border of the patella. The reference electrode is placed over the patella.

Scalp (fourth channel): Same as for tibial nerve SEPs.

Options: The infrapatellar branch of the saphenous nerve could also be stimulated to obtain saphenous SEPs.

Ground: The ground electrode is placed as close as possible to the first pair of recording electrodes over the medial aspect of the knee, avoiding contact with either the recording electrodes or the electrode paste under the electrodes.

Stimulation:

Lower leg: The cathode of the stimulator is placed 15 cm below the active recording electrode at a point just medial to the tibia. The anode is placed 4 cm distal to the cathode.

Equipment settings:
• Analysis time: 50–100 msec
• Gain: 10 μV
• Frequency bandwidth: (a) The peripheral sensory nerve action potential, 10–3,000 Hz; (b) scalp recordings, 0–2,000 Hz
• Averager (sweeps averaged): 500–1,000 sweeps

Normal values: (N = 11) Adult values, 19–45 years; height, 140–188 cm

---

Synek VM, Cowan JC: Saphenous nerve evoked potentials and the assessment of intraabdominal lesions of the femoral nerve. *Muscle Nerve* 6:453–456, 1983.

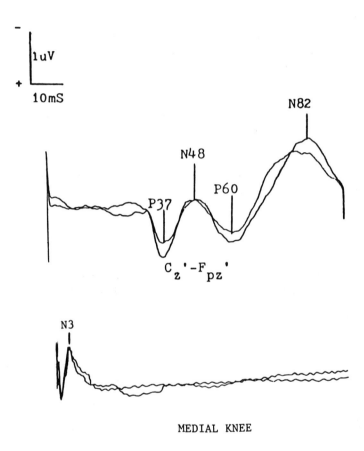

MEDIAL KNEE

Figure 10.32. Saphenous nerve stimulation (shin).

Lower leg stimulation:

	Peak latency (msec) (mean ± 1 SD)	Side-to-side latency difference (range, msec)
Knee	2.6 ± 0.3	0.15–0.79
Scalp		
P1	37.1 ± 2.8	0.32–2.81
N1	47.3 ± 4.6	0.47–5.62
P2	59.1 ± 6.8	1.76–8.21
N2	74.5 ± 9.2	2.64–10.26

	Peak amplitude (μV) (mean ± 1 SD)	Side-to-side amplitude difference (range, μV)
Knee	0.64–0.18	0.06–0.39
Scalp		
P1	0.43 ± 0.12	0.15–0.36
P1–N1	0.94 ± 0.23	0.21–0.76
N1–P2	1.17 ± 0.54	0.24–1.19
P2–N2	1.46 ± 0.63	0.31–1.52

Interpeak latency (msec): knee/scalp P1, 32.5 ± 1.9 m/sec.

Comments: The peripheral sensory nerve action potential frequently is difficult to obtain. (The above values are from E. Baran et al., *unpublished data.*)

PUDENDAL SOMATOSENSORY EVOKED POTENTIALS

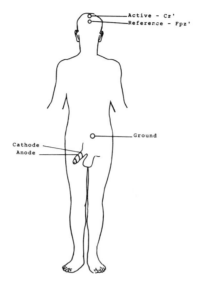

Figure 10.33. Pudendal SEPs. Penile stimulation with scalp recordings.

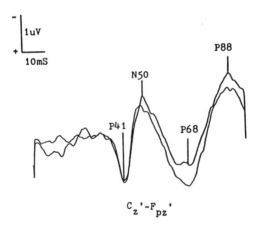

Figure 10.34. Dorsal nerve of penis stimulation.

Figures 10.33 and 10.34

Stimulation/Recording Technique

Pickup (one site):

Scalp (first channel): The dorsal nerve of the penis is stimulated with ring electrodes placed 4 cm apart. The anode is placed distally and the cathode proximally. Stimulus intensity is three times sensory threshold, and stimulus rates of 1–4.7 Hz with a stimulus duration of 0.1 or 0.2 msec can be used.

Equipment settings:
- Analysis time: 100 msec
- Gain: 10 μV
- Frequency bandwidth: scalp recordings, 0–2,000 Hz
- Averager (sweeps averaged): 200–500 sweeps

Normal values: (Taken from Haldeman et al.) Peak latency values (mean ± 1 SD msec); amplitude measurements were not provided.

	P1 onset	P1 peak	N1 peak
Men	35.2 ± 3.0	42.3 ± 1.9	52.6 ± 2.6
Women	32.9 ± 2.9	39.8 ± 1.3	49.1 ± 2.3

Comments: A spinal response at the root entry level (conus level) can be recorded in some men. Haldeman reports a peak latency of 9.9 ± 1.37 msec of the spinal response when present.

Haldeman S, Bradley WE, Bhatia NN, Johnson BK: Pudendal evoked responses. *Arch Neurol* 39:280–283, 1982.
Haldeman S, Bradley WE, Bhatia NN: Evoked responses from the pudendal nerve. *J Urol* 128:974–980, 1982.

TRIGEMINAL SOMATOSENSORY EVOKED POTENTIALS

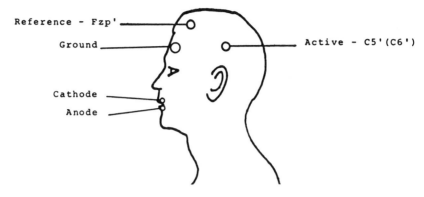

Figure 10.35. Trigeminal SEPs. Upper and lower lip stimulation and scalp recordings.

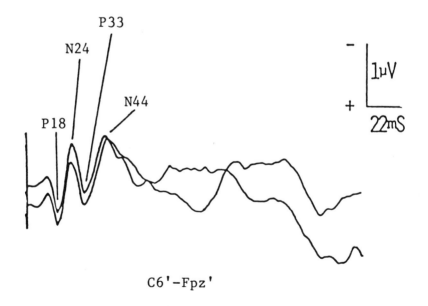

Figure 10.36. Left trigeminal nerve stimulation (lips).

Figures 10.35 and 10.36

Stimulation/Recording Technique

Pickup (one site):

Scalp (first channel): The active electrode is placed 2 cm behind C5 (when stimulating the right trigeminal nerve) or C6 (when stimulating the left trigeminal nerve). C5 and C6 positions are located midway between C3/T3 and C4/T4, respectively. A reference electrode is placed over Fpz'.

Options: None.

Ground: The ground electrode is placed over the inion midsagitally.

Stimulation: The upper and lower lips are stimulated simultaneously by placement of the anode over the lower lip 1 cm from the angle of the mouth. The cathode is placed over the upper lip 1 cm from the angle of the mouth. Stimulus intensity should be approximately three times sensory threshold, and the stimulation rate is 1–2 Hz. Stimulus duration is 0.2 msec.

Equipment settings:
- Analysis time: 50–200 msec
- Gain: 10 μV
- Frequency bandwidth: 0–3,000 Hz
- Averager (sweeps averaged): 128–500 sweeps

Normal values: (Taken from Stohr et al.) Peak latency values (mean ± 1 SD msec); amplitude (mean ± 1 SD μV)

	P1 latency (msec)	N1–P1 amplitude (μV)
Ipsilateral stimulation	18.5 ± 1.51	2.6 ± 1.1
Side-to-side difference	0.55 ± 0.55	0.51 ± 0.54

Bennett MH, Jannetta PJ: Trigeminal evoked potentials in humans. *Electroencephalogr Clin Neurophysiol* 48:517–526, 1980.

Findler G, Feinsod M: Sensory evoked response to electrical stimulation of the trigeminal nerve in humans. *J Neurosurg* 56:545–549, 1982.

Stohr M, Petruch F, Scheglmann K: Somatosensory evoked potentials following trigeminal nerve stimulation in trigeminal neuralgia. *Ann Neurol* 9:63–66, 1981.

Comments: Trigeminal SEPs can also be elicited by electrical stimulation of the tongue, gingiva, and teeth. Forms of natural stimulation of the face, such as taps to the face, puffs of air to the face, or nostrils also can generate trigeminal SEPs. Stimulus artifact may be a problem because of the proximity of the stimulus source and recording electrodes. When stimulating the first division of the fifth cranial nerve, muscle artifact from the blink reflex may contaminate the recordings.

CHAPTER 11

Movement-Related Potentials

GENERAL GUIDELINES

The study of potentials recorded before and immediately after a self-paced voluntary movement was first successfully undertaken using reverse data averaging techniques.[1,2] These signals subsequently become known as movement-related potentials (MRPs). MRPs have been studied extensively with scalp recordings and occasionally with subdural recordings. Their purpose is to elucidate the neural mechanisms in the brain responsible for the initiation, control, and execution of voluntary movement.

Research[3-5] has indicated the involvement of the supplementary motor area in voluntary movement initiation and the production of the earliest MRP component, the Bereitschaftspotential (BP). The sensorimotor area is thought to be the origin of a later MRP component, the Negative Slope (NS').[6] The BP, NS' and other slow, endogenous potentials have been shown to be dependent on physical factors (force, ability, extraneous movements) and also are affected by the psychological aspects of movement, that is, intention, motivation, and attention.[7-10] Therefore, to record MRPs successfully, the patient must be able to minimize eye and body movements throughout the testing and concentrate on repeating simple movements, usually of the eyes, head, or limbs.

Typically, MRPs are analyzed with respect to the latencies and amplitudes of the various components. Although the measurements of latencies and amplitudes in other event-related potentials can be quite reproducible,[4] these measures, particularly latency, are somewhat arbitrary in MRPs.

Although valuable information has been derived from these signals, the clinical significance of MRPs is in question. The potentials have been examined in studies of patients with known localized neurophysiological disorders and subsequently compared with normal signals. Distribution deficits or amplitude and latency variations in clinical evaluations, along with previous knowledge of the mechanisms of neural motor control, have enabled researchers to speculate as to the origins of the various potential shifts. As a diagnostic tool, the recordings are too diffuse to localize deficits, but they may be used as an indication of unilateral dysfunction.[11,12]

Acknowledgment. Nancy Stagliano, MSBME, aided in the writing of this chapter.

REFERENCES

1. Kornhuber HH, Deecke L: Hirnpotentialanderungen beim Menschen vor undenach-Willkurbewegungen, dargestellt mit Magnetbandspeicherung und Ruckwartsanalyze. *Pflugers Arch Physiol Gesamte Menschen Tiere* 282:52, 1964.
2. Kornhuber HH: Attention, readiness for action, and stages of decision—some electrophysiological correlates in man. *Exp Brain Res* 9(Suppl):420–429, 1984.
3. Goldberg G: Supplementary motor area structure and function: review and hypothesis. *Behav Brain Sci* 8:567–615, 1985.
4. Shibasaki H: Movement-associated cortical potentials in unilateral cerebral lesions. *J Neurol* 209:189–198, 1975.
5. Shibasaki H, Barrett G, Halliday E, Halliday AM: Components of the movement-related cortical potential and their scalp topography. *Electroencephalogr Clin Neurophysiol* 49:213–226, 1980.
6. Taylor MJ, Davis CM: The Bereitschaftspotential before voluntary and instructed serial movements. In: *Cerebral Psychophysiology: Studies in Event-Related Potentials* (EEG Suppl. 38).
7. Chisholm RC, Karrer R: Movement-related potentials and control of associated movements. *Int J Neurosci* 42:131–148, 1988.
8. Kresch EN, Baran EM, Mandel S, Whitenack S, Betz RR, Bess HH: Correlation analysis of somatosensory evoked potential waveforms. *Arch Phys Med Rehabil* 73:829–834, 1992.
9. Porter R: The Kugelberg Lecture: Brain mechanisms of voluntary motor commands—a review. *Electroencephalogr Clin Neurophysiol* 76:282–293, 1990.
10. Stagliano N, Baran E, Kresch E, Freedman W: Quantitative analysis of the Bereitschaftspotential. *Muscle Nerve* 14:895–896, 1991. (Abstract)
11. Kristeva R, Cheyne D, Lang W, Lindinger G, Deecke L: Movement-related potentials accompanying unilateral and bilateral finger movements with different inertial loads. *Electroencephalogr Clin Neurophysiol* 75:410–418, 1990.
12. Stagliano N, Baran E, Kresch E, Freedman W: Correlation analysis of movement-related potentials. *Muscle Nerve* 14:895, 1991. (Abstract)

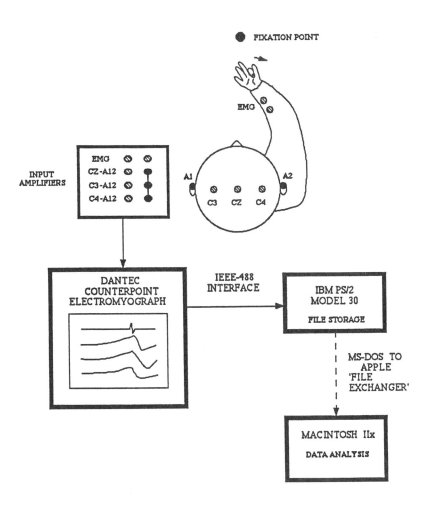

Figure 11.1. RP: experimental design.

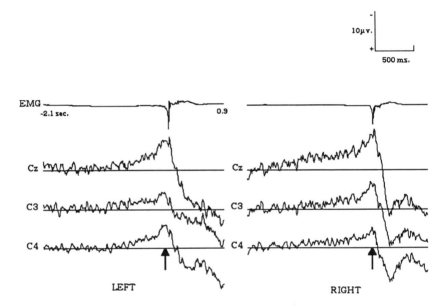

Figure 11.2.   RPs from index finger flexion.

Figures 11.1 and 11.2

Testing/Recording Technique

Pickup (four sites):

EMG (first channel): The surface EMG is recorded over the contracting muscle for the particular movement. The active electrode is placed 3 cm distal to the reference electrode.

Vertex (Cz) (second channel): The active electrode is placed at Cz. The reference electrodes are linked earlobes, A1–A2. The location of these scalp positions can be found in Figure 11.1.

Left Motor Area (third channel) (C4 for finger movement studies): The active electrode is placed at C4 and the reference electrodes are linked earlobes, A1–A2. The location of these scalp positions can be found in Figure 11.1.

Right Motor Area (fourth channel) (C3 for finger movement studies): The active electrode is placed at C3 and the reference electrodes are linked earlobes, A1–A2. The location of these scalp positions can be found in Figure 11.1.

Ground: The ground electrode is placed close to the electromyography (EMG) electrodes, avoiding contact with either the recording electrodes or the paste under the electrodes.

Movements: Simple self-paced voluntary movements usually are performed such as finger flexion or extension, wrist flexion or extension, or saccadic eye movements.

Equipment settings:
- Analysis time: ≥ 2 sec pretrigger
                     ≥ 1 sec posttrigger
- Gain: 1. EMG recording 200 μV.
           2. EEG recording 20 μV.
- Frequency bandwidth: 1. EMG recording 10 Hz to 1 kHz
                               2. EEG recordings 0.01 Hz to 100 Hz
- Averager (sweeps averaged): 200–500 sweeps

Comments: The intersubject and intrasubject variability of these data is large.

CHAPTER 12

Intraoperative Monitoring Using Somatosensory Evoked Potentials

The basic techniques for performing evoked potentials (EPs) are the same whether they are recorded in the operating room or in the more familiar clinical setting. Therefore, the individual experienced with upper and lower extremity EPs, including the ability to record from nonscalp locations, already has mastered the basics and needs only to adapt these skills to a somewhat different environment. In addition, this individual should have no difficulty mastering other procedures as well, such as performing epidural recordings.

To succeed during surgery, the clinician needs to:

1. work as part of the operating team
2. work in a "hostile" electrical environment
3. learn to distinguish nonneurologic from neurologic causes for variation in EP parameters.

WORKING AS PART OF THE OPERATING TEAM

Scalp-recorded EPs, that is, classic near-field somatosensory evoked potentials (SSEP), are influenced by many physiologic and nonphysiologic factors that are not related to impending neurologic damage. Obviously, then, to avoid alerting a surgeon to false-positive findings, the individual doing the monitoring must be aware of the multitude of nonneurologic causes of variability and how to recognize them. Among these are such factors as depth of anesthesia, type of anesthetic given, blood pressure, core temperature, pCO_2, rate of stimulation, and stimulator malfunction.[1-6]

The team member most responsible for tracking the physiologic variables (as opposed to the technical ones) is the anesthesiologist, and it is with the anesthesiologist that the person doing the monitoring must be in regular communication. Most of the time, variations in the amplitude, shape, and latencies of the different SSEP peaks can be "explained" by changes in one or more of these physiologic factors (Figures 12.1 and 12.2).

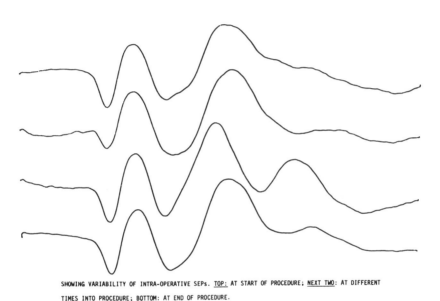

SHOWING VARIABILITY OF INTRA-OPERATIVE SEPs. TOP: AT START OF PROCEDURE; NEXT TWO: AT DIFFERENT TIMES INTO PROCEDURE; BOTTOM: AT END OF PROCEDURE.

Figure 12.1. Variability of intraoperative SSEPs during Harrington instrumentation for idiopathic scoliosis. In this fairly typical example, P1, N1, and P2 were relatively stable throughout the procedure, whereas the later deflections varied considerably. Potentials after P2 usually are unreliable for monitoring (200 msec analysis time; upward deflection indicating negativity of Cz' referenced to Fz; 100 repetitions each trace. From Spielholz, Engler, and Merkin, *Bull Am Soc Clin Evoked Potentials* 4:12–16, 1986, with permission).

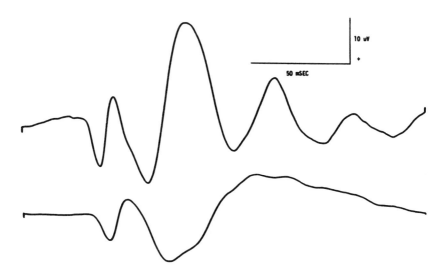

Figure 12.2. Effect of anesthesia (nitrous oxide, oxygen, barbiturate, and muscle relaxant) on SSEP. *Top:* Preoperative study with patient awake, stimulating posterior tibial nerve at ankle. *Bottom:* During surgery, with stimulus intensity twice that when awake. Note the marked prolongation of the second negative deflection *(N2)* and the disappearance of all deflections subsequent to it. Also, the initial three deflections (P1, N1, and P2) are lower in amplitude and slightly longer in latency than when awake.

WORKING IN A HOSTILE ELECTRICAL ENVIRONMENT

Because of the many electrical devices present in modern operating rooms, there are many sources of electrical "noise"; these are in addition to the common sources of interference in routine clinical practice, such as poor grounding of outlets, electrical lines in the ceilings or walls, radio transmissions, etc.

  I recommend that before doing intraoperative monitoring, trial runs be performed in the room(s) that will be used to determine how "friendly" they are. This can be accomplished by instrumenting a patient on the operating table, but with no other monitors turned on or even plugged in (including the operating table itself). Perform a run to determine if any interference is present under these "ideal" conditions. If it is, try changing the outlet from which the recording system is drawing power. In my experience, outlets on walls that border a corridor are superior to walls that separate adjacent operating rooms. If interference (especially 60 cycle) is still present, there may be either a general grounding problem or electrical conductors in the walls or ceiling that are acting as antennas. Have your engineering department help determine the source and how to eliminate it.

If, on the other hand, this preliminary trial run is free of artifact, plug in the other monitors to see if their addition causes problems. Deal with each if they arise.

Cautery frequently generates large artifacts. If possible, do not perform runs when you know the surgeon will be cauterizing bleeders. You might save a preamplifier now and then if you get the surgeon accustomed to warning you ahead of time and you put the preamplifiers in "Cal." mode to reduce possible damage to them. Some preamplifiers are equipped with "protection diodes" (or some other device) for this purpose, but even these could fail. If in doubt, check with the manufacturer of the equipment you're using.

Also, test all electrical devices at least twice a year for chassis leakage currents and to assure that patient connections remain adequately isolated. This requirement is mandated by the Joint Commission on Accreditation of Hospitals and the National Fire Protection Association.[7] If equipment has been assembled "in-house," be especially certain that all safety standards have been met.

DISTINGUISHING NEUROLOGIC LESIONS FROM NONNEUROLOGIC CAUSES OF VARIABILITY

Regardless of whether EPs are recorded from the scalp or spinal cord, neurologic dysfunction presumably would be heralded by:
1. loss of the EP
2. marked drop in amplitude of the EP
3. increases in latency of the EP.

Should any of these occur, the monitoring team must consider the following causes:

a) *The problem is "technical,"* that is, caused by stimulator malfunction (including dislodgement of stimulator electrodes or stimulator leads), problems with recording electrodes (such as dislodgement or changes in impedance), or recording circuit malfunction (such as a "blown" preamplifier). It is the responsibility of the monitoring team to be able to identify these problems when they occur and correct them when possible.

b) *The problem is "systemic,"* that is, due to a physiologic change, such as those mentioned previously. The anesthesiologist should be alerted to the change to determine if (s)he can throw any light on the matter. Another option is to monitor a nerve entering the cord *above* the level of surgery, such as the median nerve when performing Harrington instrumentation in the thoracolumbar region for scoliosis.[4,8] In this way, a systemic cause would be reflected in a change in both the median and (for example) posterior tibial EPs, whereas a focal neurologic change should affect only the EP from either one or both lower extremities.[4,8]

Indeed, it is because scalp-recorded SSEPs are so sensitive to systemic variables that some monitoring teams have either abandoned them in favor of some other recording site or have added another recording site that is not so sensitive to these nonneurologic factors. Examples of the latter are spinal potentials recorded either by epidural electrodes or from needles placed into the interspinous ligaments or from spinous processes.

c) *The problem is "neurologic,"* but its location is uncertain. This is because a change in the EP does not, by itself, distinguish between a developing spinal cord lesion or one involving the peripheral nerve being stimulated. The latter must be considered in the "differential diagnosis" since the conduction pathway to the spinal cord is a long length of peripheral nerve. For example, when monitoring EPs from the posterior tibial nerve at the ankle, it is theoretically possible (although not likely) for a conduction defect to occur somewhere between the site of stimulation and the cauda equina.

To determine that the peripheral volley is indeed reaching the spinal cord properly, a recording site distal to the spinal cord is required. Reported methods include from the interspinous ligament over-lying the cauda equina,[9] and from the sciatic nerve in the gluteal fold.[10] Note that the continued presence of such recordings also rules out the possibility of stimulator malfunction should an EP from the scalp or proximal spinal cord deteriorate.

d) *The problem is within the spinal cord.* Assuming that a marked change in the EP has occurred, the monitoring team should:

1. repeat a few more runs over the next 5 to 10 minutes to make sure that the change is not transient.

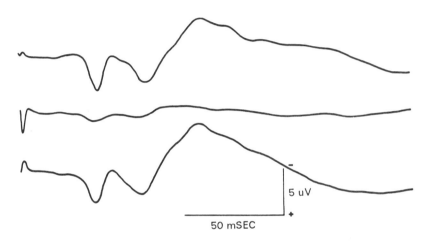

Figure 12.3. Demonstrating a patient with idiopathic scoliosis undergoing Harrington instrumentation in whom the posterior tib-ial SSEP disappeared almost completely within a few minutes after distraction. *Top:* Representative recording during predistraction phase. *Middle:* SSEP markedly reduced about 5 min after distrac-tion with no improvement over the next 10 min. *Bottom:* Reappear-ance of SSEP 2–3 min after removing the rod. SSEP then used to "titrate" how much distraction could be applied before the poten-tial began to deteriorate again. Patient awoke with no neurological deficits. (Reprinted from Spielholz, Engler, and Merkin, *Bull Am Soc Clin Evoked Potentials,* 4:12–16, 1986, with permission.)

2. if all peaks remain reduced and/or latencies remain prolonged, inform the anesthesiologist to determine if some physiologic change has occurred (*Note:* this could be "ruled out" if EPs from a proximal nerve also were being recorded as indicated above).
3. determine that the peripheral indicator of conduction into the spinal cord is unchanged (this will rule out a problem with the peripheral nerve and with the stimulator).
4. if none of these procedures reveal a "cause" for the change, inform the surgeon. What happens next is up to him or her.
5. the surgeon can elect to a) wait a little longer to see if the EP returns "spontaneously," b) perform a wake-up test, or c) reduce distraction and see if the EP returns (Figure 12.3).

SCALP RECORDINGS

The electrodes can be either surface discs or subdermal 1-cm electroencephalogram (EEG) needles (bare, not Teflon-coated!). For the long-term recordings required during surgery, I prefer needles. This is because it is easier to reinsert needles should they become dislodged than it is to reapply surface electrodes. However, if surface discs are used, collodion helps maintain them in place. Impedances should not be greater than 5,000 ohms.

For lower extremities: Cz' referenced to Fz' (i.e., the classical near-field montage for either lower extremity)

For upper extremities: C3' (for right upper extremity) or C4' (for left upper extremity) referenced to Fz' (*Note:* Fz' is a common reference both for upper and lower extremities)

Bandwidth:
for surface electrodes, 10–500 Hz (-3 dB)
for needle electrodes, 10–1,000 Hz (-3 dB)
The above values are approximations and depend, in part, on the choices different manufacturers build into their machines. Note though, that SSEPs, especially when recorded with surface electrodes, are primarily low frequency signals, that is, their rise and fall times are rela-

tively slow, and therefore do not require the high frequency filter (or low-pass filter) to be set too high. The low frequency filter (or high-pass filter) probably should not be above 30 Hz.

Analysis time: 100–150 msec

Number of runs to be averaged: 100–200
Although not universally considered necessary, I prefer studying a patient the day before surgery to make sure that the scalp-recorded potential is obtainable *and* to use the opportunity to mark the scalp site. This facilitates replacing the electrodes the next day after the patient has been intubated and positioned prone on the operating table. Once the anesthesiologist is satisfied that all monitors and other "lines" are working properly, recording electrodes can then be placed simply by parting the hair and looking for the marks. Make sure, though, that patients are instructed NOT to wash their hair after the preoperative study is performed.

STIMULATING ELECTRODES

Lower extremities: The most commonly stimulated nerves in the legs are the posterior tibial (behind the medial malleoli) and the common peroneal (behind the head of the fibula). Either can be used. I prefer the posterior tibials because the electrodes can be positioned better (and stabilized) behind the malleoli than behind the fibular head. Block surface electrodes, coated lightly with electrode gel, are taped securely (but not tightly) over the nerves. Three lengths of inch-wide tape adequately cover the block and help reduce drying of the electrolyte gel. Unlike what was just said about placing the recording electrodes after the patient is prone, I prefer placing the stimulating electrodes *before* the patient is turned. There usually is adequate time for this while the anesthesiologist is getting in the lines, placing electrocardiogram (ECG) electrodes, etc. You (or your technician) can then help in turning the patient while at the same time making sure that the electrodes and their wires are not dislodged.

Stimulus rate: If your machine permits, choose a rate between 1 and 5 Hz, which is not a multiple of 60. I prefer rates around 2/sec (e.g.,

1.7/sec or 2.3/sec). Frequencies above 5/sec tend to diminish the amplitudes of scalp-recorded SSEPs,[6] possibly because of "synaptic fatigue."

Stimulus strength: The anesthetic protocol for many spinal operations calls for the use of muscle relaxants. This obviates the use of muscle twitchings as an index of satisfactory stimulation. Furthermore, since anesthetics also reduce the size of SSEPs anyway (Figure 12.2), intensities employed preoperatively (assuming preoperative were performed, as suggested above) can be used only as a guide during surgery. In general, employ intensities somewhat higher than in the awake state, but it is recommended not to exceed 40 mA.[7] Usually, 20 to 25 mA are sufficient. Make sure the stimulating electrodes have been coated adequately with an electrolyte and that they have been secured in place (as described above) to reduce the gel's drying out. If in doubt, check the condition of these electrodes periodically (which is done fairly easily when stimulating the posterior tibial nerves at the medial malleoli).

Upper extremities: Median or ulnar nerves can be stimulated in their usual positions at the wrists.

Protocol:

Although it is true that scalp-recorded EPs may be quite variable, it is also true that most of the time they are usable. Furthermore, unlike epidural or spinal EPs, which require surgical exposure before the recording electrodes can be placed, scalp EPs can be started before the initial incision and can be followed until the patient is ready to be turned supine before leaving the operating room. In other words, scalp EPs can be started sooner and continued longer than the other options. Therefore, when using scalp EPs, perform runs from each lower extremity before the initial incision is even made to be certain that the potentials are obtainable. If EPs were obtained preoperatively, *do not* expect them to look exactly like those during anesthesia (Figure 12.2). Remember, the preoperative study was performed to make sure that EPs were obtainable under the best of conditions and to help facilitate placing recording electrodes the next day. During surgery, comparisons of amplitudes, latencies, and waveforms are made with respect to the EPs obtained early in the procedure, that is, before the critical parts of the surgery, with those obtained during and after. Study each side independently. Although earlier papers reported using simultaneous bilateral stimulation, a unilateral lesion may be missed by doing so.

Accurate record-keeping is vitally important. Store each waveform, either on disk or hard copy, properly annotated as to side stimulated, what was occurring during surgery when the recording was obtained, and, of course, the time. If possible, both the monitoring team and the anesthesiologist should use the operating room clock for their records instead of using their individual watches. Should the sequence of events have to be compared later, using the same time reference avoids the possibility of errors introduced by unsynchronized watches.

EPIDURAL/SPINAL RECORDINGS

Recordings made from either electrodes placed into the epidural space or from other locations close to the dorsal surface of the spinal column have the advantage of being more stable despite fluctuation in level of anesthesia, variations in blood pressure, etc. Their major disadvantage is that they cannot be started until well into the operation, and that they must be stopped well before surgery is completed. In other words, the time window during which epidural or other spinal recordings can be made is limited. To get the best of both worlds, some institutions use a combination of scalp-recorded SSEPs and epidural/spinal recordings. Different techniques for recording potentials from the dorsal surface of the spinal column have been reported. These include: a) needle electrodes in interspinous ligaments,[9] b) Kirschner wires in spinous processes,[11] and c) epidurally (Figure 12.4). Recording electrodes should be placed rostral and caudal to the surgical region so that both the incoming volley, and the volley propagating through the region that is at risk, can be monitored.

Epidural electrodes can be threaded into place by the surgeon through a small laminotomy. It is recommended that the wire connecting the electrode to the preamplifier be held in place by a suture.

Stimulation rates for epidural recordings can be faster than for SSEPs. Reported frequencies have been 4–8/sec,[15] 5/sec,[16] 10–20/sec,[17] and 19.9/sec.[13]

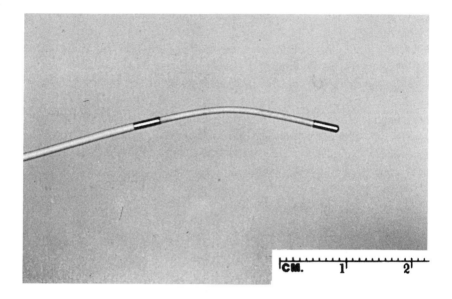

Figure 12.4. Epidural electrode modified from a dorsal column stimulator (Neuromed, Inc., Fort Lauderdale, FL. Photo courtesy of Nahid Nainzadeh, M.D.)

Recording parameters, especially with respect to bandpass settings, also have varied. The bandwidth recommended by the American Encephalographic Society[7] is:

low frequency filter: 100–200 Hz (−3 dB)
high frequency filter: 1,000–3,000 Hz (−3 dB).

As seen in Figure 12.5, the epidural potential recorded from the upper thoracic spine is a complex wave. However, the shape is not constant, being a function of the level of recording.[13] Obviously, latencies and amplitudes also will vary accordingly. Therefore, intraoperatively, each patient serves as their own "control," with potentials recorded early in the procedure being compared with those recorded later.[7]

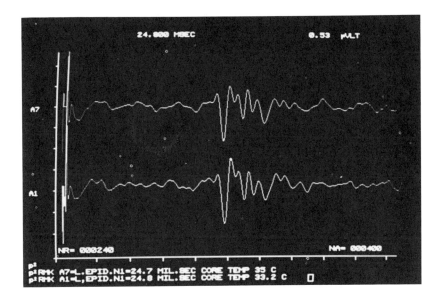

Figure 12.5.   Example of epidural recordings from the T2–T3 inter-space in response to stimulation of the right posterior tibial nerve at the medial malleolus. Note the polyphasic nature of the response at this level. (Photo courtesy of Nahid Nainzadeh, M.D.)

Summary of Recording Parameters:

Scalp recordings:

Nerve	Recording electrode Active	Reference	Stimulation site
Median or ulnar	C3' or C4'	Fz'	Wrist
Tibial or peroneal	Cz'	Fz'	Ankle (tibial) or Fibular head (peroneal)

Analysis time: 100–150 msec

Number of Runs to be averaged: 100–200

Bandwidth 10–500 Hz (− 3 dB) for surface electrode recording
10–1000 Hz (− 3 dB) for needle electrode recording

Stimulation rate: 1–5 Hz (prefer 2 Hz)

Stimulation Strength: 20–25 mA (not to exceed 40 mA)

Epidural/Spinal Recordings:

Recording electrodes are as follows: a) needle electrodes (in the interspinous ligaments), b) Kirschner wire (in the spinous process), c) epidural electrodes. The recording electrodes are placed rostral and caudal to the operating region.

Stimulation rate: Varies, 4–19.9 Hz

Bandwidth:

Low frequency: 100–200 Hz (− 3 dB)

High frequency: 1,000–3,000 Hz (− 3 dB)

REFERENCES

1. Engler GL, Spielholz NI, Bernhard WN, Danziger F, Merkin H, Wolff T: Somatosensory evoked potentials during Harrington instrumentation. *J Bone Joint Surg* 60A: 528–532, 1978.
2. Grundy BL, Nash CL Jr, Brown RH: Arterial pressure manipulation alters spinal cord function during correction of scoliosis. *Anesthesiology* 54:249–253, 1981.
3. Grundy BL, Nash CL Jr, Brown RH: Deliberate hypotension for spinal fusion: Prospective randomized study with evoked potential monitoring. *Can Anaesth Soc J* 29:452–462, 1982.
4. Nash CL Jr, Lorig RA, Schatzinger LA, Brown RH: Spinal cord monitoring during operative treatment of the spine. *Clin Orthop* 126:100–105, 1977.
5. Pathak KS, Brown RH, Cascorbi HF, Nash CL Jr: Effects of fentanyl and morphine on intraoperative somatosensory cortical evoked potentials. *Anesth Analg* 63: 833–837, 1984.
6. Spielholz NI, Benjamin MV, Engler GL, Ransohoff J: Somatosensory evoked potentials during decompression and stabilization of the spine: Methods and findings. *Spine* 4:500–505, 1979.
7. American Encephalographic Society: American Encephalographic Society Guidelines for intraoperative monitoring of sensory evoked potentials. *J Clin Neurophysiol* 4:397–416, 1987.
8. Brown RH, Nash CL Jr, Berilla JA, Amaddio MD: Cortical evoked potential monitoring: A system for intraoperative monitoring of spinal cord function. *Spine* 9: 256–261, 1984.
9. Lueders H, Gurd A, Hahn J, Andrish J, Weiker G, Klem G: A new technique for

intraoperative monitoring of spinal cord function: Multichannel recording of spinal cord and subcortical evoked potentials. *Spine* 7:110–115, 1982.

10. Veilleux M, Daube JR, Cucchiara RF: Monitoring of cortical evoked potentials during surgical procedures on the cervical spine. *Mayo Clin Proc* 62:256–264, 1987.

11. Maccabee PJ, Levine DB, Pinkhasov EI, Cracco RQ, Tsairis P: Evoked potentials recorded from scalp and spinous processes during spinal column surgery. *Electroencephalogr Clin Neurophysiol* 56:569–582, 1983.

12. Jones SJ, Edgar MA, Ransford AO, Thomas NP: A system for the electrophysiological monitoring of the spinal cord during operations for scoliosis. *J Bone Joint Surg* 65B:134–139, 1983.

13. Nainzadeh NK, Neuwirth MG, Bernstein R, Cohen LS: Direct recording of spinal evoked potentials to peripheral nerve stimulation by a specially modified electrode. In Ducker TB, Brown RH (eds): *Neurophysiology and Standards of Spinal Cord Monitoring.* New York: Springer-Verlag, 1988, 234–244.

14. Stolov WC, Slimp JC: Intraoperative monitoring of the vertebral canal. *AAEE Twelfth Annual Continuing Education Courses, 1989 AAEE Course B, Intraoperative Monitoring,* pp 27–38, 1989.

15. Morioka T, Tobimatsu S, Fujii K, et al: Direct spinal versus peripheral nerve stimulation as monitoring techniques in epidurally recorded spinal cord potentials. *Acta Neurochir* 108:122–127, 1991.

16. Roy EP, Gutmann L, Riggs JE, Jones ET, Byrd JA, Ringel RA: Intraoperative somatosensory evoked potential monitoring in scoliosis. *Clin Orthop* 229:94–98, 1988.

17. Jones SJ, Edgar MA, Ransford AO: Sensory nerve conduction in the human spinal cord: Epidural recordings made during scoliosis surgery. *J Neurol Neurosurg Psychiatry* 45:446–451, 1982.

CHAPTER 13

Auditory and Visual Evoked Potentials

BRAIN STEM AUDITORY EVOKED POTENTIALS

Auditory Evoked Potential

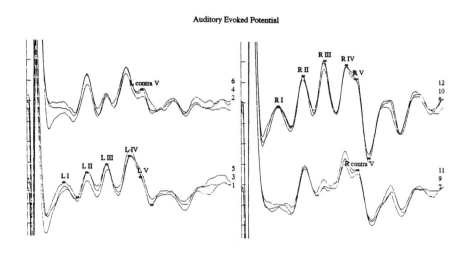

Figure 13.1. Auditory evoked potential.

Figure 13.1
Brain stem auditory evoked potentials (BAEPs) represent low amplitude for field potentials generated by successive components of the auditory pathway.

Setup:

Positioning: Supine with appropriate head propping to minimize postural muscle activity in the head and neck.

Stimulation: Click stimuli, produced by applying a 100-μsec square wave to 8-ohm impedance earphones. The stimulator should be capable of delivering either a rarefaction or a condensation click separately or in an alternating pattern. The rarefaction click phase usually is employed.
- Optimal speed of stimulation: 8–10 Hz
- Usually presented (stimulus intensity) 60–70 dB above the patient's own sensory level (dB SL), or above the average hearing level of a group of normal patients (db HL)
- Stimuli usually monaurally with contralateral masking using white noise at 30 dB SL; 30 dB below the stimulus intensity (70 dB intensity and 40 dB masking noise)
- Average 100–300 sweeps

Recording: EEG electrodes are placed over the earlobes (A1, A2, or Ai, Ac) (i and c referring to ipsilateral or contralateral), or over the mastoids (M1, M2). These are referred to the vertex (Cz).
Determine and record on worksheet the hearing threshold to nearest 5 dB for each ear with "noise" in opposite ear; use +5 dB option if needed.
Stimulate at 60 dB above threshold to obtain computer recording; record from side with better hearing first.
Turn click stimulator on at 10 Hz frequency with "click" in ear to be tested and "Noise" in opposite ear.

Ground: Frequently at Fz, but the contralatral ear (Az) or the mastoid (Mc) also can be conveniently used. One can use the forehead or chin.

Filters: 10–30 Hz
2500–3000 Hz

Montage:

Two-channel:
1. Cz-Ai (or Mi)
2. Cz-Ac (or Mc)

but usually one channel is sufficient.

Measurements:
1. The normal BAEP has seven waveforms, but only five have proven neurogenerators. These correspond to the following neural generators:

   Wave I   8th nerve potential

   Wave II   Cochlear nucleus or more proximal segment of the 8th nerve

   Wave III Superior olivary complex

   Wave IV   Lateral lemniscus

   Wave V   Inferior colliculus or more recently still the lateral lemniscus

   Wave VI   Medical geniculate body (not proved)

   Wave VII Auditory radiation (not proved)

2. Absolute latency: measured from stimulus to the positive peak of each wave.
3. Interpeak latency: measured from between the peaks of the two waves.
4. Where a peak is not well defined, a midpoint of the wave is an estimate.
5. Amplitudes are measured from the positive peak of the wave to the following negative one.
6. Ratio of IV, V/I is calculated. IV and V usually are on one slope; choose the higher amplitude.
7. Record the latencies of all identifiable waves (I through VII) as well as the I–III, III–V, and I–V interpeak latencies.
8. It is considered abnormal if:
   a. all or some of the waves are absent sequentially
   b. the interpeak latencies are prolonged (I–V)
   c. the absolute latency of a particular wave, mainly V, is prolonged
   d. decrease in the V/I ratio is suspicious
   e. decrease in interear differences is suspicious.

Normal values: (s = 55; 15–51 years)

Latency (msec)		Interpeak latency (msec)		R–L difference (msec)
		10 Hz		
I	1.7 ± 0.15	I–III	2.1 ± 0.15	0.10 ± 0.09
II	2.8 ± 0.17	I–V	4.0 ± 0.23	0.13 ± 0.10
III	3.9 ± 0.19	III–IV	1.2 ± 0.26	0.12 ± 0.14
IV	5.1 ± 0.24	III–V	1.9 ± 0.18	0.10 ± 0.11
V	5.7 ± 0.25	IV–V	0.7 ± 0.19	0.15 ± 0.14
VI	7.3 ± 0.29	V–VI	1.5 ± 0.25	0.22 ± 0.19
		30 Hz		
I	1.9 ± 0.26	I–III	2.2 ± 0.15	0.18 ± 0.15
II	2.9 ± 0.23	I–V	4.0 ± 0.21	0.15 ± 0.09
III	4.0 ± 0.26	III–IV	1.2 ± 0.22	0.19 ± 0.17
IV	5.2 ± 0.29	III–V	1.9 ± 0.25	0.20 ± 0.25
V	5.9 ± 0.34	IV–V	0.8 ± 0.21	0.21 ± 0.23
VI	7.7 ± 0.46	V–VI	1.7 ± 0.30	0.24 ± 0.22
		70 Hz		
I	1.8 ± 0.21	I–III	2.3 ± 0.29	0.18 ± 0.13
II	2.9 ± 0.19	I–V	4.3 ± 0.24	0.18 ± 0.14
III	4.2 ± 0.35	III–IV	1.3 ± 0.28	0.23 ± 0.20
IV	5.4 ± 0.30	III–V	2.0 ± 0.26	0.19 ± 0.19
V	6.2 ± 0.30	IV–V	0.8 ± 0.24	0.15 ± 0.08
VI	7.8 ± 0.42	V–VI	1.7 ± 0.39	0.35 ± 0.24

Amplitude (μV)	
	10 Hz
I	0.28 ± 0.14 (0.06–0.85)
III	0.23 ± 0.12 (0.03–0.55)
IV (pre-IV)	0.25 ± 0.12 (0.04–0.63)
IV (post-V)	0.40 ± 0.13 (0.08–0.88)
IV–V (highest)	0.47 ± 0.16 (0.14–0.88)
V	0.43 ± 0.16 (0.15–0.86)

Amplitude (µV)	
30 Hz	
I	0.16 ± 0.09 (0.04–0.39)
III	0.14 ± 0.10 (0.03–0.47)
IV–V (highest)	0.40 ± 0.15 (0.20–0.82)
70 Hz	
I	0.13 ± 0.09 (0.01–0.38)
III	0.10 ± 0.08 (0.01–0.45)
IV–V (highest)	0.37 ± 0.14 (0.08–0.73)

Amplitude Ratio (%)	
10 Hz	
III/V	50 ± 23
I/IV (pre-IV)	132 ± 75
I/IV (post-V)	75 ± 39
I/IV–V (highest)	62 ± 30
I/V	73 ± 48
30 Hz	
III/IV–V	35 ± 29
I/IV–V	41 ± 23
70 Hz	
III/IV–V	29 ± 22
I/IV–V	40 ± 31

Latency of Wave V (msec)	
60dB	5.8 ± 0.35
50dB	6.0 ± 0.36
40dB	6.4 ± 0.40
30dB	6.8 ± 0.50
20dB	7.3 ± 0.61

The above values were taken from Chiappa, Gladstone, and Young (1979).

Comments:

1. Usually average 200–300 sweeps.
2. Rarefaction stimuli usually provide better wave separation than condensation clicks. Alternate may be helpful if you have a large shock artifact.
3. Best location of the active recording electrodes is on the back of the earlobe.
4. Errors:
   a. Absent BAEP:
      1. check stimulator—click should be audible in ear being tested
      2. check electrode impedance
      3. excessive background noise—ask patient to close ears, relax jaw, keep room quiet
      4. if above fails to improve response, repeat recording at maximum intensity click (95 dB) with an average of 2,000 stimuli.
   b. Response inverted—recording and reference electrodes are reversed.

REFERENCES

Chiappa KH, Gladstone KJ, Young RR: Brain stem auditory evoked responses: Studies of waveform variations in 50 normal human subjects. *Arch Neurol* 36:81–87, 1979.

Jerger J, Hall J: Effects of age and sex on auditory brainstem response. *Arch Otolaryngol* 106:387–391, 1980.

Kjaer M: Recognizability of brain stem auditory evoked potential components. *Acta Neurol Scand* 62:20–23, 1980.

McClelland RJ, McCrea RS: Intersubject variability of the auditory-evoked brain stem potentials. *Audiology* 18:462–471, 1979.

Michalewski HJ, Thompson LW, Patterson JV, Bowman TE, Litzelman D: Sex differences in the amplitudes and latencies of the human auditory brain stem potential. *Electroencephalogr Clin Neurophysiol* 48:351–356, 1980.

Rowe MJ III: Normal variability of the brain-stem auditory evoked response in young and old adult subjects. *Electroencephalogr Clin Neurophysiol* 44:459–470, 1978.

Starr A, Achor LJ: Auditory brain stem responses in neurological disease. *Arch Neurol* 32:761–768, 1975.

Stockard JJ, Sharbrough FW, Tinker JA: Effects of hypothermia on the human brainstem auditory response. *Ann Neurol* 3:368–370, 1978.

VISUAL EVOKED POTENTIALS

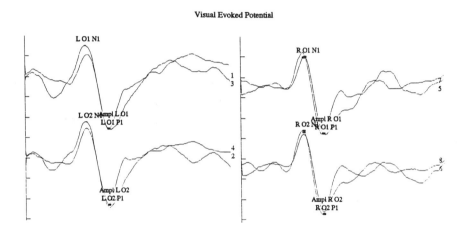

Figure 13.2.   Visual evoked potential.

Figure 13.2
Visual evoked potentials (VEPs) provide a qualitative and quantitative measure of the optical pathway in that they indicate a degree of function of the optic nerve, optic chiasm and tracts, lateral geniculate bodies, and geniculocalcarine projection to the visual cortex.

Setup:
Visual correction must be 20/200 or better
The pupil should not be dilated within 12 hours of the study
No amblyopia exanopsia

Stimulation:
- Pattern reversal studies: Checkerboard pattern is presented monocularly—large (56') or small (28') checks in a checkerboard pattern over a screen the size of a television set occupying a visual field of 12.3° (stimulation and testing protocols differ and each lab should develop its own normals).
- Hemifield stimulation: large checks (50 min to 1.5°) are presented to each eye. The total field should be 10–16°.
- Flash-evoked:
1. Responses should be presented 30–45 cm in front of the patient's eyes.
2. Ganzfield stimulator is preferable.
3. This less sensitive procedure is used when there are uncorrectable refractive errors or opacity of the ocular media, or if the patient is uncooperative.
- Luminance should be standard
- Check sizes should be a standardized size since smaller checks often increase the amplitude

Stimulation rate: 2 Hz

Recording/montage: Disk EEG electrodes are placed over the midocciput (0z) and 5 cm lateral to this on each side (01 and 02). These can be referred to as midfrontal lead (Fz). The ground can be placed at the vertex (e.g., Cz). A recommended montage is:
I: 02–Fz
II: 0z–Fz
III: 01–Fz

Only one channel montage (I) is sufficient in most cases.

For hemifield studies, two additional electrodes should be placed 10 cm lateral to the midline on both temporal regions (RT and LT). In that case, two additional channels are appropriate:

IV: LT–Fz

V: RT–Fz

The ipsilateral temporal channel can be omitted if necessary.

For flash-evoked studies, the usual leads can be used with reference to interconnected ears (A1A2).

Filter settings: 0.2–1.0 Hz
200–300 Hz

Data collection:

1. P100 is the most important peak to identify. It is often preceded by an N75, and followed less reliably by an N145 peak.
2. Hemifield studies: contralateral waves are measured (P75, N105, P135). The only secure abnormalities are absence of the waves or significantly delayed latencies.
3. In flash-evoked studies, alternating positive and negative waves appear.

Values:

Hughes et al. (1987):
(N = 19) Age, 14–65 years (mean, 40.2 years)

Latency (msec)

	P100			
28 'PR 49.7 ± 8.2	62.3 ± 11.7	98.6 ± 4.9	145.8 ± 17.8	192.7 ± 20.9
56 'PR 47.9 ± 8.0	59.0 ± 10.9	100.3 ± 6.5	144.7 ± 16.3	188.5 ± 21.8
Flash 49.3 ± 6.6	64.6 ± 10.5	103.9 ± 9.2	141.3 ± 17.6	177.8 ± 18.8

Amplitude (μV)

	P100			
28 'PR 0.62 ± 0.67	−0.24 ± 0.85	3.82 ± 2.66	−2.52 ± 1.75	0.55 ± 1.18
56 'PR 0.31 ± 0.63	−0.37 ± 0.79	4.55 ± 3.12	−2.24 ± 2.34	0.09 ± 1.02
Flash 0.17 ± 1.48	−2.93 ± 2.25	5.28 ± 3.27	−1.33 ± 2.88	3.89 ± 2.49

Normal limits of P100

	Both sexes 10–19 years	Males 20–49 years	Males 50–69 years	Females 20–59 years	Females 60–69 years
Latency (msec)	<115	<110	<120	<107	<110
L–R difference	all groups	<6 msec			
Minimal L/R ratio	all groups	>0.66			

Latency (msec)

Age (years)	P55 Male	P55 Female	N70 Male	N70 Female	P100 Male	P100 Female	L–R P100 Difference Male	L–R P100 Difference Female
10–14	51.5	51.6	69.7	67.0	102.4	104.8	2.1	1.1
15–19	52.3	54.1	69.3	69.2	98.5	99.1	2.5	6.1
20–29	56.3	52.3	73.3	68.5	101.2	96.9	2.4	8.0
30–39	54.8	53.2	71.4	71.4	98.9	97.1	1.3	2.2
40–49	55.5	53.9	69.9	70.2	99.1	96.7	2.0	7.1
50–59	56.8	54.9	73.6	70.6	103.9	97.5	3.7	0.2
60–69	59.8	57.4	74.3	71.5	107.0	101.5	2.5	9.1

Age (years)	Amplitude (μV) Male	Amplitude (μV) Female	L/R Ratio Male	L/R Ratio Female
10–14	20.3	16.4	0.88	0.94
15–19	12.5	14.6	0.85	0.88
20–29	6.5	18.2	0.87	0.95
30–39	6.5	9.8	0.91	0.88
40–49	9.9	10.9	0.88	0.92
50–59	8.3	10.7	0.91	0.89
60–69	7.4	7.8	0.86	0.95

Comments:
1. Room should be darkened or the background subdued.
2. The patient should be seated or slightly supine with the head elevated.
3. Visual acuity should be tested before performing pattern reversal and corrective lenses used if necessary.
4. For pattern reversal the patient is seated 1 m away and fixates at a central rate slightly off 2 Hz. Each eye should be tested separately.
5. For a flash, a 10-μsec stroboscopic pulse is presented from a distance of 10 cm (using an intensity of 8 on the Grass PS22 stimulator).
6. Hemifield tests can be accomplished by having the patient fixate on the right edge of the target for left field stimulation, and on the left edge for right field stimulation. In this case, surface recording should be taken from electrodes placed 5 and 10 cm lateral to the midline.
7. The primary response is best recorded 5 cm above the inion.

REFERENCES

Celesia GG: Steady-state and transient visual evoked potentials in clinical practice. *Ann NY Acad Sci* 388:290–307, 1982.

Celesia GG, Kaufman D, Cone S: Effects of age and sex on pattern electroretinograms and visual evoked potentials. *Electroencephalogr Clin Neurophysiol* 68:161–171, 1987.

Celesia GG, Daly RF: Visual electroencephalographic computer analysis (VECA). A new electrophysiologic test for the diagnosis of optic nerve lesions. *Neurology* 27: 637–641, 1977.

Celesia GG, Daly RF: Effects of aging on visual evoked responses. *Arch Neurol* 34: 403–407, 1977.

Halliday AM, McDonald WI, Mushin J: Delayed visual evoked response in optic neuritis. *Lancet* 1:982–985, 1972.

Halliday AM: The visual evoked potential in healthy subjects. In: Halliday AM (ed): *Evoked Potentials in Clinical Testing.* New York: Churchill Livingstone, 1982; 71–120.

Hughes JR, et al: Usefulness of different stimuli in visual evoked potentials. *Neurology* 37:656–662, 1987.

Kjaer M: Visual evoked potentials in normal subjects and patients with multiple sclerosis. *Acta Neurol Scand* 62:1–13, 1980.

Kaufman D, Celesia GG: Simultaneous recording of pattern electroretinogram and visual evoked responses in neuro-opthalmologic disorders. *Neurology* 35:644–651, 1985.

Pitt MC, Daldry SJ: The use of weighted quadratic regression for the study of latencies of the P100 component of the visual evoked potential. *Electroencephalogr Clin Neurophysiol* 71:150–152, 1988.

Shaw NA, Cant BR: Age-dependent changes in the latency of the pattern visual evoked potential. *Electroencephalogr Clin Neurophysiol* 48:237–241, 1980.

CHAPTER 14

Magnetoelectric Stimulation[1]

GENERAL GUIDELINES

The first work of transcranial magnetoelectric stimulation (TMS) was published by Barker and his coworkers in 1985. Since then, the technique of magnetoelectric stimulation (MS) has been used extensively in the study of both the central and peripheral nervous systems but mostly in a research setting. Figure 14.1 is a schematic representation of the principle of MS. The magnetic stimulator has three basic components: a high voltage source with charging circuit, storage capacitors and a high-current, high-voltage, solid-state switch. The capacitors are charged up to a high DC voltage by the voltage source. Then they are discharged rapidly through a copper coil by closing the solid-state switch. The rapid discharge of current in the coil creates a rapidly time-varying magnetic field. The intensity of the magnetic field generated could be as high as 2.2 teslas (T) or more. Faraday's law says that a changing magnetic field would induce a secondary electric field that impedes the changing magnetic field. Hence, a secondary electric field would be induced in the nearby biologic tissue such that, if it is of the appropriate amplitude and duration, the neuromuscular tissue could be stimulated just as in the case of electric stimulation. The magnitude of the induced electric field is proportional to the time rate of change of the magnetic field, not to the absolute magnitude of the magnetic field itself. The above probably is an oversimplification of MS. The actual mechanism also depends on a number of other parameters, such as the orientation of neuronal tissues relative to the induced electric field and the design of the magnetic coil, just to name a few.

Magnetic coils usually are available commercially in two basic configurations: the rounded coils and figure-of-eight coils (also called but-

---

[1] At the time of publication of this book in the United States, cortical magnetoelectric stimulation was approved only under research protocols.

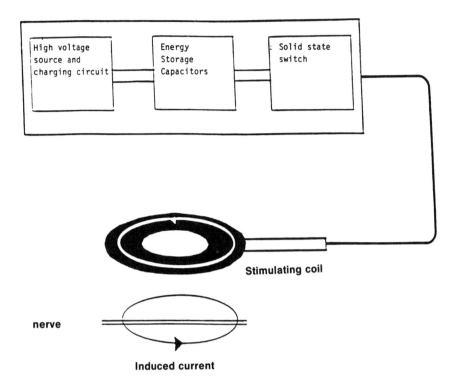

Figure 14.1. Schematic representation of the principle of magnetoelectric stimulation.

terfly coils) (Figure 14.2). The rounded coils come in different sizes of diameter. The smaller rounded coil is believed to deliver a slightly more focal stimulus and hence penetrate a deeper depth than the larger one. Some rounded coils have an angulated extension that, supposedly, increases the focalization of the coil (Figure 14.3). However, all these may not show any significant difference in the performance of the coil. The butterfly coil is composed of two rounded coils (wings of the butterfly) in series, arranged side by side so that the current in each foil flows in an opposite direction.

The induced electric field for the rounded coil is maximal close to the rim of the coil and decreases toward the center of the coil and outward away from the rim. However, the area of maximum electric

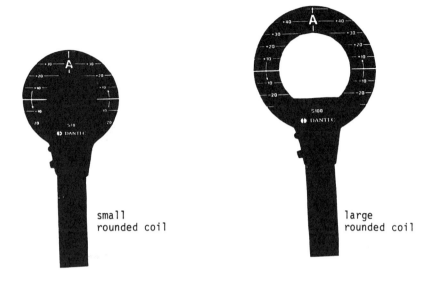

small
rounded coil

large
rounded coil

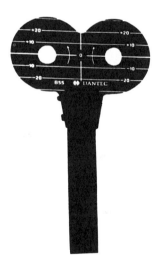

figure-of-eight coil

Figure 14.2. Different configurations of magnetic coil.

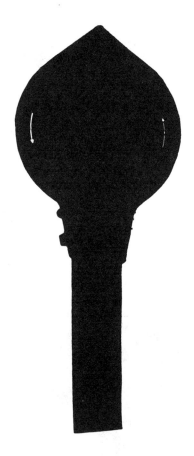

Figure 14.3.   Rounded magnetic coil with an angulated extension.

field for the butterfly coil is under its center where the two wings meet, with a smaller peak at the outer edges of the wings. In addition, the current flows in clockwise direction at one wing and counterclockwise direction at the other wing; therefore, there is twice the amount of current flowing in the center of the coil. Hence, the butterfly coil delivers the largest, most directional, and most focal stimulus.

Not all the magnetic coils have the same design even though they may look alike. For example, some rounded coils are made of tightly wound copper coils and some have spinal copper coils. Their internal wiring configuration is different and, therefore, their stimulation characteristics would be different. Similarly, not all the magnetic stimulators are the same. Magnetic stimulators produced by various manufacturers generate different pulse characteristics and hence induce different electric field waveforms. For example, some produce a polyphasic, decaying current pulse and some produce monophasic pulse stimuli (Figure 14.4). It is also important to know the direction of current in the coil and to know what type of current pulse your magnetic stimulator produces because reversing the coil current direction would shift the site of nerve stimulation with the monophasic magnetic stimulator but not with the polyphasic magnetic stimulator.[1] Hence, in the author's opinion, when you compare the data of your MS study with the published normal values of other laboratories, it is crucial that the equipments used in both studies be comparable with each other.

The specific site of nerve depolarization with MS has never been determined as well as that with conventional percutaneous electric stimulation. In peripheral nerve stimulation, the site of stimulation seems to be distributed under the part of the rounded coil circumference placed over and parallel to the nerve. For a smaller rounded coil, the area of stimulation may even extend outside the coil.[2] For the butterfly coils, the site of stimulation is definitely near the center of the coil where the wings meet. However, this site would be displaced with reversal of the current direction, acting like cathode-like and anode-like behaviors.[3] In the case of cortical stimulation, most likely it does not stimulate the motor cortex directly. It probably activates the corticospinal neurons transynaptically near the level of the gray–white matter junction (layer VI of cerebral cortex).[4] In summary, the actual site of stimulation would depend on a number of parameters including the design of the coil, the orientation and position of the coil, the orientation and position of the neural tissues and the properties of the surrounding volume conductors.

The motor cortex is sensitive to the direction of the induced current in TMS. It has a lower threshold when the current flows perpendicularly to the central sulcus, diagonally from back to front. That would be clockwise for the left hemisphere stimulation and counterclockwise for the right hemisphere stimulation with a large rounded coil centered at the vertex when viewed from above. However, this directional phe-

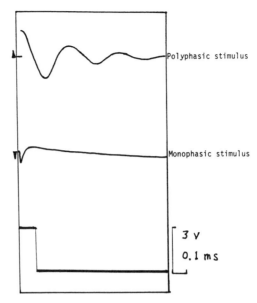

Figure 14.4. Stimuli of two different magnetic stimulators measured at the coil center. The DC voltage was measured by a small measuring coil held parallel to the stimulation coil. Note the difference in wave forms of the stimuli.

nomenon is seen only with monophasic current pulse and not with polyphasic current pulse.[5]

The newest generation of magnetic coil and stimulator has an active cooling system for the coil to keep the coil temperature down without overheating. Hence, repetitive MS becomes truly possible. Without the active cooling system, the fastest rate of stimulation at submaximal stimulus intensity is about 0.33 Hz for most magnetic coils and stimulators.

In TMS, the central conduction time from the motor cortex to the lumbar region is highly correlated with the height of the patient whereas that from the motor cortex to the cervical region is not.[6] Motor evoked potential latency does not seem to depend significantly on the sex, age, or weight of the patient.[7] Hence, in defining normality, height is an important variable.

In MS of peripheral nerves in the limbs with rounded coil, the magnitude of the induced electric field is smallest when the coil is perpendicular to the skin surface and it is largest when it is parallel to the skin. These findings are consistent with clinical experience and are supported by theoretical modeling as well.[8] Furthermore, computer modeling suggests that nerve fibers running parallel to the skin surface would have less stimulating threshold than those running obliquely and that nerve fibers running perpendicularly to the skin would have the highest stimulating threshold (i.e., most difficult to stimulate).[9]

When compared with conventional electric stimulation at Erb's point for brachial plexus, supraclavicular MS is considered to be less effective with only 16% of the time when its compound muscle action potential (CMAP) amplitude is greater than those obtained with electric stimulation.[10]

In general, it is more difficult to obtain an H reflex with MS. This may be due to the much higher threshold for sensory fibers than for motor fibers in MS. In the case of conventional electric stimulation with long duration electric stimuli (1.0 msec), the threshold for sensory fibers is lower than that for motor fibers.[11]

SAFETY ISSUES

MS is a relatively safe technique, with no significant short-term side effects. However, its long-term side effects require further investigation. Some possible side effects from TMS in normal volunteers may include headache and short-term memory impairment. However, none of these seems to be contributed directly to TMS. The risk of inducing seizures in normal healthy volunteers is very low unless high-frequency (>1 Hz) TMS is used.[12] It is known that low-frequency (0.33 Hz) single-pulse TMS can induce seizures in patients with recent stroke, multiple sclerosis, and epilepsy. However, adequately treated epileptic patients are considered to be safe for low-frequency TMS.[13] On the other hand, the risk of inducing seizures in epileptic patients with high-frequency, high-intensity (100% output) TMS is real.[14] The presence of implanted metallic structure in the brain should be a contraindication to TMS. Similarly, the magnetic coil should never be placed near cardiac pacemakers or any kind of bioelectronic implants because the circuits may be affected by MS. The question of whether TMS may induce secondary cerebral hemorrhage requires further study.

Even though MS is considered to be a relatively safe technique for the stimulation of neural tissues, its clinical safety is still being investigated. The impact of transcranial MS on the blood–brain barrier was studied in rats.[15] It was concluded that the permeability of the blood–brain barrier remained intact under pulsed MS. However, Matsumiya and his coworkers[16] showed that with high stimulus intensity (2.8 T) and 100 or more stimulations, it could produce clearly defined microvascular changes in the neuropil portion of the cortex from layers II to VI in rats. Gates and his coworkers[17] reported the first histopathologic studies of human brains after transcranial MS in two epileptic patients, each of whom had received 2,000 stimuli. They found no lesions in the surgical specimens attributable to TMS in these two patients.

Changes in several pituitary hormones were reported in relation to seizures and electroconvulsive therapy. The plasma levels of prolactin, follicle-stimulating hormone (FSH), luteinizing hormone (LH), human growth hormone (hGH), thyroid-stimulating hormone (TSH), and cortisol were studied before and after TMS.[18,19] No specific changes in the plasma levels of these pituitary hormones as a direct result of TMS could be found.

The rapid discharge of electricity through the magnetic coil in TMS produces an intense impulse noise artifact. This magnetic coil acoustic artifact (MCAA) may range from 145 to 157 dB peak sound pressure level at the eardrum with stimulation intensity of 50% to 100%. The international standards for damage risk criteria consider a level of 110 to 140 dB to be unsafe. Hence, it is of concern that the MCAA may cause permanent hearing loss to patients, especially when doing TMS and cranial nerve stimulation. It was shown to cause permanent threshold shifts in unprotected ears of rabbits.[20] Even though audiologic studies before and after TMS in humans has shown little risk of hearing loss from MCAA,[21] it is recommended to use ear protectors for the patient and clinician during MS to prevent hearing damage.[22]

The rapid discharge of electricity through the magnetic coil also produces heat in the coil that, when placed in direct contact with skin, can cause a first degree burn under the area of coil if multiple stimulations are performed and if there is no active cooling system in the magnetic coil. However, nowadays, most magnetic simulators would have a temperature sensor in the coil that automatically shuts off the circuit when it reaches a certain preset temperature so as to prevent overheating of the coil. With the introduction of new magnetic stimulators capable of stimulating at rates up to 60 Hz, there is another safety hazard if a metal electrode is near the coil during repetitive stimulation. The skin temperature under a silver/silver-chloride cup electrode can be raised by 4.4°C with 160 stimuli at 100% output intensity and 1 Hz frequency.[23]

Out of concern about the possibility of cerebral effects by TMS, Bridgers and his coworkers[24] performed cognitive and motor tests before and after TMS on 30 healthy adults. They found no detrimental effects on test performance. However, in a study of influence of TMS on memory function, there was a small but significant reduction in short-term memory performance after TMS at 100% field intensity (2 T) in a group of 21 healthy volunteers[25]; however, this effect on memory function was thought not due to cortical effect of TMS. Therefore, TMS was considered to be safe with respect to memory function.

Last but not least, the effect of TMS on epilepsy has been studied quite extensively. Hufnagel and coworkers[26] showed that cortical threshold intensities were markedly elevated and peripheral latencies were prolonged in patients treated with antiepileptic drugs for medically intractable temporal lobe epilepsy. The cortical threshold intensities and peripheral latencies would decrease toward control values after the reduction of anticonvulsant drugs. The central motor conduction time increased when the patient was treated with multiple anticonvulsant drugs instead of a single agent.

FACILITATION

Motor evoked potentials can be enhanced in TMS by certain maneuvers. This phenomenon is called "facilitation." For example, mild voluntary contraction of the target muscle would reduce the threshold stimulus intensity, increase the amplitude, and decrease the latency of the CMAP. A voluntary contraction between 2% and 6% of maximal surface electromyography (EMG) activity[27] or 10% to 20% root mean square maximal integrated electrical muscle activity[28] would be sufficient to produce the optimal effects. No significant gain occurs when contraction increases beyond this level. In addition, there have been observations of facilitation by contracting a nearby ipsilateral muscle and/or a contralateral homologous muscle. A lesser facilitating effect also can be induced by nonspecific maneuvers such as sticking out the tongue or counting aloud. However, these spreads of facilitation needs further investigation.[29,30] Facilitation produced by voluntary contraction can be explained in part by the recruitment of the faster conducting neurons at the cortical level and in part by the lowering of the motoneuron threshold at the spinal level.[31] MS of peripheral nerves usually does not require facilitation.

Motor evoked potentials also can be influenced (facilitated) by the posture of the patient. For example, in TMS of the lower limb muscles, the amplitude of the CMAP is increased significantly with the patient standing upright rather than lying supine.[32] However, the mechanism of postural facilitation probably is different from that of voluntary contraction because it does not shorten the onset latency of the CMAP. More interestingly, facilitation also can be induced by percutaneous electric stimulation of the peripheral nerve or the dermatone.[33,34] This method of electrical facilitation potentially may provide an easy, reproducible, and quantitative way to standardize facilitation in the future.

MAGNETOELECTRIC STIMULATION TO UPPER AND LOWER LIMBS

Terminology

A few words about terminology. The total motor conduction time (TMCT) is the time from the triggering of TMS to the initial onset of the motor evoked potential (MEP) at the target muscle (i.e., from cortex to muscle). The peripheral motor conduction time (PMCT) is the time from the triggering of spinal root MS to the initial onset of the MEP at the target muscle (i.e., from root to muscle). However, the PMCT also can be obtained by the F-wave method as calculated from the formula: (F + M − 1)/2, where F is the shortest latency of the F wave in milliseconds and M is the latency of the M wave in milliseconds. Hence, central motor conduction time (CMCT) can be determined by the subtraction of latencies between the TMCT and the PMCT using either the spinal root stimulation or the F-wave formula. To prevent confusion, we designate the CMCT obtained by the latency difference between TMCT and PMCT from spinal root stimulation as CMCT(r) and that obtained by the latency difference between TMCT and PMCT from F-wave formula as CMCT(F). Therefore, CMCT(r) is the sum of the conduction times in the corticospinal fibers, of the spinal synaptic delay and in the proximal part of the motor roots, up to the site of depolarization whereas CMCT(F) is the conduction time from the motor cortex to the motor neurons. When a patient exerts a voluntary muscle contraction during TMS, the MEP, besides having a facilitating effect, typically ends with a silent or inhibitory period (Figure 14.5). The time between the end of the MEP and the resumption of background EMG is called the inhibitory period.

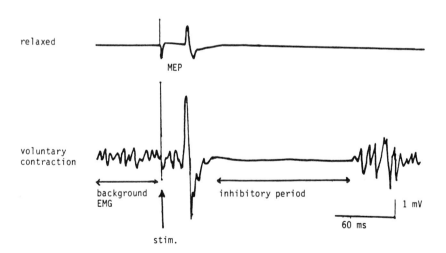

Figure 14.5. Inhibition study.

CERVICAL STIMULATION

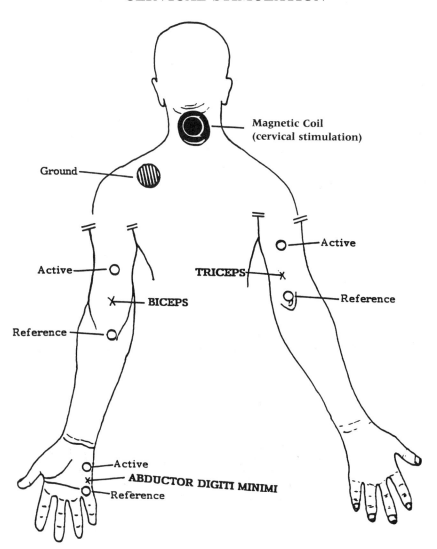

Figure 14.6. Cervical stimulation.

Cros et al. Study (1990)

Pickup: MEPs were recorded with 10-mm silver disk electrodes at the abductor digiti minima (ADM), the biceps brachii (biceps), and the triceps brachii (triceps) muscles bilaterally using a tendon-belly montage and simultaneously using a multichannel EMG machine.

Reference Site: See Pickup.

Ground: The position of ground electrode was not given in the study.

Stimulation: The magnetic coil was placed in a tangential position to the back of the neck centered on the midline with its center on the spinous processes of C3, C4, C5, and C6 levels subsequently. MS at each level with 100% maximum intensity was repeated twice to obtain reproducible tracings. The onset latency was determined from the CMAP of maximum amplitude.

Equipment: A Novametrix Magstim 200 magnetic stimulator that delivered a monophasic pulse and maximum magnetic field of 1.5 T was used with a rounded magnetic coil consisting of 19 turns of concentric copper wire (diameter range, 5.5–12.5 cm). The mean diameter of the coil was 9 cm.

Patient position: During the study, patients were seated comfortably, with their neck in 45° flexion, their arms relaxed, and their elbows in semiflexion.

Normal values:

For biceps, mean onset latency = 5.9 msec (SD = 0.8; range: 7.45–8.1)

side-to-side mean latency difference (right minus left) = 0.2 msec (SD = 0.65; range: −0.6–1.8)

mean amplitude = 9,800 μV (SD = 5,500; range: 2,800–22,350)

side-to-side mean amplitude difference = 650 μV (SD = 2,500; range: −3,900–5,400)

Cros D, Chiappa KH, Gominak S, Fang J, Santamaria J, King PJ, Shahani BT: Cervical magnetic stimulation. *Neurology* 40:1751–1756, 1990.

For triceps, mean onset latency = 6.1 msec (SD = 0.85; range: 4.7–7.8)
side-to-side mean latency difference = 0.03 msec
(SD = 1.03; range: –0.23–1.2)
mean amplitude = 8,900 μV (SD = 5,350; range: 2,200–18,300)
side-to-side mean amplitude difference = 1,200 μV
(SD = 2,800; range: –1,500–8,100)
For ADM, mean onset latency = 14.1 msec (SD = 1.5; range: 11.6–17.4)
side-to-side mean latency difference = –0.51 msec
(SD = 0.94; range: –2.5–0.5)
mean amplitude = 7,700 μV (SD = 2,500; range: 1,800–10,900)
side-to-side mean amplitude difference = 780 mV
(SD = 2,500; range: –2,400–8,600)

The authors did not specify whether the CMAP amplitudes were measured from baseline to peak or from peak to peak.

Comments:
1. Twenty normal volunteers (age, 21–47 years) were studied. No further information on the volunteers was given.
2. The muscles were studied at rest without facilitation.
3. The authors found that the coil current should flow counterclockwise to obtain the largest amplitudes on the right side and clockwise to obtain the largest amplitudes on the left side.
4. The levels of stimulation for maximum amplitudes were C3 or C4 for biceps, C4 for triceps, and C5 for ADM.
5. The latency to a target muscle would not shift significantly when the coil was moved longitudinally from level to level. However, the CMAP amplitude would differ markedly with suboptimal coil placement.
6. When compared with PMCT derived from the F-wave formula, the average PMCT to ADM by cervical magnetoelectric stimulation was 0.1 msec longer.

7. The authors also performed near-nerve "root" needle stimulation. When compared with electric needle stimulation, the latencies for MS were 0.5 and 0.6 msec longer for biceps and triceps, respectively, and 0.3 msec shorter for ADM. The CMAP amplitudes, however, were always larger with electric needle stimulation.

8. No temperature of the room or of the volunteer's skin was given.

LUMBOSACRAL STIMULATION

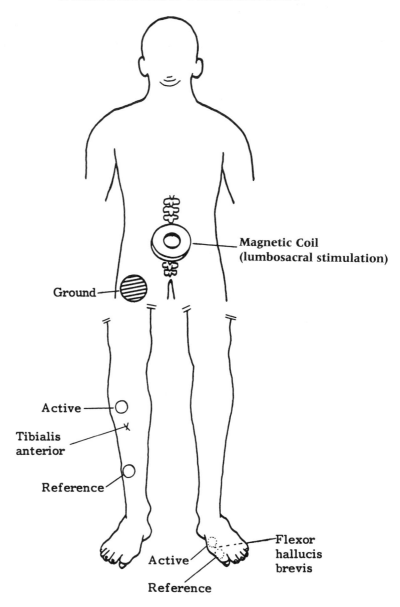

Figure 14.7.   Lumbosacral stimulation.

Macdonell et al. Study (1992)

Pickup: Ag-AgCl electroencephalogram (EEG) electrodes were placed 3 cm apart over the tibialis anterior (TA) and flexor hallucis brevis (FHB) muscles bilaterally. CMAPs were recorded bilaterally and simultaneously with four-channel Mystro EMG machine (Teca Corp).

Reference site: See Pickup.

Ground: Not given in the study.

Stimulation: The magnetic coil was placed tangentially to the low back surface with its center over the L5 and S1 spinous processes subsequently. The coil handle was perpendicular to the vertebral column. Stimulation was performed with 100% maximum intensity using both clockwise and counterclockwise directions of coil current.

Equipment: A 7-cm diameter Novametrix magnet coil was used with a Magstim 200 stimulator that gave a monophasic current pulse of 75 μsec rise time. The maximum magnetic field strength was 1.5 T at the center of the coil. A four-channel Teca Mystro EMG machine was used for recording. The filter bandwidth was set at 10 Hz to 10 kHz with a gain of 200 μV to 5 mV/cm and a sweep duration of 50 msec.

Patient position: The patient was seated comfortably with the back straight and legs extended.

MacDonell RA, Cros D, Shahani BT: Lumbosacral nerve root stimulation comparing electrical with surface magnetic coil techniques. *Muscle Nerve* 15:885–890, 1992.

Normal values:

For TA, mean latency = 13.6 msec (SD = 1.2; range: 11.2–15.8)
side-to-side mean latency difference = 0.6 msec (SD = 0.6)
mean amplitude (as % of peripheral supramaximal M response)
= 36% (SD = 25; range: 9–92)
side-to-side mean amplitude difference = 21% (range: 2–70)
For FHB, mean latency = 24.7 msec (SD = 2.2; range: 20.6–28.9)
side-to-side mean latency difference = 0.7 msec (SD = 0.6)
mean amplitude = 25% (SD = 17.4; range: 2–61)
side-to-side mean amplitude difference = 10% (range: 0–25)
The authors did not specify whether the CMAP amplitudes were measured from baseline to peak or from peak to peak.

Comments:

1. Eighteen persons with no history or evidence of peripheral nervous disorder were studied (age: 25–72 years; 10 males and 8 females).
2. There was no significant difference in latency and CMAP amplitude from both muscles comparing L5 with S1 stimulation.
3. Reversal of current direction of the coil did not affect the latency or the amplitude. The coil current direction that produces the largest amplitude at each side was unpredictable.
4. The CMAP amplitude from MS was expressed as a percentage of the CMAP amplitude evoked by distal supramaximal stimulation to the same muscle.
5. The CMAP latencies by MS had a positive correlation with patient height.

6. The authors also performed needle electric stimulations to TA and FHB muscles with a monopolar needle electrode. There was no significant difference in CMAP latency between the magnetic and electric techniques. However, the CMAP amplitude was always larger in needle root stimulation.

7. Comparison of F-wave latencies with those of MS suggested that the site of MS of spinal motor nerve roots was within the spinal canal before the entry of the root into intervertebral foramen.

TRANSCRANIAL STIMULATION TO MUSCLES OF UPPER LIMB

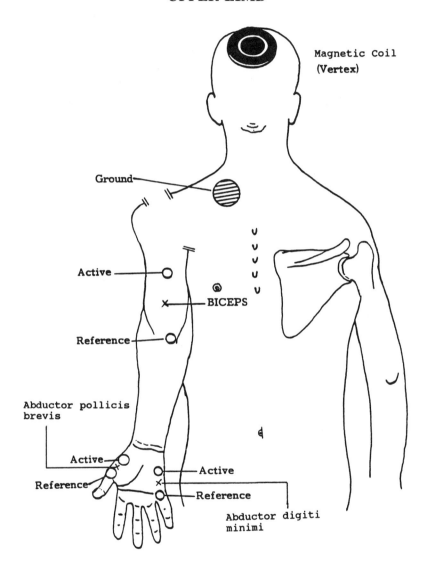

Figure 14.8. Transcranial stimulation to muscles of upper limb.

Dvorak et al. Study (1990)

Pickup: Surface electrodes were placed over the muscle bellies of the long head of biceps brachii (Bi), the abductor pollicis brevis (APB), and the abductor digiti minimi (ADM) muscles.

Reference site: Surface electrodes were placed over the distal tendons of the above muscles.

Ground: Not given in the study.

Stimulation:

Transcranial Stimulation: The center of the magnetic coil was placed above the vertex to activate the upper limb muscles. The latency measured was called cortical latency (CL).

Cervical Stimulation: The center of the coil was positioned in midline over the C7 vertebra. The latency measured was called root latency (RL).

Proximal Nerve Trunk Stimulation: The center of the coil was placed ventral to the coracoid process. The latency measured was called peripheral latency (PL).

Dvorak J, Herdmann J, Theiler R: Magnetic transcranial brain stimulation: Painless evaluation of central motor pathways. Normal values and clinical application in spinal cord diagnostics: Upper extremities. *Spine* 15:155–160, 1990.

The coil was in physical contact with the skin during stimulation. For TMS, stimuli of 50% intensity above threshold were used. Patients were asked to hold both arms in front of them and to spread their fingers to achieve an equivalence of about 10% maximal voluntary contraction for facilitation purpose. For cervical and proximal stimulations, the muscles were tested at rest and with minimal stimulus intensity to avoid the spread of the magnetic field. At least five consecutive stimulations were given to each site of stimulation. The shortest reproducible latency and the largest MEP amplitude were measured. Furthermore, in each patient the shortest F-wave latency was measured for the median and ulnar nerves.

Equipment: Both a Dantec Magnetic Stimulator and a Novametrix Magstim ME 200 magnetic stimulator were used with their respective rounded coils. The Dantec magnetic coil had 14 copper windings and a maximum winding diameter of 12 cm. The Novametrix coil had 19 copper windings and similar maximum winding diameter. MEPs were recorded with a Dantec Counterpoint EMG machine with filters set at 2 Hz and 10 kHz.

Patient position: Patients flexed their neck during cervical stimulation.

Normal values: N = 50: 30 men, 20 women; age: 18–75 years (mean 42 ± 15 years)
For the biceps muscle,
mean TMCT = 13.0 msec (SD = 1.4)
mean PMCT = 7.9 msec (SD = 1.3)
mean CMCT(r) = 5.1 msec (SD = 1.0; range: 3.5–6.2)
For the APB muscle,
mean TMCT ≈ 20.7 msec (SD = 1.3)
mean PMCT = 15.6 msec (SD = 1.2)
mean CMCT(r) = 5.2 msec (SD = 0.6; range: 4.0–6.3)
mean CMCT(F) = 4.3 msec (SD = 0.8; range: 3.2–5.7)
mean PML (proximal motor latency, RL–PL)
= 2.2 msec (SD = 0.4; range: 1.4–2.7
For the ADM muscle,
mean TMCT = 20.0 msec (SD = 1.5)
mean PMCT = 14.9 msec (SD = 1.5)
mean CMCT(r) = 5.2 msec (SD = 0.9; range: 3.5–6.7)
mean CMCT(F) = 4.0 msec (SD = 0.8; range: 3.0–5.5)
mean PML (proximal motor latency, RL–PL)
= 2.6 msec (SD = 0.8; range: 1.5–3.9)

Comments:
1. Height of subjects ranged from 150 to 191 cm (mean 172; SD 9) and weight ranged from 47 to 95 kg (mean 70; SD 13).
2. The authors did not find any statistically significant dependence of CMCT(r), CMCT(F), and PML on age, sex, size, or body weight.
3. The authors used both the Dantec and Novametrix stimulators in their study and found no statistically significant differences between the results obtained using either of the two stimulators.
4. Since maximum stimulation intensity was not used in cervical stimulation, the PMCT obtained might not be from that of the fastest conducting axons.
5. Room temperature and skin temperature were not given in the study.

Ghezzi et al. Study (1991)

Pickup: Surface electrode was placed over the thenar muscle.

Reference site: Not given in the study.

Ground: Not given in the study.

Stimulation:

Transcranial Stimulation: The center of the coil was placed at the vertex. The stimulation intensity was adjusted at 10% above the motor threshold. The patient was asked to contract the thenar muscle slightly.

Cervical Stimulation: The center of the coil was placed over the C5, C7, and T2 spinous process. The stimulation intensity was also set at 10% above the motor threshold. Contraction of the muscle was not necessary.

At least four stimulations were obtained at each site and the shortest latency and largest MEP amplitude measured. The shortest F-wave latency to the thenar eminence was obtained by conventional electrical stimulation to the median nerve at the wrist.

Equipment: MS was performed with a Novametrix Magstim stimulator and a rounded magnetic coil. The diameter of the coil was not mentioned in the study. The bandpass of the EMG machine was set at 1–2000 Hz.

Patient position: Not given in the study.

Ghezzi A, Callea L, Zaffaroni M, Zibetti A, Montanini R: Study of central and peripheral motor conduction in normal subjects. *Acta Neurol Scand* 84:503–506, 1991.

Normal values: (N = 25; 14 women, 11 men) Ages, 15–58 years (mean: 32.3 years). Height: 153–185 cm (mean, 167.2 cm). Arm length (C7 to thenar eminence); mean was 71.2 cm (range: 61–90 cm).

For the thenar muscle,

mean TMCT = 20.5 msec (SD = 2.0; range: 16.7–25.0)

mean PMCT (at C5 level) = 13.6 msec (SD = 1.0; range: 10.9–15.6)

mean CMCT(r) = 6.9 msec (SD = 1.3; range: 4.5–9.4)

In cervical stimulation,

for the right thenar muscle, stimulated at C5 with clockwise coil current,

mean amplitude = 4.6 mV (SD = 2.5)

for the left thenar muscle stimulated at C5 with counterclockwise coil current,

mean amplitude = 5.0 mV (SD = 2.5)

The author did not specify whether the amplitude was measured from baseline to peak or from peak to peak.

Comments:

1. The mean difference between PMCT obtained by root stimulation and that by the F-wave method was 0.5 msec shorter.
2. In cervical stimulation to the right upper limb, clockwise coil current was used. In cervical stimulation to the left upper limb, counterclockwise coil current was used.
3. Total motor conduction time and central motor conduction time both correlated positively with patients height and arm length. However, the R coefficient was higher with patients height than with arm length. Therefore, the authors suggested using the body height as a clinical variable.
4. The TMCT and PMCT did not correlate statistically to age and sex.
5. No room temperature or skin temperature was given in the study.

Eisen et al. Study (1991)

Pickup: Surface disk electrodes (filled with conductive gel) were placed over the motor end plate regions of the thenar and hypothenar muscles.

Reference site: Surface disk electrodes (filled with conductive gel) were placed over the distal tendons of the muscles mentioned above.

Ground: Not given in the study.

Stimulation: The center of the magnetic coil was placed over the vertex. This position was adjusted to obtain the largest MEP amplitude. Twenty consecutive stimulations were given at stimulus intensity of 20% above threshold and at intervals varied from 1.5 to 4 sec. The patient was asked to contract the target muscle at between 15% and 20% of maximum force, which was monitored by a force transducer. The MEP amplitude was measured from peak to peak. Both the maximum MEP amplitude (MAXMEP) and the mean MEP amplitude (AVMEP) of 20 consecutive MEPs were determined. The CMAP amplitudes of the thenar and hypothenar muscles also were determined by supramaximal electrical stimulation of the median and ulnar nerves at the wrist, respectively.

Equipment: TMS was performed with a Dantec magnetic stimulator and a Dantec rounded coil, which had an outer diameter of 14 cm and a central hole of 2 cm.

Patient position: The patient was seated comfortably in a temperature-controlled room at 20–22°C.

Eisen A, Siejka S, Schulzer M, Calne D: Age-dependent decline in motor evoked potential (MEP) amplitude: With a comment on changes in Parkinson's disease. *Electroencephalogr Clin Neurophysiol* 81:209–215, 1991.

Normal values:
For thenar muscle,
in young patient group (age <40 years; mean age, 33.1 years),
    mean CMAP = 13.4 mV (SD = 1.6; range: 11.6–17)
    mean MAXMEP = 12.1 mV (SD = 1.4; range: 10–14.5)
    mean AVMEP = 9.0 mV (SD = 1.1; range: 7.8–11.5)
    mean MAXMEP/CMAP = 90.3% (SD = 14.7; range: 71–122)
    mean AVMEP/CMAP = 67.2% (SD = 11.9; range: 53–97)
    frequency of MAXMEP (per 10 consecutive stimuli) = 1.8
        (SD = 1.0; range: 1–4)
in older patient group (age >45 years; mean age, 63.3 years),
    mean CMAP = 8.0 mV (SD = 1.4; range: 5.8–11.8)
    mean MAXMEP = 7.5 mV (SD = 2.5; range: 3–11.8)
    mean AVMEP = 6.2 mV (SD = 2.4; range: 2–10.6)
    mean MAXMEP/CMAP = 93.7% (SD = 23.8; range: 34–139)
    mean AVMEP/CMAP = 77.5% (SD = 27.9; range: 25–134)
    Frequency of MAXMEP (per 10 consecutive stimuli) = 2.2
        (SD = 1.2; range: 1–5)
in all ages group,
    mean MAXMEP/CMAP = 92.6% (SD = 25.8)
    mean AVMEP/CMAP = 73.7% (SD = 23.1)
For hypothenar muscle,
in young patient group (age <40 years; mean age, 38.4 years),
    mean CMAP = 15.8 mV (SD = 1.4; range: 14–18)
    mean MAXMEP = 9.6 mV (SD = 2.7; range: 8–14.4)
    mean MAX MEP/CMAP = 60.8% (SD = 9.6; range: 49.7–67.8)
in older patient group (age >45 years; mean age, 68.7 years),
    mean CMAP = 10.7 mV (SD = 1.8; range: 8.3–15.2)
    mean MAXMEP = 4.9 mV (SD = 3.1; range: 2.5–9.4)
    mean MAXMEP/CMAP = 51.0% (SD = 10.2; range: 35.7–62.0)
in all ages group,
    mean MAXMEP/CMAP = 54.8% (SD = 12.3).
Using the linear regression method for the thenar muscle,
    CMAP (mV) (all ages) = $-0.165 \times$ age (years) + 18.639
    MAXMEP (mV) (all ages) = $-0.148 \times$ age (years) + 16.980
    MAXMEP (mV) (>45 years) = $-0.194 \times$ age (years) + 19.830
    AVMEP (mV) (all ages) = $-0.099 \times$ age (years) + 12.392
    AVMEP (mV) (>45 years) = $-0.164 \times$ age (years) + 16.607

Comments:

1. Forty-one healthy volunteers (7 males, 34 females) were studied in this work. Their ages ranged from 23 to 82 years (mean 51.7 years).
2. All the amplitudes, including those of CMAPs, were measured from peak to peak.
3. The usage of force transducer was not necessary for routine clinical testing because as long as the muscle contraction was maintained above 10% of maximum contraction force, there was little influence on MEP amplitude.
4. Ten consecutive stimuli probably were sufficient to bring out the largest MEP response, although 20 would be ideal.
5. The authors considered thenar MAXMEP <3.6 mV, thenar AVMEP <2.3 mV, and hypothenar MAXMEP <3.0 mV as abnormal.
6. The hypothenar MAXMEP/CMAP ratio was about 40% less than the thenar MAXMEP/CMAP ratio. It was explained by the coactivation of ulnar-supplied thenar muscles.
7. The fact that the thenar MAXMEP/CMAP ratio for all ages was about 90% suggested that not all the relevant cortical motor neurons were excited by TMS in most normal persons.
8. The authors concluded that MEP amplitude was a better indicator than MEP/CMAP amplitude ratio.
9. The authors had studied 18 patients with Parkinson's disease; seven of them (39%) had larger than normal age-corrected thenar MAXMEPs.

TRANSCRANIAL STIMULATION TO MUSCLES OF LOWER LIMB

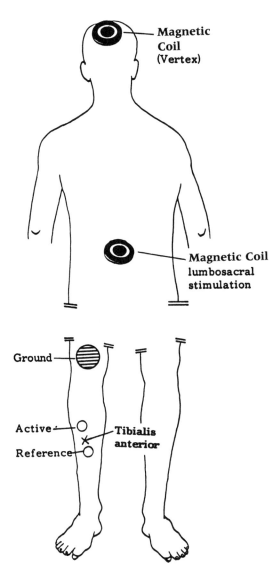

Figure 14.9. Transcranial stimulation to muscles of lower limb.

Booth et al. Study (1991)

Pickup: The recording surface electrode was placed over the tibialis anterior (TA) muscle at the junction of the upper third and lower two-thirds of the line between the tibial tuberosity and the tip of the lateral malleolus.

Reference site: The reference electrode was on the medial aspect of the tibia at 4 cm distal to the recording electrode.

Ground: The ground electrode was placed on the subcutaneous surface of the tibia, 4 cm distal from the reference.

Stimulation: The Cadwell MES-10 magnetic stimulator and a 9.5-cm diameter magnetic coil were used in the study. The stimulator produced a maximum intensity output of 2.3 T. The magnetic coil was held in the investigator's right hand, tangential to the body surface and with current flowing counterclockwise. The peroneal nerve was stimulated magnetoelectrically at the fibular head (FH). For lumbosacral stimulation, the center of the coil was placed over the L4–5 intervertebral space at midline. For TMS, the coil was placed over the scalp with its center near the vertex, 15 cm rostral to the inion. If there was no response at the vertex, the coil was moved in 1-cm increments posterior or lateral to the vertex. Some patients were tested with voluntary facilitation (ankle dorsiflexion at 5–10% maximum contraction) and some with nonvoluntary facilitation (TA at rest with vibration of the TA tendon). The nonvoluntary facilitation was done by applying a hand-held vibrator (Oster, No. 396-08B) at 120 Hz over the TA tendon at the ankle, ipsilateral to the recording site, beginning at 5 sec before TMS and during the recording of the MEP. The total period of vibration was about 10 sec. Each site was stimulated 3 times and the mean onset latency and amplitude were determined. The MEPs were recorded with a Teca TD-10 EMG machine with a sweep of 50–100 msec and a sensitivity of 0.5–1.0 mV/division.

Booth KR, Streletz LJ, Raab VE, Kerrigan JJ, Alaimo MA, Herbison GJ: Motor evoked potentials and central motor conduction: Studies of transcranial magnetic stimulation with recording from the leg. *Electroencephalogr Clin Neurophysiol* 81:57–62, 1991.

Patient position: For TMS and FH stimulation, the patient was in a supine and resting position. For lumbosacral stimulation, the patient's position was not given. During the study, the skin temperature over the TA was $\geq 34°C$.

Normal value: ($N = 30$) Age, 19–50 years (mean age, 32.3 ± 8.4 years) Height 150–198 cm (mean height, 174.1 ± 11.3 cm)

For TA muscle in TMS,

Muscle at rest,

mean TMCT (onset latency = 30.3 msec (SD = 2.2; range: 25.6–34.2)

mean baseline to peak amplitude = 1.3 mV (SD = 1.4; range: 0.1–5.7)

For TA muscle in lumbosacral stimulation,

mean PMCT = 14.2 msec (SD = 2.5; range: 11.0–21.6)

Mean CMCT (r) for TA muscle = 16.2 msec (SD = 1.7; range: 12.6–19.3)

Mean CMCT (F) for TA muscle = 13.8 msec (SD = 1.8; range: 9.7–17.5)

Comments:

1. The F wave was obtained by MS of the peroneal nerve at FH instead of by conventional electrical stimulation. The F-wave latency was selected from the shortest F-wave response from the three stimulations.

2. There was a statistically significant correlation between the MEP latencies and the height of the patients, but not their age.

3. A smaller group of patients ($n = 12$) was studied for the effects of voluntary and nonvoluntary facilitation. With voluntary facilitation, the MEP latency was shortened by about 2 msec and the amplitude was increased fourfold, compared with the resting responses. In contrast, with nonvoluntary facilitation, MEP latency was not significantly changed but the amplitude was increased by about threefold.

TRANSCRANIAL STIMULATION TO UPPER AND LOWER LIMBS

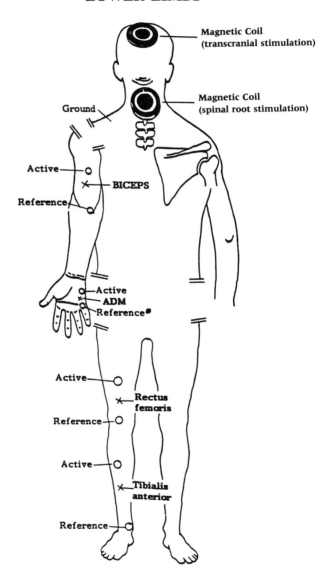

Figure 14.10. Transcranial stimulation to upper and lower limbs.

Furby et al. Study (1992)

Pickup: Surface Ag/AgCl electrodes were placed over the motor points of the biceps brachii (Bi), abductor digiti minim (ADM), tibialis anterior (TA), and rectus femoris (Quad) muscles bilaterally.

Reference site: The reference electrodes were placed on the lateral epicondyl for Bi, the fifth digit for ADM, the medial condyle of tibia for TA, and the patella for Quad.

Ground: Not given in the study.

Stimulation:

Transcranial Stimulation: The center of the coil was placed tangentially over Cz for stimulation of the upper limb muscles. For lower limb muscles, the coil was moved 3 cm forward from Cz along midline. Both clockwise and counterclockwise coil currents were used. The muscles were tested with 100% maximum stimulation output intensity both at rest and at slight sustained voluntary contraction of the target muscle at about 10% maximal tension.

Spinal Root Stimulation: For cervical root stimulation, the center of the coil was placed tangential to the skin 2 cm lateral to the T3 spinal process so that the C8–T1 roots were under the upper quadrant of the coil. At this position, the response was optimal for ADM. For lumbosacral root stimulation, the center of the coil was placed 2 cm lateral to the S2 spinous process with the upper quadrant of the coil over the L4 L5 roots. At this position, the response was largest for TA. The muscles were tested at rest with 100% maximum stimulation intensity.

In both stimulations, three responses were obtained from each muscle for each stimulation condition (such as current direction, muscle at rest, or in contraction). The shortest onset latency, largest MEP amplitude, and area of the first negative peak were measured, all of which might not be from the same response.

Furby A, Bourriez JL, Jacquesson JM, Mounier-Vehier F, Guieu JD: Motor evoked potentials to magnetic stimulation: Technical considerations and normative data from 50 subjects. *J Neurol* 239:152–156, 1992.

Furthermore, conventional electrical stimulations were done to the ulnar nerve at the wrist and the peroneal nerve at the knee for supramaximal responses of ADM and TA respectively. At the same time, the minimal F-wave latency was obtained after a train of 10 stimulations.

Equipment: The Novametrix Magstim 200 stimulator with a 9-cm mean diameter magnetic coil was used in the study. The MEPs and CMAPs were recorded from the upper and lower limb muscles simultaneously with a Nicolet Viking EMG machine at a bandpass of 20 Hz to 2 kHz.

Patient position: Not given in the study.

Normal values: (N = 50; 27 men, 23 women) Age: 21–54 years (mean, 28 ± 6)

    For ADM muscle in TMS,
        muscle at rest, mean TMCT = 22.1 msec (SD = 1.5)
        muscle with contraction, mean TMCT = 20.5 msec
          (SD = 1.2; side-to-side mean difference = 0.69)
          mean amplitude = 3.6 mV (SD = 1.1)
    For ADM muscle in cervical stimulation,
        mean PMCT = 13.5 msec (SD = 1.0; side-to-side mean difference = 0.50)
    Mean CMCT (r) for ADM muscle = 7.0 msec
        (SD = 0.9; side-to-side mean difference = 0.66)
    Mean CMCT(F) for ADM muscle = 6.1 msec
        (SD = 1.0; side-to-side mean difference = 0.72)
    For Bi muscle in TMS,
        muscle at rest, mean TMCT = 14.2 msec (SD = 1.2)
        muscle with contraction, mean TMCT = 12.5 msec
          (SD = 1.2; side-to-side mean difference = 0.65)
          mean amplitude = 3.8 mV (SD = 2.3)
    For Bi muscle in cervical stimulation,
        mean PMCT = 5.4 msec (SD = 0.6; side-to-side mean difference = 0.31)
    Mean CMCT (r) for Bi muscle = 7.1 msec
        (SD = 1.1; side-to-side mean difference = 0.60)
    For TA muscle in TMS,
        muscle at rest, mean TMCT = 28.2 msec (SD = 2.1)
        muscle with contraction, mean TMCT = 26.1 msec

(SD = 1.9; side-to-side mean difference = 0.82)
mean amplitude = 2.3 mV (SD = 1.1)
For TA muscle in lumbosacral stimulation,
mean PMCT = 12.3 msec (SD = 1.2; side-to-side mean difference = 0.44)
Mean CMCT(r) for TA muscle = 13.8 msec (SD = 1.5; side-to-side mean difference = 0.93)
Mean CMCT(F) for TA muscle = 9.9 msec (SD = 1.8; side-to-side mean difference = 0.99)
For Quad muscle in TMS,
muscle at rest, mean TMCT = 23 msec (SD = 1.8)
muscle with contraction, mean TMCT = 21.5 msec
(SD = 1.7; side-to-side mean difference = 0.88)
mean amplitude = 2.7 mV (SD = 2.0)
For Quad muscle in lumbosacral stimulation,
mean PMCT = 7.3 msec (SD = 0.9; side-to-side mean difference = 0.48)
Mean CMCT(r) for Quad muscle = 14.2 msec
(SD = 1.5; side-to-side mean difference = 0.93)

Comments:

1. To obtain the largest and shortest MEPs in TMS, the coil current had to flow counterclockwise for the right limb and clockwise for the left limb.
2. For cervical and lumbosacral stimulations, CMAPs were larger on the side where the induced current flowed proximally.
3. There were no statistical differences in side-to-side comparison of the CMCTs, PMCTs, and TMCTs.
4. There was positive correlation between the CMCTs to the lower limb muscles and patients heights. The upper limit of normal value (mean + 2.5 SD) of CMCT to TA muscle could be estimated by the formula:
   CMCT (msec) = 0.83 × height (cm) + 3.28
5. CMCTs to the lower limb were significantly longer in men than in women.
6. The room temperature and skin temperature were not given in the study.

Ravnborg et al. Study (1991)

Pickup: Surface Ag/AgCl electrodes were placed over the bellies of the brachial biceps (Bi), the flexor carpal radialis (FCR), the first dorsal interosseus (FDI), the vastus medialis of the quadriceps (VM), the tibialis anterior (TA), and the abductor hallucis (AH) muscles.

Reference site: Reference electrodes were placed over the distal tendons of the muscles mentioned above.

Ground: Not given in the study.

Stimulation:

Transcranial Stimulation: The magnetic coil was placed in the coronal plane with its center in the midline 1 cm in front of the vertex. The stimulus threshold was determined by increasing or decreasing the stimulator output in steps of 5% during a standard facilitation so that at least three crossings of the no-response/response limit were made. The threshold was determined for both clockwise and counterclockwise coil currents. The coil current direction of the lower threshold was then used for subsequent cortical stimulation. Once the lowest threshold and its current direction had been determined, MEPs were recorded with a stimulator output of 20% above threshold. At least three MEPs by cortical stimulation were recorded from each muscle bilaterally. The shortest latency and the largest amplitude were chosen for analysis.

Root Stimulation: The coil was held in the frontal plan in the midline over the spine with the coil current flowing proximally in the part of the coil over the root. For Bi, the C5–6 roots were stimulated; C6–7 roots for FCR; C8–T1 roots for FDI; L3–4 roots for VM; L4–5 roots for TA, and S1 root for AH. At least two MEPs by root stimulation were recorded at each level using 100% stimulator output. Threshold was not deter-

Ravnborg M, Dahl K: Examination of central and peripheral motor pathways by standardized magnetic stimulation. *Acta Neurol Scand* 84:491–497, 1991.

mined. The MEP with the largest amplitude was used for analysis. If the MEP was not optimal, the position of the coil could be adjusted in small steps along the spine.

Facilitation was standardized by the root mean square (RMS) of the EMG signal. For threshold determination, facilitation was set at 10% of the RMS of the maximum voluntary contraction (10% RMS max). For cortical stimulations of the Bi, FDI, and VM, 15% RMS max was used. For cortical stimulations of the FCR, TA, and AH, 10% RMS max was used.

Equipment: A Dantec magnetic stimulator was used with a magnetic coil that contained 14 copper windings from 2 cm to 6 cm from the center and had an outer diameter of 14 cm. The Dantec stimulator delivered a monophasic pulse with a rise time of 160 μsec. The EMG was recorded with a Dantec Counterpoint EMG machine with a filter bandpass of 10 Hz to 5 kHz. The RMS of the EMG signal was determined by an RMS meter (Bruel & Kjaer, Denmark), which was connected to a time-Y plotter. The latency of the MEP was determined at a gain of 0.5 mV/cm.

Patient position: Not given in the study. However, the patient was in a room at 22°C. The skin temperature was not measured.

Normal Value: (*N* = 50; 25 men, 25 women) Age: 18–60 years Height: 155–195 cm (mean, 174.7 cm)
　For Bi muscle, mean TMCT = 11.2 msec (SDr = 0.6)
　　L-R mean TMCT difference = 0.3 msec (SD = 0.3)
　　mean PMCT = 5.4 msec (SDr = 0.4)
　　L-R mean PMCT difference = 0.3 msec (SD = 0.3)
　　mean CMCT(r) = 5.8 msec (SDr = 0.6)
　　L-R mean CMCT(r) difference = 0.5 (SD = 0.4)
　　median cortical MEP (cMEP) amplitude = 4 mV (range: 1.1–10.9)
　　median root MEP (rMEP) amplitude = 3.7 mV (range: 1.2–7.6)
　For FCR muscle, mean TMCT = 14.4 msec (SDr = 0.7)
　　L-R mean TMCT difference = 0.3 msec (SD = 0.3)
　　mean PMCT = 8.1 msec (SDr = 0.5)

L-R mean PMCT difference = 0.3 msec (SD = 0.2)
mean CMCT(r) = 6.3 msec (SDr = 0.6)
L-R mean CMCT(r) difference = 0.4 msec (SD = 0.4)
median cMEP amplitude = 4 mV (range: 1.4–8.7)
median rMEP amplitude = 8.8 mV (range: 1.6–15.3)
For FDI muscle, mean TMCT = 21.7 msec (SDr = 0.9)
L-R mean TMCT difference = 0.6 msec (SD = 0.5)
mean PMCT = 14.5 msec (SDr = 0.8)
L-R mean PMCT difference = 0.4 msec (SD = 0.3)
mean CMCT(r) = 7.2 msec (SDr = 0.8)
L-R CMCT(r) difference = 0.6 msec (SD = 0.5)
median cMEP amplitude = 4.1 mV (range: 0.9–8.0)
median rMEP amplitude = 4.3 mV (range: 0.1–14.9)
For VM muscle, mean TMCT = 22.3 msec (SDr = 1.4)
L-R mean TMCT difference = 0.8 msec (SD = 0.7)
mean PMCT = 8.7 msec (SDr = 0.6)
L-R mean PMCT difference = 0.5 msec (SD = 0.4)
mean CMCT(r) = 13.7 msec (SDr = 1.3)
L-R mean CMCT(r) difference = 0.8 msec (SD = 0.7)
median cMEP amplitude = 2.6 mV (range: 0.6–10.9)
median rMEP amplitude = 3.7 mV (range: 0.5–12.3)
For TA muscle, mean TMCT = 29.5 msec (SDr = 1.5)
L-R mean TMCT difference = 1.1 msec (SD = 1.1)
mean PMCT = 13.9 msec (SDr = 0.8)
L-R mean PMCT difference = 0.7 msec (SD = 0.6)
mean CMCT(r) = 15.5 msec (SDr = 1.3)
L-R mean CMCT(r) difference = 1.2 msec (SD = 0.9)
median cMEP amplitude = 2.3 mV (range: 0.4–4.4)
median rMEP amplitude = 1.3 mV (range: 0.2–6.3)
For AH muscle, mean TMCT = 41.5 msec (SDr = 1.9)
L-R mean TMCT difference = 1.8 msec (SD = 1.5)
mean PMCT = 23.4 msec (SDr = 1.5)
L-R mean PMCT difference = 1.1 msec (SD = 0.9)
mean CMCT(r) = 18.0 msec (SDr = 1.3)
L-R mean CMCT(r) difference = 2.2 msec (SD = 1.6)
median cMEP amplitude = 1.5 mV (range: 0.3–6.6)
median rMEP amplitude = 2.3 mV (range: 0.2–9.0)

Note: SDr: standard deviation of the residuals; L-R difference: left-right difference.

Comments:

1. Regarding age and side-to-side difference, the correlation with the conduction times were insignificant statistically. However, significant correlation was found between height and conduction time, except for the CMCT(r) to the upper limb.
2. No correlation between amplitude and height or age was found.
3. For cortical stimulation to the upper limb, the lowest threshold was obtained when the coil current flowed posteriorly over the contralateral hemisphere. For cortical stimulation to the lower limb, the lowest threshold was obtained in 21 of the 300 muscles when it flowed anteriorly over the contralateral side. For root stimulation, the most effective coil current direction was centripetal. (The current direction was defined as the direction of electron movement.) These findings were opposite to other studies. The authors contributed it to the fact that they used the Dantec stimulator and the other studies did not.
4. Some of the side effects, reported by the patients, included headache (5 cases), dizziness for several hours (1 case), feeling sick for 1 hour (1 case), and neck pain lasting several days (2 cases).

INHIBITORY PERIOD STIMULATION

Uozumi et al. Study (1991)

Pickup: Surface electrode placed over the abductor pollicis brevis (APB) muscle.

Reference site: Not given in the study.

Ground: Not given in the study.

Stimulation: The center of the magnetic coil was placed over the vertex. TMS was given with stimulus intensity ranging from 800–900 V. Two to four stimulations were given to each patient for reproducibility. The shortest onset latency was measured. If the onset was not well defined because of the background EMG, three to four responses were averaged. The patient was asked to do maximum voluntary contraction of the APB muscle before and during TMS.

Equipment: TMS was performed with a Nihon Kohden magnetic stimulator and a flat rounded coil with an inner diameter of 12 cm and an outer diameter of 14.5 cm. The maximum magnetic field was 0.4 T at the maximum output intensity of 1,000 V. MEPs were recorded with the Neuropack machine (Nihon Kohden) at a filter setting of 20–3000 Hz.

Patient position: Not given in the study.

Normal values: (N = 20) Ages: 20–74 years (mean, 42 years)
    For APB in maximum voluntary contraction,
    mean onset latency = 17.4 msec (SD = 1.3)
    mean peak-to-peak amplitude = 7.33 mV (SD = 1.47)
    mean MEP/M wave amplitude ratio = 91.5% (SD = 7.2)
    mean period of inhibitory period = 126.6 msec (SD = 29.5)

Comments:
    1. The M-wave amplitude was obtained by conventional electric stimulation of the median nerve at the elbow.

Uozumi T, Tsuji S, Murai Y: Motor potentials evoked by magnetic stimulation of the motor cortex in normal subjects and patients with motor disorders. *Electroencephalogr Clin Neurophysiol* 81:251–256, 1991.

2. The mean inhibitory period duration in this study was much longer than that reported by Amassian et al. (20–50 msec).*

3. The mean inhibitory period was much reduced in patients with cerebral infarction, amyotrophic lateral sclerosis, cervical spondylitic radiculomyelopathy, Parkinson's disease, and multiple sclerosis. The authors used mean value ± 3 SD as the normal limits of MEP parameters.

---

* Amassian VE, Cracco RQ, Maccabee PJ: Focal stimulation of human cerebral cortex with the magnetic coil: A comparison with electrical stimulation. *Electroencephalogr Clin Neurophysiol* 74:401–416, 1989.

PHRENIC NERVE STIMULATION

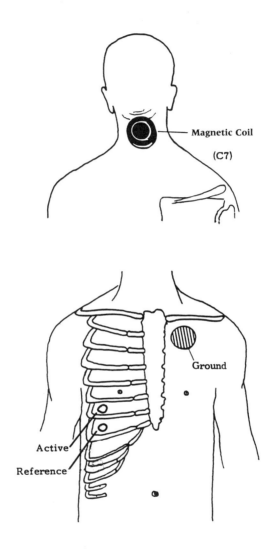

Figure 14.11.   Phrenic nerve stimulation.

Similowski et al. Study (1989)

Pickup: Surface electrode was placed at the sixth or seventh right and left intercostal spaces, approximately on the anterior axillary line. The skin was prepared with a mild abrasion. Conductive gel was placed between the electrode and the skin to improve conductivity.

Reference site: The reference electrode was placed on the corresponding lower rib.

Ground: The position of the ground electrode was not mentioned in the study.

Stimulation: The magnetic coil was placed behind the central back of the neck, parallel to the frontal plane of the patient, with the center of the coil above the C7 spinous process so that bilateral phrenic nerves could be stimulated with a single magnetic stimulus. The magnetic stimuli were 0.1-msec duration pulses of modulable intensity and were always delivered while the patient was at functional residual capacity. The optimal stimulus intensity and the actual position of the coil were adjusted for each patient to obtain maximal stimulation.

Equipment: Novametric Magstim 200 magnetic stimulator (Novametric, UK) was used with a 9-cm diameter magnetic rounded coil with a central hole. The maximum magnetic field at the center of the coil was 1.5 T. Diaphragmatic EMG activity was recorded with a Dantec 2000 EMG machine (Dantec Electronik, Denmark) of a sweep speed of 5 mpa. Disa 7-mm diameter silver chloride discs were used to record the surface EMG activity.

Patient position: The patient was seated in a semi-recumbent posture with abdomen unbound and head bent forward at 30° ahead of the vertical plane and hands over the head.

Similowski T, Fleury B, Launois S, Cathala HP, Bouche P, Derenne JP: Cervical magnetic stimulation: A new painless method for bilateral phrenic nerve stimulation in conscious humans. *J Appl Physiol* 67:1311–1318, 1989.

Normal value: Bilateral phrenic nerve stimulation at C7 level, mean right latency of M wave = 6.42 msec (SD = 0.55) mean right compound diaphragmatic action potential (CDAP) amplitude = 273.89 μV (SD = 79.56) mean left latency of M wave = 6.99 msec (SD = 0.72) mean left CDAP amplitude = 233.77 μV (SD = 66.12)

Comments:

1. There were four patients (one woman and three men), aged 24 to 27 years old; their heights were 166–187 cm and their body weights were 65–80 kg.

2. The optimal position of the magnetic coil was adjusted for maximal CDAP response. In all the patients studied, this position was found to be at the level of C7 or in the C6–C7 intervertebral space.

3. In most patients, the stimulus intensity was 90–98% of the maximal output for maximal CDAP responses.

4. For each patient, a series of 10–25 MSs was performed. Intervals between stimulations ranged between 30 sec and 2 min. To perform the MS at constant lung volume, the patient was stimulated at functional residual capacity with the air openings occluded manually.

5. There was no significant difference between right and left CDAP. However, the right phrenic nerve latency was slightly shorter than that of the left, on the average, which was explained by the slightly longer length of the left phrenic nerve. In addition, the direction of the coil current was not specified in the study.

6. TMS to activate the diaphragm was reported by Maskill and his coworkers.[1] They used a figure-of-eight coil over the right motor cortex. The center of the figure-of-eight coil was placed approximately 3 cm to the right of the midline of the scalp and 2–3 cm anterior to the auricular plane for maximal CMAP recorded over the left diaphragm. Surface electrodes were

---

[1] Maskill D, Murphy K, Mier A, Owen M, Guz A: Motor cortical representation of the diaphragm in man. *J Physiol* 443:105–121, 1991.

placed at either the seventh or eighth intercostal spaces 3 cm lateral to the anterior costal margin. The effectiveness of the magnetic stimulus was facilitated by having the patient inspired through a restricted airway with peak mouth pressure ranging from -10 to -20 cm H_2O. They had found that the amplitude of the CMAP depended on the angulation of the figure-of-eight coil. However, they did not report their data on the cortex-to-diaphragm conduction time and the CMAP amplitude of the diaphragm.

7. No complaint of abnormal or painful feeling was reported by the patients other than the mild and nondisturbing hiccup perception at stimulation.

PUDENDAL NERVE STIMULATION

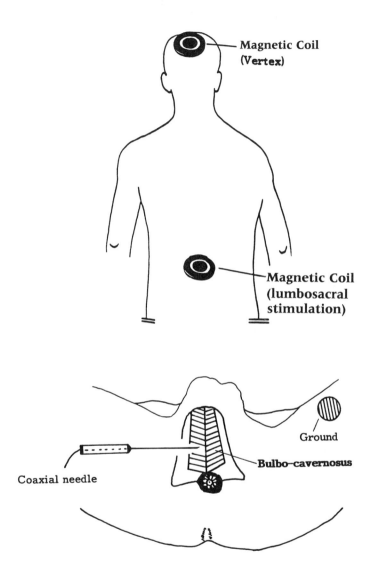

Figure 14.12. Pudendal nerve stimulation.

Ghezzi et al. Study (1991)

Pickup: The MEP was recorded from the bulbocavernosus muscle using a surface Ag/AgCl electrode (see comment).

Reference site: Reference was made to S_1 (see comment).

Ground: The placement of the ground electrode was not mentioned in the study.

Stimulation: The magnetic coil was placed over the vertex or slightly anterior to it to obtain the optimal transcranial stimulation. For lumbar stimulation, the coil was placed over the L1 spinous process.

Equipment: A Novametrix Magstim magnetic stimulator was used. No information of the type of magnetic coil used was given. The EMG machine was set at 2–2000 Hz band pass for MEP recording.

Patient position: The position of the patient was not mentioned in the study.

Normal values: Cortical stimulation at 90–100% of maximal output and with facilitation, onset latency of bulbocavernosus MEP = 22.9 msec (SD = 1.8), peak latency of bulbocavernosus MEP = 27.7 msec (SD = 3.6), peak-to-peak amplitude of bulbocavernosus MEP = 353 μV (SD = 205)

  Lumbar stimulation at 70–80% of maximal output and without facilitation,
    onset latency of bulbocavernosus SMAP = 5.9 msec (SD = 0.4)
  Central conduction time (CCT) = 17.0 msec (SD = 2.5)

Comments:

1. The number of patients in the study was 17 (all healthy male volunteers). The mean age was 47.8 years (range: 22–80) and

Ghezzi A, Callea L, Zaffaroni M, Montanini R, Tessera G: Motor potentials of bulbocavernosus muscle after transcranial and lumbar magnetic stimulation: Comparative study with bulbocavernosus reflex and pudendal evoked potentials. *J Neurol Neurosurg Psychiatry* 54:524–526, 1991.

the mean height was 169.2 cm (range: 161–188). All patients had normal sphincteric and sexual functions, with no neurologic deficit.

2. The authors did not give details of the placement of the recording and reference electrodes. However, in an article* to which the authors referred, it was given that the active recording surface electrode was placed over the bulbocavernosus muscle beneath the sacrum and the reference electrode was placed over the iliac crest.

3. For cortical stimulation, the intensity was started at 70% of maximal output and was increased gradually up to 100% for maximal response. The patients were asked to relax and then to contract the perineal muscles slightly for facilitation. At least eight stimulations were performed in the two conditions. For lumbar stimulation, an intensity of 70–80% of maximal output was sufficient for maximal response and no facilitation was necessary.

Opsomer et al. Study (1989)

Pickup: Coaxial needle electrodes were inserted to the right bulbocavernosus muscle (BC) and the anal sphincter (AS) to record their MEPs.

Reference site: Coaxial needle electrode was used.

Ground: Its position was not given in the study.

Stimulation: For TMS, the circular coil was placed with its posterior edge 2 cm behind the Cz point of the international 10–20 system. For sacral root stimulation, the center of the coil was applied 5 cm laterally to the spine at the level of the right iliac crest. Five stimuli delivered at a 0.2/sec repetition rate were given and the average was taken as the final value.

---

* Haldeman S, Bradley W, Bhatia NN, Johnson BK: Pudendal evoked responses. *Arch Neurol* 39:280–283, 1982.

Opsomer RJ, Caramia MD, Zarola F, Pesce F, Rossini PM: Neurophysiological evaluation of central-peripheral sensory and motor pudendal fibres. *Electroencephalogr Clin Neurophysiol* 74:260–270, 1989.

Equipment: MS was performed with a Cadwell MES-10 magnetic stimulator and a round coil of 5-cm internal diameter applied directly in contact to the skin. MEP was analyzed with a filter bandpass of 1.6–1600 Hz and a time span of 100 msec.

Patient position: It was not given in the study.

Normal values: For right BC muscle, at rest,
   mean TMCT
   = 28.8 msec (SD = 2.6; range: 26.8–30.8)
   mean PMCT
   = 7.2 msec (SD = 1.0; range: 6.5–7.9)
   mean CMCT
   = 22.4 msec (SD = 1.7; range: 20.8–24.0)
   For right BC muscle with facilitation,
      mean TMCT
      = 22.5 msec (SD = 2.7; range: 20.9–24.1)
      mean CMCT
      = 15.1 msec (SD = 3.1; range: 12.9–17.3)
   For right AS at rest,
      mean TMCT
      = 30.0 msec (SD = 4.4; range: 25.9–34.1)
      mean PMCT
      = 7.9 msec (SD = 2.1; range: 5.7–10.1)
      mean CMCT
      = 21.2 msec (SD = 4.6; range: 15.5–26.9)
   For right AS with facilitation,
      mean TMCT
      = 22.8 msec (SD = 3.6; range: 20.0–25.6)
      mean CMCT
      = 12.4 msec (SD = 2.9; range: 8.8–16.0)

Comments:
   1. Fifteen healthy male volunteers participated in this study. Their mean age was 46.5 years (range: 23–60 years) and their mean height was 171.4 cm (range: 155–187 cm).
   2. The transcranial MEP was first recorded in the muscle(s) with the patient at rest. It was then repeated at the same stimulation

intensity with moderate voluntary contraction of the target muscles. The sacral root stimulation required no facilitation.

3. All the latencies were measured at the onset of the first steady deflection from the base line.

4. An intensity of 80–90% of the maximum output was required for transcranial stimulation.

REFERENCES

1. Claus D: Magnetic stimulation: Technical aspects. *Electroencephalogr Clin Neurophysiol* 43(Suppl):249–254, 1991.
2. Odderson IR, Halar EM: Localization of nerve depolarization with magnetic stimulation. *Muscle Nerve* 15:711–715, 1992.
3. Nilsson J, Panizza M, Roth BJ, et al: Determining the site of stimulation during magnetic stimulation of a peripheral nerve. *Electroencephalogr Clin Neurophys* 85:253–264, 1992.
4. Epstein CM, Schwartzberg DG, Davey KR, Sudderth DB: Localizing the site of magnetic brain stimulation in humans. *Neurology* 40:666–670, 1990.
5. Chiappa KH, Cros D, Cohen D: Magnetic stimulation: Determination of coil current flow direction. *Neurology* 41:1154–1155, 1991.
6. Chu NS: Motor evoked potentials with magnetic stimulation: Correlations with height. *Electroencephalogr Clin Neurphysiol* 74:481–485, 1989.
7. Toleikis JR, Sloan TB, Ronai AK: Optimal transcranial magnetic stimulation sites for the assessment of motor function. *Electroencephalogr Clin Neurophysiol* 81:443–449, 1991.
8. Roth BJ, Cohen LG, Hallett M, Friauf W, Basser PJ: A theoretical calculation of the electric field induced by magnetic stimulation of a peripheral nerve. *Muscle Nerve* 13:734–741, 1990.
9. Tofts PS: The distribution of induced currents in magnetic stimulation of the nervous system. *Phys Med Biol* 35:1119–1128, 1990.
10. Cros D, Gominak S, Shahani B, Fang J, Day B: Comparison of electric and magnetic coil stimulation in the supraclavicular region. *Muscle Nerve* 15:587–590, 1992.
11. Panizza M, Nilsson J, Roth BJ, Basser PJ, Hallett M: Relevance of stimulus duration for activation of motor and sensory fibers: Implications for the study of H-reflexes and magnetic stimulation. *Electroencephalogr Clin Neurophysiol* 85:22–29, 1992.
12. Pascual-Leone A, Valls-Sole J, Brasil-Neto JP, Cohen LG, Hallett M: Seizure induction and transcranial magnetic stimulation. *Lancet* 339:997, 1992 (Letter).
13. Tassinari CA, Michelucci R, Forti A, et al: Transcranial magnetic stimulation in epileptic patients: Usefulness and safety. *Neurology* 40:1132–1133, 1990.
14. Dhuna A, Gates J, Paxcual-Leone A: Transcranial magnetic stimulation in patients with epilepsy. *Neurology* 41:1067–1071, 1991.
15. Ravnborg M, Knudsen GM, Blinkenberg M: No effect of pulsed magnetic stimulation on the blood-brain barrier in rats. *Neuroscience* 38:277–280, 1990.
16. Matsumiya Y, Yamamoto T, Yarita M, Miyauchi S, Kling JW: Physical and physiological specification of magnetic pulse stimuli that produce cortica damage in rats. *J Clin Neurophysiol* 9:278–287, 1992.
17. Gates JR, Dhuna A, Pascual-Leone A: Lack of pathologic changes in human temporal lobes after transcranial magnetic stimulation. *Epilepsia* 33:504–508, 1992.

18. Thomas S, Merton WL, Boyd SG: Pituitary hormones in relation to magnetic stimulation of the brain. *J Neurol Neurosurg Psychiatry* 54:89–90, 1991. (Letter)

19. Masur H, Ludolph AC, Hilker E, Hengst K, Knuth U, Rolf LH, Bals-Pratsch M: Transcranial magnetic stimulation: Influence on plasma levels of hormones of the anterior pituitary gland and of cortisol? *Funct Neurol* 6:59–63, 1991.

20. Counter SA, Borg E, Lofqvist L, Brismar T: Hearing loss from the acoustic artifact of the coil used in extracranial magnetic stimulation. *Neurology* 40:1159–1162, 1990.

21. Pascual-Leone A, Cohen LG, Shotland LI, et al: No evidence of hearing loss in humans due to transcranial magnetic stimulation. *Neurology* 42:647–651, 1992.

22. Counter SA, Borg E: Analysis of the coil generated impulse noise in extracranial magnetic stimulation. *Electroencephalogr Clin Neurophysiol* 85:280–288, 1992.

23. Pascual-Leone A, Dhuna A, Roth BJ, Cohen L, Hallett M: Risk of burns during rapid-rate magnetic stimulation in presence of electrodes. *Lancet* 336:1195–1196, 1990 (Letter).

24. Bridgers SL, Delaney RC: Transcranial magnetic stimulation: An assessment of cognitive and other cerebral effects. *Neurology* 39:417–419, 1989.

25. Ferbert A, Mussmann N, Menne A, Buchner H, Hartje W: Short-term memory performance with magnetic stimulation of the motor cortex. *Eur Arch Psychiatry Clin Neurosci* 241:135–138, 1991.

26. Hufnagel A, Elger CE, Marx W, Ising A: Magnetic motor-evoked potentials in epilepsy: Effects of the disease and of anticonvulsant medication. *Ann Neurol* 28:680–686, 1990.

27. Lim CL, Yiannikas C: Motor evoked potentials: A new method of controlled facilitation using quantitative surface EMG. *Electroencephalogr Clin Neurophysiol* 85:38–41, 1992.

28. Ravnborg M, Blinkenberg M, Dahl K: Standardization of facilitation of compound muscle action potentials evoked by magnetic stimulation of the cortex. Results in healthy volunteers and patients with multiple sclerosis. *Electroencephalogr Clin Neurophysiol* 81:195–201, 1991.

29. Chiappa KH, Cros D, Day B, Fang JJ, Macdonell R, Mavroudakis N: Magnetic stimulation of the human cortex: Ipsilateral and contralateral facilitation effects. *Electroencephalogr Clin Neurophysiol* 43(Suppl):186–201, 1991.

30. Hufnagel A, Jaeger M, Elger CE: Transcranial magnetic stimulation: Specific and nonspecific facilitation of magnetic motor evoked potentials. *J Neurol* 237:416–419, 1990.

31. Thompson PD, Day BL, Rothwell JC, et al: Further observations on the facilitation of muscle responses to cortical stimulation by voluntary contraction. *Electroencephalogr Clin Neurophysiol* 81:397–402, 1991.

32. Ackermann H, Scholz E, Koehler W, Dichgans J: Influence of posture and voluntary background contraction upon compound muscle action potentials from anterior tibial and soleus muscle following transcranial magnetic stimulation. *Electroencephalogr Clin Neurophysiol* 81:71–80, 1991.

33. Date M, Schmid UD, Hess CW, Schmid J: Influence of peripheral nerve stimulation on the responses in small hand muscles to transcranial magnetic cortex stimulation. *Electroencephalogr Clin Neurophysiol* 43(Suppl):212–223, 1991.

34. Kasai T, Hayes KC, Wolfe DL, Allatt RD: Afferent conditioning of motor evoked potentials following transcranial magnetic stimulation of motor cortex in normal subjects. *Electroencephalogr Clin Neurophysiol* 85:95–101, 1992.

CHAPTER 15

Motor Unit Action Potential Analysis

Electromyography is used widely in the study of neuromuscular disorders. On routine examination, individual motor units are examined qualitatively. However, quantitative analysis is useful in specific cases, where abnormalities are minimal or equivocal in nature, to increase the diagnostic certainty of neuromuscular disorders.[1-4] A motor unit consists of an anterior horn cell (motor neuron), its axon, and the muscle fibers innervated by its axon. The muscle fibers innervated by a single motor neuron are scattered over a cross-sectional area with a diameter of 5 to 10 mm (motor unit territory). When the muscle is activated voluntarily, motor unit action potentials (MUAPs) are recorded. The MUAP is the summated electrical activity of the skeletal muscle fibers in a motor unit that are within the recording range of the recording electrode. A MUAP is characterized by its shape and size. This includes duration, number of phases, amplitude, rate of rise of the fast component, and variability of shape at consecutive discharges.[2] The MUAP spike consists of a few fibers in immediate proximity to the leading-off area of the needle. The early and late slow components of the MUAP represent more distant fibers.[1,2] The quantitative analysis of MUAP usually is performed in the muscle that appears to be the most abnormal. The amplitude and duration of MUAP recorded with a monopolar needle are slightly larger and longer than those recorded with a concentric needle.

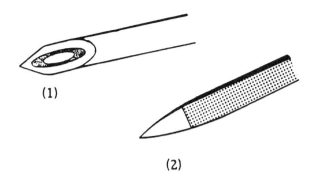

Figure 15.1. Concentric (1) and monopolar (2) needle electrode.

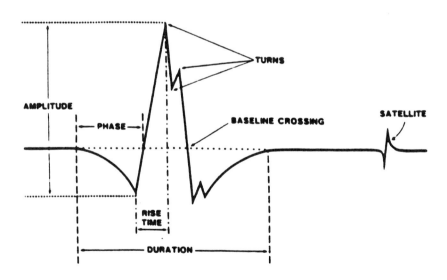

Figure 15.2. A schematic motor unit potential with characteristics that can be measured. (From Daube, ref. 4, with permission.)

Figure 15.1:

Recording electrodes:

	Concentric	Monopolar
Recording	Central core Stainless wire 0.15 mm in diameter 0.07 mm²	Monopolar Teflon-coated 0.56–0.80 mm²
	Connected to positive terminal	Same
Reference	Cannula of the needle connected to negative terminal	Surface or subcutaneous needle connected to negative terminal

EMG settings for MUAP recording:
 • Filters: 2 Hz and 10 kHz (concentric needle)
       20 Hz and 10 kHz (monopolar needle)
 • Sweep speed: 5 or 10 msec/div (sweep time 50 or 100 msec)
 • Gain: 100 μV or more

Sampling MUAP (isolation of individual MUAP):
 • Rise time: about 500 μsec (0.5 msec)
 • Contraction of muscle: minimum, weak voluntary
 • Collection of different MUAPs: minimum 20 from 20 different
   needle positions

Figure 15.2:

MUAP parameters:
Duration, amplitude, and phases

Duration:
The duration of a MUAP is defined as the interval from the beginning of the first deflection from the baseline to its final return to the baseline. It is the most sensitive parameter of abnormality. The duration increases with age and with decreasing temperatures.[1,2]

Concentric Needle Electrode Recordings

Mean duration (msec) of MUAPs (From ref. 2, with permission from Rosenfalck):

Age (years)	Frontalis	Temporalis	Sterno-cleido-mastoid	Rhomboid	Infra-spinatus
0	4.1	5.6	6.5	8.3	8.6
3	4.4	6.2	6.9	8.9	9.2
5	4.5	6.7	7.1	9.2	9.5
8	4.7	7.3	7.5	9.6	9.9
10	4.8	7.7	7.6	9.8	10.2
15	5.1	8.4	8.1	10.4	10.6
20	5.3	8.6	8.4	10.8	11.2
25	5.3	8.6	8.7	11.1	11.5
30	5.4	8.7	8.9	11.4	11.9
35	5.4	8.7	9.2	11.8	12.2
40	5.5	8.7	9.3	12.0	12.4
45	5.5	8.8	9.4	12.1	12.6
50	5.6	8.8	9.6	12.3	12.8
55	5.6	8.8	9.8	12.5	13.0
60	5.7	8.9	10.0	12.9	13.3
65	5.7	8.9	10.2	13.2	13.7
70	5.8	8.9	10.2	13.4	13.9
75	5.8	8.9	10.6	13.6	14.1
80	5.9	8.9	10.8	13.8	14.3

Age (years)	Deltoid	Biceps	Triceps	Flexor digitorum sublimis	Extensor digitorum communis	Brachio-radialis
0	7.8	7.7	9.0	7.4	7.1	7.3
3	8.3	8.2	9.6	7.9	7.6	7.8
5	8.6	8.5	9.9	8.2	7.8	8.1
8	9.0	8.9	10.3	8.5	8.2	8.5
10	9.3	9.1	10.6	8.7	8.4	8.6
15	9.8	9.6	11.2	9.1	8.8	9.1
20	10.2	10.0	11.6	9.6	9.2	9.5
25	10.5	10.3	11.9	9.9	9.5	9.8
30	10.7	10.6	12.0	10.2	9.8	10.1
35	11.1	10.9	12.1	10.5	10.0	10.4
40	11.3	11.1	12.2	10.7	10.2	10.5
45	11.4	11.2	12.3	10.8	10.3	10.6
50	11.6	11.4	12.4	11.0	10.5	10.8
55	11.8	11.6	12.5	11.1	10.7	11.0
60	12.1	11.9	12.6	11.4	11.0	11.3
65	12.1	12.2	12.7	11.7	11.2	11.6
70	12.1	12.4	12.8	11.9	11.4	11.8
75	12.8	12.6	12.8	12.1	11.6	12.0
80	13.0	12.8	12.8	12.3	11.8	12.2

Age (years)	Flexor carpi ulnaris	Opponens pollicis	Abductor pollicis brevis	Dorsal. interosseous	Abductor digitis minimi
0	8.6	6.1	6.2	7.7	6.2
3	9.2	6.7	6.8	8.2	6.8
5	9.5	7.2	7.3	8.5	7.3
8	10.0	7.8	7.9	8.9	7.9
10	10.2	8.2	8.3	9.1	9.0
15	10.8	8.9	9.0	9.6	9.2
20	11.2	9.1	9.2	10.0	9.2
25	11.5	9.1	9.2	10.3	9.2
30	11.9	9.2	9.3	10.6	9.3
35	12.2	9.2	9.3	10.9	9.3
40	12.4	9.2	9.3	11.1	9.3
45	12.5	9.3	9.4	11.2	9.4
50	12.8	9.3	9.4	11.4	9.4
55	13.0	9.3	9.4	11.6	9.4
60	13.3	9.4	9.5	11.9	9.5
65	13.7	9.4	9.5	12.2	9.5
70	13.9	9.4	9.5	12.4	9.5
75	14.1	9.4	9.5	12.6	9.5
80	14.3	9.4	9.5	12.8	9.5

Age (years)	Gluteus maximus	Biceps femoris	Rectus femoris	Vastus medialis	Vastus lateralis	Tibialis anterior	Peroneus longus
0	9.2	8.5	8.7	7.9	9.7	9.5	7.6
3	9.8	9.1	9.2	8.4	10.3	10.1	8.1
5	10.2	9.4	9.6	8.7	10.7	10.5	8.4
8	10.7	9.9	10.0	9.1	11.2	11.0	8.7
10	10.9	10.1	10.3	9.3	11.5	11.2	8.9
15	11.5	10.6	10.7	9.8	12.1	11.7	9.4
20	12.0	11.1	11.3	10.2	12.6	12.3	9.8
25	12.4	11.4	11.6	10.5	13.0	12.7	10.1
30	12.7	11.8	12.0	10.8	13.4	13.1	10.4
35	13.1	12.1	12.3	11.1	13.7	13.3	10.7
40	13.3	12.3	12.6	11.3	14.0	13.6	10.9
45	13.4	12.4	12.7	11.4	14.1	13.8	11.0
50	13.7	12.7	12.9	11.6	14.4	14.0	11.2
55	13.9	12.9	13.1	11.8	14.6	14.3	11.4
60	14.3	13.2	13.5	12.1	15.0	14.7	11.7
65	14.6	13.5	13.7	12.4	15.4	15.0	12.0
70	14.9	13.8	14.0	12.6	15.6	15.3	12.2
75	15.1	14.0	14.2	12.8	15.9	15.5	12.4
80	15.4	14.2	14.4	13.0	16.1	15.7	12.6

Age (years)	Gastrocnemius	Soleus	Extensor digitorum brevis	Abductor hallucis
0	7.2	7.7	7.2	6.5
3	7.7	8.2	7.7	7.0
5	8.0	8.5	8.0	7.2
8	8.4	8.9	8.4	7.6
10	8.6	9.1	8.6	7.7
15	8.9	9.6	8.9	8.2
20	9.4	10.0	9.4	8.5
25	9.7	10.3	9.7	8.8
30	10.0	10.6	10.0	9.0
35	10.2	10.9	10.2	9.3
40	10.4	11.1	10.4	9.4
45	10.5	11.2	10.5	9.5
50	10.7	11.4	10.7	9.7
55	10.9	11.6	10.9	9.9
60	11.2	11.9	11.2	10.2
65	11.5	12.2	11.5	10.4
70	11.7	12.4	11.7	10.6
75	11.8	12.6	11.8	10.8
80	12.0	12.8	12.0	11.0

Values deviating less than 20% are considered normal.

Monopolar Needle Recordings (From Chu-Andrews, ref. 6, with permission)
Duration (msec):

Age (years)	Deltoid	Biceps	Extensor digitorum communis	Triceps	Vastus lateralis	Tibialis anterior	Gastrocnemius	Adductor longus
<60	12.4 ± 1.9 (5.6–18.1)	14.6 ± 3.8 (4.2–26.0)	14.1 ± 4.4 (4.8–27.3)	10.8 ± 2.2 (6.0–17.4)	13.4 ± 2.8 (6.2–21.8)	15.8 ± 4.9 (5.4–30.5)	10.2 ± 1.9 (4.0–15.9)	
>60	13.8 ± 1.9 (8.0–19.5)	16.2 ± 4.5 (4.2–29.7)	16.1 ± 6.5 (6.8–35.6)	11.6 ± 1.8 (8.2–17.0)	14.5 ± 3.4 (6.4–24.7)	18.1 ± 6.3 (7.0–37.0)	11.4 ± 2.6 (7.0–19.2)	
All ages	12.7 ± 1.9 (5.6–18.4)	14.9 ± 3.9 (4.2–26.0)	14.5 ± 4.9 (4.8–29.2)	11.0 ± 2.1 (6.0–17.3)	13.7 ± 2.9 (6.2–22.4)	16.2 ± 5.2 (5.4–31.8)	10.5 ± 2.1 (4.0–13.8)	14.3 ± 5.7 (3.8–31.4)
20–29		15.1 ± 4.1 (4.2–27.4)	14.5 ± 4.2 (4.8–27.1)			15.5 ± 4.8 (6.0–29.9)		14.3 ± 5.7 (3.8–31.4)
30–39		14.0 ± 3.2 (5.6–23.6)	13.8 ± 2.6 (5.6–24.6)			15.1 ± 3.7 (7.2–26.2)		
40–49		14.7 ± 4.2 (5.8–27.1)	13.8 ± 4.9 (7.0–28.5)			16.1 ± 5.6 (5.4–32.9)		
50–59		14.7 ± 3.6 (7.6–25.5)	14.3 ± 4.9 (7.0–29.0)			16.4 ± 5.2 (6.8–32.0)		

Amplitude:
The amplitude is measured maximum peak-to-peak and is determined by (a) the diameter of the muscle fibers, (b) the number of fibers, (c) the temporal distribution of the action potential closest to the recording electrode, and (d) the leading-off area of the electrode. With a given leading-off area, MUAP amplitude is determined by one to three muscle fibers closest to the tip of recording electrode.[1,2]

Motor Unit Action Potential Amplitudes

Concentric needle recordings (from ref. 2, with permission from Rosenfalck):

Muscle	Amplitude (μV) (mean $\pm$ SD)	Range
Deltoid	212 $\pm$ 147	150–304
Triceps	340	
Biceps	180	120–390
Extensor digitorum communis	210 $\pm$ 115	
Abductor digitorum quinti	350	
Abductor pollicis brevis	260	
Vastus medialis	230	150–360
Vastus lateralis	260	210–370
Rectus femoris	170	130–215
Tibialis anterior	220	
Gastrocnemius	160 $\pm$ 95	
Extensor digitorum brevis	460	

Monopolar Needle Recordings (From Chu-Andrews, ref. 6, with permission)
Amplitude (mV):

Age (years)	Deltoid	Biceps	Extensor digitorum communis	Triceps	Vastus lateralis	Tibialis anterior	Gastro-cnemius	Adductor longus
<60	0.9 ± 0.5 (0.2–2.4)	0.7 ± 0.3 (0.2–1.6)	0.9 ± 0.5 (0.2–2.4)	1.4 ± 0.8 (0.3–3.8)	1.1 ± 0.5 (0.3–2.6)	1.1 ± 0.6 (0.2–2.9)	1.3 ± 0.6 (0.3–3.1)	
>60	0.9 ± 0.4 (0.2–2.1)	0.9 ± 0.4 (0.2–2.1)	1.1 ± 0.7 (0.2–3.1)	1.4 ± 1.7 (0.5–3.5)	1.4 ± 0.8 (0.3–3.8)	1.4 ± 0.9 (0.3–4.1)	1.7 ± 0.7 (0.3–3.8)	
All ages	0.9 ± 0.5 (0.2–2.4)	0.7 ± 0.4 (0.2–1.9)	1.0 ± 0.6 (0.2–2.8)	1.4 ± 0.7 (0.5–3.5)	1.2 ± 0.6 (0.3–3.0)	1.2 ± 0.7 (0.2–3.3)	1.4 ± 0.6 (3.0–3.2)	0.7 ± 0.4 (0.2–1.9)
20–29		0.6 ± 0.3 (0.2–1.5)		1.0 ± 0.5 (0.2–2.5)		1.0 ± 0.6 (0.3–1.8)		0.7 ± 0.4 (0.2–1.9)
30–39		0.6 ± 0.3 (0.2–1.5)	1.0 ± 0.6 (0.2–2.8)			1.0 ± 0.5 (0.3–2.5)		
40–49		0.7 ± 0.3 (0.2–1.6)	0.9 ± 0.6 (0.2–2.7)			1.3 ± 0.7 (0.2–3.4)		
50–59		0.8 ± 0.4 (0.3–2.0)	1.0 ± 0.5 (0.3–2.5)			1.2 ± 0.6 (0.2–3.0)		

Phases:
The number of baseline crossings plus one is called the number of phases. MUAP with more than four phases is called polyphasic.[5]

Turns:
These represent the points of change in direction in the MUAP form and the magnitude of the voltage change after the turning point. It is not necessary to pass through the baseline.[5] The normal magnitude of the amplitude criterion has not been determined. In the tibialis anterior muscle turns increase with age but phases do not.[1]

Satellite:
The satellite is a small action potential separated from the main MUAP but it fires in a time-locked relationship to the main MUAP. It may originate from single fibers. It also is called late component, parasite potential, linked potential, and coupled discharge. The satellites are not included in the MUAP duration measurement.[1,3,4,5]

Interference pattern[5]:
The interference pattern refers to the electric activity recorded from a muscle with a needle electrode during maximal voluntary effort. It is a qualitative and/or quantitative description of the sequence of MUAP activity with increasing strength of voluntary muscle contraction. It can be described by a degree of electric activities recorded in the monitor screen as follows:

Full Interference Pattern: No individual MUAPs can be identified.

Reduced Interference Pattern: Some individual MUAPs may be identified whereas other individual MUAPs cannot be identified because of overlap.

Discrete Activity Pattern: Each of several different MUAPs can be identified.

Single Unit Pattern: A single MUAP fires rapidly during maximum voluntary effort.

REFERENCES

1. Stalberg E, Andreassen S, Falck B, Lang H, Rosenfalck A, Trojaborg W: Quantitative analysis of individual motor unit potentials: A proposition for standardized terminology and criteria for measurement. *J Clin Neurophysiol* 3:313–348, 1986.
2. Buchthal F: Electromyography in the evaluation of muscle diseases. *Meth Clin Neurophysiol* 2:25–45, 1991. (Electromyography in normal subjects of different ages compiled by P. Rosenfalck.)
3. Kelly JJ, Stolov WC: Motor unit potential quantitation. An American Association of Electromyography and Electrodiagnosis workshop. May, 1984.
4. Daube JR: AAEM Minimonograph #11: Needle examination in clinical electromyography. *Muscle Nerve* 14:685–700, 1991.
5. Nomenclature Committee, AAEE: Glosary of Terms in Clinical Electromyography. Supplement 10:G5–G60, 1987.
6. Chu-Andrews J, Johnson RJ: *Electrodiagnosis: An Anatomical and Clinical Approach.* Philadelphia: JB Lippincott, 1986.

CHAPTER 16

Single Fiber Electromyography

Single fiber electromyography (SFEMG) is a technique for selectively recording individual muscle fiber action potentials within a small recording surface using a concentric needle electrode.[1,2] The recording surface of the needle is 25 μm in diameter (500 μm²). Its small leading-off surface was found to be most satisfactory for recording the single muscle fiber action potentials.[1,2] The diameter of these fibers normally is 50–80 μm. The electrode has a 0.5-mm steel cannula with the leading-off surface of the shaft 3–5 mm from the tip (Figure 16.1). This platinum recording surface faces away from the bevel of the needle to avoid recording action potentials (APs) from mechanically damaged muscle fibers during needle insertions. In practice, the SFEMG measures neuromuscular jitter, fiber density, and blocking.

The characteristics of the single-fiber action potential are[1:]
Amplitude: 0.5–5 mV (may reach 25 mV)
Duration: 1–2 msec
Rise time: 100–200 μsec

Equipment settings[1]:
Filter: 500 Hz to 10 kHz (or higher)
Sweep speed: 0.5–1 msec/div (Jitter measurement) or slow enough
to cover 5 msec after the trigger spike (fiber density measurement)
Gain: 0.2–1 mV
Delay line: At least 0.5 msec delay
Signal-triggering oscilloscope
The muscle tissue acts as a low-pass filter, in which the action potential loses its high frequency components more quickly than its low frequency (LF) components. By increasing the high-pass filter (LF 500

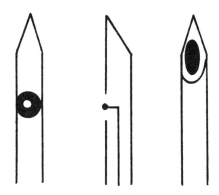

Figure 16.1. Single fiber EMG electrode.

Hz), the amplitude of the distant fiber action potential is markedly attenuated in comparison to its adjacent fiber. The AP amplitude depends on the high frequency components, so that the high frequency (low-pass) filter should be 10 kHz or more.[1,2]

Technique:

Needle Into the Muscle: Usually placed perpendicularly through the skin and into the minimally contracting muscle (e.g., extensor digitorum communis) or horizontally from a lateral position (e.g., frontalis).

Muscle Contraction: Minimum voluntary contraction, so that the firing frequencies maintain between 8 and 15 Hz to keep them firing steadily.

The extremity to be tested should be well supported in a comfortable position so that the muscle to be tested will be relaxed. SFEMG can be performed in any extremity muscles but the extensor digitorum communis (EDC) usually is tested first.[2]

MEASUREMENT OF JITTER

Jitter is the variability with consecutive discharges of the interpotential interval (IPI) between two muscle fiber action potentials belonging to the same motor unit.[3] This may result from fluctuations in the time it takes for end plate potentials at the neuromuscular junction to reach the threshold for impulse propagation (Figure 16.2). Jitter usually is

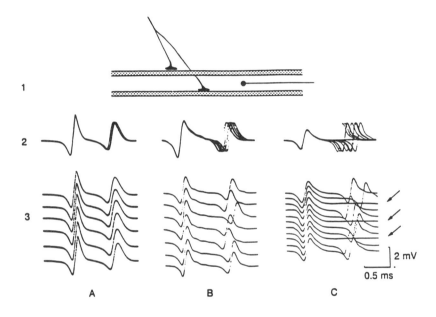

Figure 16.2. Single fiber electromyography—jitter. Schematic representation of the location of the recording surface of single fiber needle electrode recording from two muscle fibers innervated by the same motor neuron *(row 1)*. Consecutive discharges of a potential pair are shown in a superimposed display *(row 2)* and in a raster display *(row 3)*. The potential pairs were recorded from the extensor digitorum communis of a patient with myasthenia gravis and show normal jitter *(column A)*, increased jitter *(column B)*, and increased jitter and impulse blocking *(column C, arrows)*. (With permission from the American Association of Electromyography and Electrodiagnosis.)

expressed as the mean value of the consecutive differences of successive discharges (MCD). The MCD is calculated by the following formula[2,3]:

$$MCD = \frac{[IPI1 - IPI2] + [IPI2 - IPI3] + \cdots + [IPIn\text{-}1 - IPIn]}{n - 1},$$

where   IPI = interpotential interval and n = numbers of IPIs measured.

Most of the IPI are less than 1 msec in normal muscle. In certain conditions the IPI is influenced by the preceding interdischarge interval (IDI). This case introduces an additional variability because of the velocity recovery function effect on the action potential propagation in the muscle fibers. This effect may be eliminated by sorting the measured IPIs in the preceding IDIs in increasing order. The MCD then is measured in this new sequence. In this situation the jitter is expressed as the mean sorted-data difference (MSD).[1]
If the ratio MCD/MSD is:

>1.25: use MSD as representing the jitter
0.8–1.25: use MCD
<0.8: use MCD.

Normal Jitter Values; age, 10–70 years (From Stalberg and Trotelj, ref. 1, with permission)

Muscles	MCD mean ± SD (μsec)	Upper normal limit mean + 3 SD (μsec)
Frontalis	20.4 ± 8.8	45
Biceps	15.6 ± 5.9	35
EDC	24.6 ± 10.6	55
Rectus femoris	31.0 ± 12.6	60
Tibialis anterior	32.1 ± 15.0	60
EDB	85.3 ± 68.6	none

Criteria of Abnormal Jitter[2]

	Upper limit, mean jitter (μsec)	Upper limit, individual mean jitter (μsec)
EDC	34	55
Biceps/deltoid	30	35
Frontalis	30	45

A study is considered abnormal if either of the following criteria is met:
1. the mean jitter of all potential pairs recorded exceeds the upper limit of mean jitter for that muscle
2. 10% or more of potential pairs have jitter that exceeds the upper limit of normal for paired jitter in that muscle.

Mean MCD—95% Upper Normal Limits, Ad Hoc Committee of the AAEM Special Interest Group (From Gilchrist et al., ref. 8, with permission)

Age	Frontalis	EDC	Orbicularis oculi	Muscle Orbicularis oris	Biceps	Deltoid	Tibialis anterior	Quadri- ceps
5	33.6	34.9	39.8	34.6	29.5	32.9	49.4	35.8
10	33.6	34.9	39.8	34.7	29.5	32.9	49.4	35.9
15	33.7	34.9	39.8	34.7	29.5	32.9	49.4	35.9
20	33.9	34.9	39.8	34.7	29.6	32.9	49.3	36.0
25	34.1	35.0	39.9	34.8	29.6	32.9	49.3	36.2
30	34.4	35.1	40.0	34.9	29.6	32.9	49.2	36.5
35	34.9	35.2	40.2	35.1	29.7	32.9	49.1	36.9
40	35.5	35.4	40.4	35.3	29.8	32.9	48.9	37.5
45	36.3	35.6	40.6	35.6	29.9	32.9	48.7	38.2
50	37.3	35.9	40.9	36.0	30.1	33.0	48.5	39.0
55	38.6	36.2	41.3	36.4	30.2	33.0	48.2	40.1
60	40.0	36.6	41.8	37.0	30.5	33.0	47.9	41.3
65	41.8	37.1	42.4	37.6	30.7	33.1	47.5	42.8
70	43.8	37.7	43.0	38.3	31.0	33.1	47.0	44.6
75	46.2	38.3	43.7	39.2	31.4	33.2	46.4	46.6
80		39.1		40.2			33.2	45.8
85		39.9		41.3			33.3	45.1
90		40.9		42.5			33.3	

Abnormal criteria: mean MCD above the 95% upper limit for age for that muscle.

Jitter—95% Upper Normal Limits, Ad Hoc Committee of the AAEM Special Interest Group (From Gilchrist et al., ref. 8, with permission)

Age	Frontalis	EDC	Orbicularis oculi	Muscle Orbicularis oris	Biceps	Deltoid	Tibialis anterior	Quadriceps
5	49.7	50.0	54.6	52.5	45.1	44.4	80.0	47.9
10	49.7	50.0	54.6	52.5	45.2	44.4	80.0	47.9
15	49.9	50.1	54.6	52.6	45.2	44.5	79.9	48.0
20	50.1	50.1	54.7	52.7	45.2	44.5	79.8	48.0
25	50.6	50.3	54.7	52.9	45.3	44.5	79.6	48.1
30	51.3	50.5	54.7	53.2	45.4	44.5	79.3	48.2
35	52.2	50.8	54.8	53.6	45.5	44.6	78.9	48.3
40	53.5	51.3	54.8	54.1	45.7	44.6	78.3	48.5
45	55.2	51.8	54.9	54.8	45.9	44.7	77.6	48.8
50	57.5	52.5	55.0	55.7	46.2	44.8	76.8	49.1
55	60.3	53.4	55.2	56.8	46.5	45.0	75.7	49.5
60	63.9	54.4	55.3	58.2	46.9	45.1	74.5	50.0
65	68.4	55.7	55.5	59.8	47.4		73.1	50.5
70	74.1	57.2	55.8	61.8	48.0		71.4	51.2
75	81.3	59.0	56.0	64.2	48.7		69.6	52.0
80	90.3	61.1		67.0			67.5	
85		63.6		70.3			65.3	
90		66.5		74.2			62.9	

Abnormal criteria: jitter greater than the 95% upper normal limit for action potential pairs in a muscle (or >10% of pairs if more than 20 action potential pairs are analyzed).

Mean of mean MCDs (from Gilchrist et al., ref. 8, with permission)

27–28 μsec	30–38 μsec	23–25 μsec
EDC	Tibialis anterior	Frontalis
Orbicularis oculi	Quadriceps	Biceps
Orbicularis oris	Extensor digiti quinti	Sternocleidomastoid
Tongue		
Deltoid		

MEASUREMENT OF FIBER DENSITY

To measure the fiber density (FD), the SFEMG needle is inserted randomly into the muscle as the patient voluntarily contracts the muscle. The action potential amplitude from one muscle fiber is made maximal by slight axial and rotational movements of the electrode (Figure 16.3). As this potential triggers the oscilloscope, the number of synchronized action potentials are counted. It is. different from the technique for recording the jitter, in which the needle is adjusted to record the action potentials from the two muscle fibers of one motor unit with optimal amplitudes.[1,2,4] To qualify for counting, the AP amplitude optimally

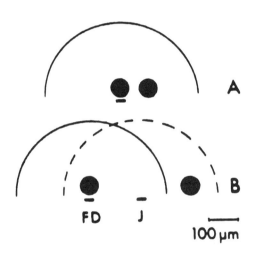

Figure 16.3. Different recording positions for fiber density and jitter measurements. For fiber density measurement the electrode must be as close as possible to one active muscle fiber, indicated in *A* and as FD position in *B*. In B only one fiber is then recorded. In jitter measurements the electrode position is adjusted to obtain recordings from potential pairs. This is achieved in A with the same position as for fiber density measurement but in B another position must be used *(J)*. If this position were used for fiber density measurement the value would be erroneously high. Semicircles indicate the uptake area of the electrode. (From Stalberg and Trotelj, ref. 1, with permission.)

should be 200 μV and the rise time should be shorter than 300 μsec.[5] Action potentials are obtained in 20 sites with at least four separate skin penetrations within a muscle. In the normal extensor digitorum communis, only single AP is recorded in 65–70% of the time. Only 25% of the recording sites show pairs of potentials.[6] The FD is expressed as the mean value of APs counted in 20 different recording sites. Normal FD is different among different muscles and ranges from 1.3 to 1.8 in normal individuals under the age of 70 years. FD represents the fiber density of one motor unit within the recording area (300 μm in radius). It increases with any disorder that might result in histologic regrouping of muscle fibers. It is seen with reinnervations and muscle diseases associated with fiber splitting, such as muscular dystrophies or polymyositis. The FD also increases with age after 60 years, particularly in the tibialis anterior and extensor digitorum brevis muscles.

Blocking:
Blocking is seen in transmission disorders affecting myoneural junction. Whenever the ratio between the action potential threshold and the end plate potential is greater than normal, the nerve impulse may fail to evoke the muscle action potentials (Figure 16.2). In this case the SFEMG demonstrates AP blocking. When blockings are significant in a muscle, there is clinical weakness.[2,7] Blocking can be seen when the jitter is increased to 80–100 μsec.[1]

Fiber Density in Different Muscles of Normal Persons (From Stalberg and Trotelj, ref. 1, with permission)

Muscles	Age (years)			
	10–25	26–50	51–75	Above 75
Frontailis	1.61 ± 0.21	1.72 ± 0.21		
Deltoid	1.36 ± 0.16	1.40 ± 0.11		
Biceps	1.25 ± 0.09	1.33 ± 0.07		
EDC	1.47 ± 0.16	1.49 ± 0.16	1.57 ± 0.17	2.13 ± 0.41
First dorsal interosseous	1.33 ± 0.13	1.45 ± 0.12		
Rectus femoris	1.43 ± 0.18	1.57 ± 0.23		
Tibialis anterior	1.57 ± 0.22	1.56 ± 0.22	1.77 ± 0.12	3.8
EDB	2.07 ± 0.42	2.62 ± 0.30		

Ad Hoc Committee of the AAEM Special Interest Group (From Gilchrist et al., ref. 8, with permission)

Age	EDC	Frontalis	Biceps	Deltoid	Muscle Tibialis anterior	Quadriceps	Soleus
5	1.77	1.67	1.52	1.56	1.94	1.93	1.56
10	1.77	1.67	1.52·	1.56	1.94	1.93	1.56
15	1.77	1.67	1.52	1.56	1.94	1.93	1.56
20	1.78	1.67	1.52	1.56	1.94	1.94	1.56
25	1.78	1.67	1.52	1.56	1.95	1.94	1.56
30	1.80	1.68	1.53	1.57	1.96	1.96	1.56
35	1.81	1.68	1.53	1.57	1.97	1.97	1.57
40	1.83	1.69	1.54	1.57	1.98	1.99	1.57
45	1.86	1.69	1.55	1.57	2.00	2.02	1.58
50	1.90	1.70	1.57	1.58	2.02	2.05	1.59
55	1.94	1.71	1.58	1.58	2.04	2.09	1.61
60	1.99	1.73	1.60	1.59	2.07	2.14	1.62
65	2.05	1.74	1.63	1.59	2.11	2.20	1.64
70	2.12	1.76	1.65	1.60	2.15	2.26	1.66
75	2.20	1.78	1.68	1.61	2.20	2.34	
80	2.29		1.72	1.62	2.26	2.43	1.68
85	2.39		1.76	1.63	2.32	2.53	1.71
90	2.51		1.80	1.65			1.74

Recommended criteria of abnormality: if FD exceeds the 95% upper limit for the patient's age or action potential counts greater than 4 at a single recording site.

REFERENCES

1. Stalberg E, Trontelj JV: *Single Fibre Electromyography*. Old Working, Surrey U.K.: Mirvalle Press, 1979.
2. Sanders DB: Single fiber electromyography. An American Association of Electrodmyography and Electrodiagnosis Workshop, October 1988.
3. Ekstedt J, Nilsson G, Stalberg E: Calculation of the electromyographic jitter. *J Neurol Neurosurg Psychiatry* 37:526–539, 1974
4. Stalberg E, Thiele B: Motor unit fibre density in the extensor digitorum communis muscle. *J Neurol Neurosurg Psychiatry* 38:874–880, 1975.
5. Sanders DB, Phillips LH: Single fiber electromyography. An American Association of Electromyography and Electrodiagnosis Workshop, October 1984.
6. Stalberg E, Ekstedt J: Single fibre EMG and microphysiology of the motor unit in normal and diseased muscle. In Desmedt JE (ed): *New Developments in Electromyography and Clinical Neurophysiology*. Basel, Switzerland: Karger, 1973;113–129.

7. Stalberg E, Thiele B: Transmission block in terminal nerve twigs: A single fibre electromyographic finding in man. *J Neurol Neurosurg Psychiatry* 35:52–59, 1972.
8. Ad Hoc Committee of the AAEM Special Interest Group on Single Fiber EMG, Gilchrist JM, Coordinator: Single fiber EMG reference values: A collaborative effort. *Muscle Nerve* 15:151–161, 1992.

CHAPTER 17

Anatomy

SEGMENTAL INNERVATION OF MUSCLES

Upper Extremity

Muscle	Peripheral nerve	Spinal segment
Sternocleidomastoid	Spinal accessory	C2, 3
Trapezius	Spinal accessory	C3, 4
Diaphragm	Phrenic	C3, 4, 5
Levator scapulae (LS)	Nerve to LS	C3, 4
Rhomboid	Dorsal scapular	C4, 5
Supraspinatus	Suprascapular	C5, 6
Infraspinatus	Suprascapular	C5, 6
Teres major	Subscapular	C6, 7
Teres minor	Axillary	C5, 6
Serratus anterior	Long thoracic	C5, 6, 7
Latissimus dorsi	Thoracodorsal	C6, 7, 8
Pectoralis major	Lateral and Medial pectoral	C5, 6, 7, 8, and T1
Deltoid	Axillary	C5, 6
Biceps	Musculocutaneous	C5, 6
Coracobrachialis	Musculocutaneous	C5, 6
Brachialis	Musculocutaneous	C5, 6
Triceps	Radial	C6, 7, 8
Anconeous	Radial	C7, 8
Brachioradialis	Radial	C5, 6
Extensor carpi radialis	Radial	C6, 7
Extensor digitorum	Radial	C7, 8
Extensor carpi ulnaris	Radial	C7, 8
Extensor pollicis longus	Radial	C7, 8

Muscle	Peripheral nerve	Spinal segment
Abductor pollicis longus	Radial	C7, 8
Extensor indicis	Radial	C7, 8
Supinator	Radial	C5, 6
Pronator teres	Median	C6, 7
Flexor carpi radialis	Median	C6, 7
Palmaris longus	Median	C7, 8
Flexor digitorum sublimis	Median	C7, 8, and T1
Flexor digitorum profundus	Median	C8 and T1
	Ulnar	C8 and T1
Pronator quandratus	Median	C8 and T1
Flexor pollicis longus	Median	C8 and T1
Flexor carpi ulnaris	Ulnar	C7, 8
Abductor digiti minimi	Ulnar	C8 and T1
Adductor pollicis	Ulnar	C8 and T1
Interossei	Ulnar	C8 and T1
Lumbricals:		
1st and 2nd	Median	C8 and T1
3rd and 4th	Ulnar	C8 and T1
Abductor pollicis brevis	Median	C8 and T1
Opponens pollicis	Median (Ulnar)	C8 and T1

Lower Extremity

Iliopsoas	Femoral	L2, 3
Sartorius	Femoral	L2, 3
Quadriceps	Femoral	L2, 3, 4
Adductor longus	Obturator	L2, 3, 4
Adductor magnus	Obturator and Sciatic	L2, 3, 4
Gracilis	Obturator	L2, 3
Tensor fascia lata	Superior gluteal	L4, 5, and S1
Gluteus medius	Superior gluteal	L4, 5, and S1
Gluteus maximus	Inferior gluteal	L5, S1, and 2

Muscle	Peripheral nerve	Spinal segment
Biceps femoris:		
Short head	Sciatic (common peroneal)	L5, S1 and 2
Long head	Sciatic (tibial)	L5, S1 and 2
Semitendinosus	Sciatic (tibial)	L5, S1 and 2
Semimembranosus	Sciatic (tibial)	L5, S1 and 2
Tibialis anterior	Deep peroneal	L4, 5
Extensor digitorum longus	Deep peroneal	L5 and S1
Extensor hallucis longus	Deep peroneal	L5 and S1
Extensor digitorum brevis	Deep peroneal	L5, S1 and 2
Peroneus longus	Superficial peroneal	L5 and S1
Gastrocnemius	Tibial	S1, 2
Soleus	Tibial	S1, 2
Flexor digitorum longus	Tibial	L5, S1 and 2
Flexor hallucis longus	Tibial	S2, 3
Tibialis posterior	Tibial	L5 and S1
Abductor hallucis	Medial plantar	S2, 3
Flexor digitorum brevis	Medial plantar	S2, 3
Abductor digiti minimi	Lateral plantar	S2, 3
Lumbricals	Medial and Lateral plantar	S2, 3

Myotome

C5
  Deltoid
  Supraspinatus
  Infraspinatus
  Teres major
  Biceps brachii
  Brachioradialis
  Rhomboid

C6

Brachioradialis
Biceps
Pronator teres
Flexor carpi radialis
Extensor carpi radialis
Supinator
Serratus anterior

C7

Triceps
Anconeous
Extensor carpi radialis longus
Extensor digitorum
Pronator teres
Flexor carpi radialis
Flexor digitorum superficialis
Serratus anterior

C8 and T1

Extensor carpi ulnaris
Extensor indicis
Flexor carpi ulnaris
Flexor digitorum profundus
Abductor pollicis brevis
Pronator quadratus
Flexor pollicis longus
Flexor pollicis brevis
Abductor digiti minimi
First dorsal interosseous

L23

Ilicus
Vastus medialis
Vastus lateralis
Rectus femoris
Adductor longus

L4

Vastus medialis
Vastus lateralis

Rectus femoris
Tibialis anterior
Medial hamstring
Gluteus medius
Tensor fascia lata
L5
Tibialis anterior
Tibialis posterior
Peroneus longus
Extensor digitorum longus
Flexor digitorum longus
Extensor hallucis longus
Extensor digitorum brevis
Medial hamstring
Gluteus medius
Tensor fascia lata
S1
Gastrocnemius
Soleus
Tibialis posterior
Abductor hallucis
Peroneous longus
Extensor digitorum brevis
Lateral hamstring
Gluteus maximus

Root Search for Cervical Radiculopathy

Muscle	Root	Nerve
Deltoid	C5, 6	Axillary
Biceps	C5, 6	Musculocutaneous
Pronator teres	C6, 7	Median
Triceps	C6, 7, 8	Radial
First dorsi interosseous	C8, T1	Ulnar
Cervical paraspinals	Posterior ramus	

Root Search for Lumbosacral Radiculopathy

Muscle	Root	Nerve
Vastus lateralis	L2, 3, 4	Femoral
Tibialis anterior	L4, 5	Deep peroneal
Peroneous longus	L5, S1	Superficial peroneal
Gastrocnemius (medial)	S1, 2	Tibial
Gluteus maximus	S1, 2	Inferior gluteal
Lumbosacral paraspinals	Posterior ramus	

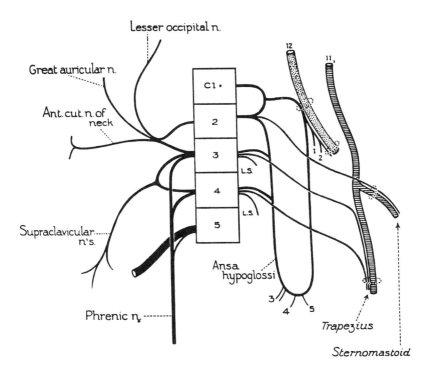

Figure 17.1. *Diagram of the cervical plexus.* The relations of branches of the plexus to hypoglossal (*12*) and accessory (*11*) nerves are indicated. The numbered branches of the ansa hypoglossi innervate the following muscles: *1*, thyrohyoid; *2*, geniohyoid; *3*, omohyoid; *4*, sternothyroid; *5*, sternohyoid. *L.S.* refers to the levator scapulae. (From Haymaker and Woodhall, with permission from the publisher.)

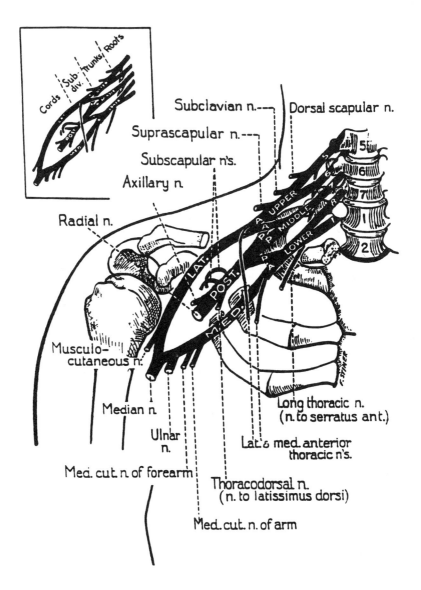

Figure 17.2. Brachial plexus. (From Haymaker and Woodhall, with permission.)

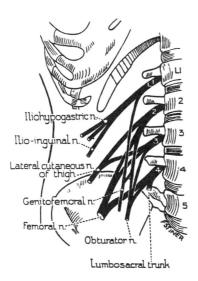

Figure 17.3. Lumbar plexus. (From Haymaker and Woodhall, with permission.)

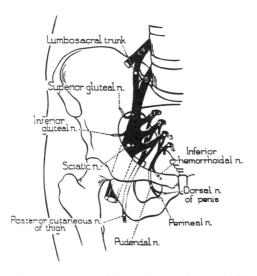

Figure 17.4. Sacral plexus. (From Haymaker and Woodhall, with permission.)

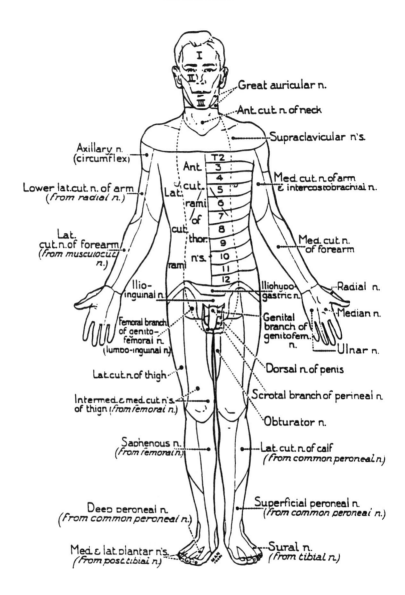

Figure 17.5. The cutaneous fields of peripheral nerves from the anterior aspect. (From Haymaker and Woodhall, with permission.)

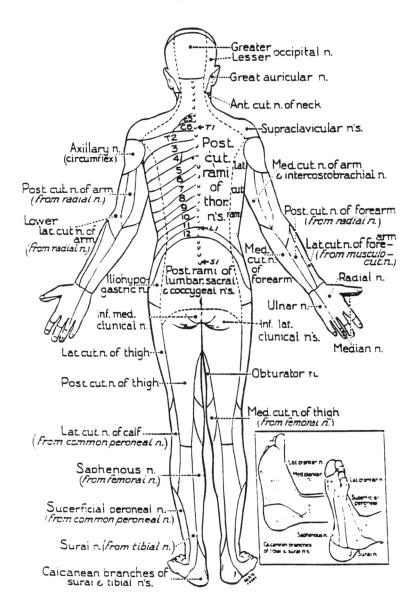

Figure 17.6. The cutaneous fields of peripheral nerves from the posterior aspect. (From Haymaker and Woodhall, with permission.)

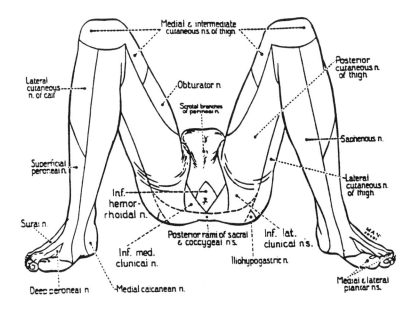

Figure 17.7. Peripheral nerve of the perineum and limbs. (From Haymaker and Woodhall, with permission.)

Glossary of Terms Used in Clinical Electromyography

SECTION I:
ALPHABETICAL LIST OF TERMS WITH DEFINITIONS

*A wave   A compound action potential evoked consistently from a muscle by submaximal electric stimuli to the nerve and frequently abolished by supramaximal stimuli. The amplitude of the A wave is similar to that of the F wave, but the latency is more constant. The A wave usually occurs before the F wave, but may occur afterwards. The A wave is due to normal or pathologic axonal branching. Compare the *F wave.*

absolute refractory period   See *refractory period.*

accommodation   True accommodation in neuronal physiology is a rise in the threshold transmembrane depolarization required to initiate a spike when depolarization is slow or a subthreshold depolarization is maintained. In the older literature, accommodation described the observation that the final intensity of current applied in a slowly rising fashion to stimulate a nerve was greater than the intensity of a pulse of current required to stimulate the same nerve. The latter may largely be an artifact of the nerve sheath and bears little relation to true accommodation as measured intracellularly.

accommodation curve   See *strength-duration curve.*

action current   The electric currents associated with an *action potential.*

---

[1] This entire glossary was reprinted from *Muscle & Nerve*, Vol. 10, No. 8s, Supplement 1987, with permission from the American Association of Electrodiagnostic Medicine (AAEM), formerly the American Association of Electromyography and Electrodiagnosis.
* Illustration in Section II.

action potential (AP) The brief regenerative electric potential that propagates along a single axon or muscle fiber membrane. The action potential is an all-or-none phenomenon; whenever the stimulus is at or above threshold, the action potential generated has a constant size and configuration. See also *compound action potential, motor unit action potential.*

active electrode Synonymous with *exploring electrode.* See *recording electrode.*

adaptation A decline in the frequency of the spike discharge as typically recorded from sensory axons in response to a maintained stimulus.

AEPs See *auditory evoked potentials.*

afterdischarge The continuation of an impulse train in a neuron, axon, or muscle fiber after the termination of an applied stimulus. The number of extra impulses and their periodicity in the train may vary depending on the circumstances.

afterpotential The membrane potential between the end of the spike and the time when the membrane potential is restored to its resting value. The membrane during this period may be depolarized or hyperpolarized.

amplitude With reference to an *action potential,* the maximum voltage difference between two points, usually baseline to peak or peak to peak. By convention, the amplitude of the *compound muscle action potential* is measured from the baseline to the most negative peak. In contrast, the amplitude of a *compound sensory nerve action potential, motor unit potential, fibrillation potential, positive sharp wave, fasciculation potential,* and most other *action potentials* is measured from the most positive peak to the most negative peak.

anodal block A local block of nerve conduction caused by *hyperpolarization* of the nerve cell membrane by an electric stimulus. See *stimulating electrode.*

anode The positive terminal of a source of electric current.

antidromic Propagation of an impulse in the direction opposite to physiologic conduction; e.g., conduction along motor nerve fibers away from the muscle and conduction along sensory fibers away from the spinal cord. Contrast with *orthodromic.*

AP See *action potential.*

artifact (also artefact) A voltage change generated by a biologic or nonbiologic source other than the ones of interest. The *stimulus artifact* is the potential recorded at the time the stimulus is applied and includes the *electric* or *shock artifact,* which represents cutaneous spread of stimulating current to the recording electrode. The stimulus and shock artifacts usually precede the activity of interest. A *movement artifact* refers to a change in the recorded activity caused by movement of the recording electrodes.

auditory evoked potentials (AEPs). Electric waveforms of biologic origin elicited in response to sound stimuli. AEPs are classified by their latency as short-latency brain stem AEPs (BAEPs) with a latency of up to 10 msec, middle-latency AEPs with a latency of 10–50 msec, and long-latency AEPs with a latency of more than 50 msec. See *brain stem auditory evoked potentials.*

axon reflex Use of term discouraged as it is incorrect. No reflex is considered to be involved. See preferred term, *A wave.*

axon response See preferred term, *A wave.*

axon wave See *A wave.*

axonotmesis Nerve injury characterized by disruption of the axon and myelin sheath, but with preservation of the supporting connective tissue, resulting in axonal degeneration distal to the injury site.

backfiring Discharge of an antidromically activated motor neuron.

BAEPs See *brain stem auditory evoked potentials.*

BAERs Abbreviation for *brain stem auditory evoked responses.* See preferred term, *brain stem auditory evoked potentials.*

baseline The potential recorded from a biologic system while the system is at rest.

benign fasciculation Use of term discouraged to describe a firing pattern of fasciculation potentials. The term has been used to describe a clinical syndrome and/or the presence of fasciculations in nonprogressive neuromuscular disorders. See *fasciculation potential.*

BERs Abbreviation for *brain stem auditory evoked responses.* See preferred term, *brain stem auditory evoked potentials.*

bifilar needle recording electrode *Recording electrode* that measures variations in voltage between the bare tips of two insulated wires cemented side by side in a steel cannula. The bare tips of the electrodes are flush with the level of the cannula. The latter may be grounded.

biphasic action potential   An *action potential* with two phases.

biphasic end plate activity   See *end plate activity (biphasic)*.

bipolar needle recording electrode   See preferred term, *bifilar needle recording electrode*.

bipolar stimulating electrode   See *stimulating electrode*.

bizarre high-frequency discharge   See preferred term, *complex repetitive discharge*.

bizarre repetitive discharge   See preferred term, *complex repetitive discharge*.

bizarre repetitive potential   See preferred term, *complex repetitive discharge*.

blink reflex   See *blink responses*.

blink response   Strictly defined, one of the *blink responses*. See *blink responses*.

***blink responses**   *Compound muscle action potentials* evoked from orbicularis oculi muscles as a result of brief electric or mechanical stimuli to the cutaneous area innervated by the supraorbital (or less commonly, the infraorbital) branch of the trigeminal nerve. Typically, there is an early compound muscle action potential *(R1 wave)* ipsilateral to the stimulation site with a latency of about 10 msec and a bilateral late compound muscle action potential *(R2 wave)* with a latency of approximately 30 msec. Generally, only the *R2 wave* is associated with a visible twitch of the orbicularis oculi. The configuration, amplitude, duration, and latency of the two components, along with the sites of recording and the sites of stimulation, should be specified. *R1* and *R2 waves* probably are oligosynaptic and polysynaptic brain stem reflexes, respectively, together called the *blink reflex,* with the afferent arc provided by the sensory branches of the trigeminal nerve and the efferent arc provided by the facial nerve motor fibers.

***brain stem auditory evoked potentials**   (BAEPs) Electric waveforms of biologic origin elicited in response to sound stimuli. The normal BAEP consists of a sequence of up to seven waves, named I to VII, which occur during the first 10 msec after the onset of the stimulus and have positive polarity at the vertex of the head.

brain stem auditory evoked responses (BAERs, BERs)   See preferred term, *brain stem auditory evoked potentials.*

BSAPs   Abbreviation for brief, small, abundant potentials. Use of term is discouraged. It is used to describe a recruitment pattern of brief-duration, small-amplitude, overly abundant motor unit action potentials. Quantitative measurements of motor unit potential duration, amplitude, numbers of phases, and recruitment frequency are to be preferred to qualitative descriptions such as this. See *motor unit action potential.*

BSAPPs   Abbreviation for brief, small, abundant, polyphasic potentials. Use of term is discouraged. It is used to describe a recruitment pattern of brief-duration, small-amplitude, overly abundant, polyphasic motor unit action potentials. Quantitative measurements of motor unit potential duration, amplitude, numbers of phases, and recruitment frequency are to be preferred to qualitative descriptions such as this. See *motor unit action potential.*

cathode   The negative terminal of a source of electric current.

central electromyography (central EMG)   Use of electromyographic recording techniques to study reflexes and the control of movement by the spinal cord and brain.

chronaxie (also chronaxy)   See *strength-duration curve.*

clinical electromyography   Synonymous with *electroneuromyography.* Used to refer to all electrodiagnostic studies of human peripheral nerves and muscle. See also *electromyography* and *nerve conduction studies.*

coaxial needle electrode   See synonym, *concentric needle electrode.*

collision   When used with reference to nerve conduction studies, the interaction of two action potentials propagated toward each other from opposite directions on the same nerve fiber so that the refractory periods of the two potentials prevent propagation past each other.

complex action potential   See preferred term, *serrated action potential.*

complex motor unit action potential   A *motor unit action potential* that is polyphasic or serrated. See preferred terms, *polyphasic action potential* or *serrated action potential.*

*complex repetitive discharge   Polyphasic or serrated action potentials that may begin spontaneously or after a needle movement. They have a uniform frequency, shape, and amplitude, with abrupt onset, cessation, or change in configuration. Amplitude ranges from 100 μV to 1 mV and frequency of discharge from 5 to 100 Hz. This term is preferred to *bizarre high frequency discharge, bizarre repetitive discharge, bizarre repetitive potential, near constant frequency trains, pseudomyotonic discharge,* and *synchronized fibrillation.*

compound action potential   See *compound mixed nerve action potential, compound motor nerve action potential, compound nerve action potential, compound sensory nerve action potential,* and *compound muscle action potential.*

compound mixed nerve action potential (compound mixed NAP)   A compound nerve action potential is considered to have been evoked from afferent and efferent fibers if the recording electrodes detect activity on a mixed nerve with the electric stimulus applied to a segment of the nerve which contains both afferent and efferent fibers. The amplitude, latency, duration, and phases should be noted.

compound motor nerve action potential (compound motor NAP)   A compound nerve action potential is considered to have been evoked from efferent fibers to a muscle if the recording electrodes detect activity only in a motor nerve or a motor branch of a mixed nerve, or if the electric stimulus is applied only to such a nerve or a ventral root. The amplitude, latency, duration, and phases should be noted. See *compound nerve action potential.*

compound muscle action potential (CMAP)   The summation of nearly synchronous muscle fiber action potentials recorded from a muscle commonly produced by stimulation of the nerve supplying the muscle either directly or indirectly. Baseline-to-peak amplitude, duration, and latency of the negative phase should be noted, along with details of the method of stimulation and recording. Use of specific named potentials is recommended, e.g., *M wave, F wave, H wave, T wave, A wave,* and *R1 wave* or *R2 wave (blink responses).*

compound nerve action potential (compound NAP)   The summation of nearly synchronous nerve fiber action potentials recorded from a nerve trunk, commonly produced by stimulation of the nerve directly or indirectly. Details of the method of stimulation and recording should be specified, together with the fiber type (sensory, motor, or mixed).

*compound sensory nerve action potential (compound SNAP)   A compound nerve action potential is considered to have been evoked from afferent fibers if the recording electrodes detect activity only in a sensory nerve or in a sensory branch of a mixed nerve, or if the electric stimulus is applied to a sensory nerve or a dorsal nerve root, or an adequate stimulus is applied synchronously to sensory receptors. The amplitude, latency, duration, and configuration should be noted. Generally, the amplitude is measured as the maximum peak-to-peak voltage, the latency as either the *latency* to the initial deflection or the *peak latency* to the negative peak, and the duration as the interval from the first deflection of the waveform from the baseline to its final return to the baseline. The compound sensory nerve action potential has been referred to as the *sensory response* or *sensory potential.*

concentric needle electrode   *Recording electrode* that measures an electric potential difference between the bare tip of an insulated wire, usually stainless steel, silver, or platinum, and the bare shaft of a steel cannula through which it is inserted. The bare tip of the central wire (exploring electrode) is flush with the level of the cannula (reference electrode).

conditioning stimulus   See *paired stimuli.*

conduction block   Failure of an action potential to be conducted past a particular point in the nervous system whereas conduction is possible below the point of the block. Conduction block is documented by demonstration of a reduction in the area of an evoked potential greater than that normally seen with electric stimulation at two different points on a nerve trunk; anatomic variations of nerve pathways and technical factors related to nerve stimulation must be excluded as the cause of the reduction in area.

conduction distance   See *conduction velocity.*

conduction time   See *conduction velocity.*

conduction velocity (CV)   Speed of propagation of an *action potential* along a nerve or muscle fiber. The nerve fibers studied (motor, sensory, autonomic, or mixed) should be specified. For a nerve trunk, the maximum conduction velocity is calculated from the *latency* of the evoked potential (muscle or nerve) at maximal or supramaximal intensity of stimulation at two different points. The distance between the two points *(conduction distance)* is divided by the difference between the corresponding latencies *(conduction time).* The calculated velocity represents the conduction velocity of the fastest fibers and is expressed as meters per second (m/sec). As commonly used, the term *conduction velocity* refers to the maximum conduction velocity. By specialized techniques, the conduction velocity of other fibers can be determined as well and should be specified, e.g., minimum conduction velocity.

contraction   A voluntary or involuntary reversible muscle shortening that may or may not be accompanied by *action potentials* from muscle. This term is to be contrasted with the term *contracture,* which refers to a condition of fixed muscle shortening.

contraction fasciculation   Rhythmic, visible twitching of a muscle with weak voluntary or postural contraction. The phenomenon occurs in neuromuscular disorders in which the motor unit territory is enlarged and the tissue covering the muscle is thin.

contracture   The term is used to refer to immobility of a joint due to fixed muscle shortening. Contrast *contraction.* The term also has been used to refer to an electrically silent, involuntary state of maintained muscle contraction, as seen in phosphorylase deficiency, for which the preferred term is *muscle cramp.*

coupled discharge   See preferred term, *satellite potential.*

cps (also c/sec)   See *cycles per second.*

*cramp discharge   Involuntary repetitive firing of *motor unit action potentials* at a high frequency (up to 150 Hz) in a large area of muscles, usually associated with painful muscle contraction. Both the discharge frequency and the number of *motor unit action potentials* firing increase gradually during development and both subside gradually with cessation. See *muscle cramp.*

c/sec (also cps)   See *cycles per second.*

CV   See *conduction velocity.*

cycles per second   Unit of frequency (cps or c/sec). See also *hertz* (Hz).

decremental response   See preferred term, *decrementing response.*

*decrementing response   A reproducible decline in the amplitude and/or area of the *M wave* of successive responses to *repetitive nerve stimulation.* The rate of stimulation and the total number of stimuli should be specified. Decrementing responses with disorders of neuromuscular transmission are most reliably seen with slow rates (2–5 Hz) of nerve stimulation. A decrementing response with repetitive nerve stimulation commonly occurs in disorders of neuromuscular transmission, but also can be seen in some neuropathies, myopathies, and motor neuron disease. An artifact resembling a decrementing response can result from movement of the stimulating or recording electrodes during repetitive nerve stimulation. Contrast with *incrementing response*.

delay As originally used in clinical electromyography, delay referred to the time between the beginning of the horizontal sweep of the oscilloscope and the onset of an applied stimulus. The term also is used to refer to an information storage device (delay line) used to display events occurring before a trigger signal.

denervation potential This term has been used to describe a *fibrillation potential*. The use of this term is discouraged because fibrillation potentials may occur in settings where transient muscle membrane instability occurs in the absence of denervation, e.g., hyperkalemia periodic paralysis. See preferred term, *fibrillation potential*.

depolarization See *polarization*.

depolarization block Failure of an excitable cell to respond to a stimulus because of depolarization of the cell membrane.

discharge Refers to the firing of one or more excitable elements (neurons, axons, or muscle fibers) and as conventionally applied refers to the all-or-none potentials only. Synonymous with *action potential*.

discharge frequency The rate of repetition of potentials. When potentials occur in groups, the rate of recurrence of the group and the rate of repetition of the individual components in the groups should be specified. See also *firing rate*.

discrete activity See *interference pattern*.

distal latency See *motor latency* and *sensory latency*.

double discharge Two action potentials *(motor unit action potential, fibrillation potential)* of the same form and nearly the same amplitude, occurring consistently in the same relationship to one another at intervals of 2–20 msec. Contrast with *paired discharge*.

doublet Synonymous with *double discharge*.

duration The time during which something exists or acts. (1) The total duration of individual potential *waveforms* is defined as the interval from the beginning of the first deflection from the baseline to its final return to the baseline, unless otherwise specified. If only part of the waveform duration is measured, the points of measurement should be specified. For example, the duration of the *M wave* may refer to the interval from the deflection of the first negative phase from the baseline to its return to the baseline. (2) The duration of a single electric stimulus refers to the interval of the applied current or voltage. (3) The duration of recurring stimuli or action potentials refers to the interval from the beginning to the end of the series.

earth electrode   Synonymous with *ground electrode.*

EDX   See *electrodiagnosis.*

electric artifact   See *artifact.*

electric inactivity   Absence of identifiable electric activity in a structure or organ under investigation. See preferred term, *electric silence.*

electric silence   The absence of measurable electric activity due to biologic or nonbiologic sources. The sensitivity and signal-to-noise level of the recording system should be specified.

electrode   A conducting device used to record an electric potential *(recording electrode)* or to apply an electric current *(stimulating electrode).* In addition to the *ground electrode* used in clinical recordings, two electrodes are always required either to record an electric potential or to apply an electric current. Depending on the relative size and location of the electrodes, however, the stimulating or recording condition may be referred to as *monopolar* or *unipolar.* See *ground electrode, recording electrode,* and *stimulating electrode.* Also see specific needle electrode configurations: *monopolar, unipolar, concentric, bifilar recording, bipolar stimulating, multilead, single fiber,* and *macro-EMG needle electrodes.*

electrodiagnosis (EDX)   The recording and analysis of responses of nerves and muscles to electric stimulation and the identification of patterns of insertion, spontaneous, involuntary, and voluntary action potentials in muscle and nerve tissue. See also *electromyography, electroneurography, electroneuromyography,* and *evoked potential studies.*

electrodiagnostic medicine A specific area of medical practice in which a physician uses information from the clinical history, observations from the physical examination, and the techniques of *electrodiagnosis* to diagnose and treat neuromuscular disorders. See *electrodiagnosis*.

electromyelography The recording and study of electric activity from the spinal cord and/or from the cauda equina.

electromyogram The record obtained by *electromyography*.

electromyograph Equipment used to activate, record, process, and display nerve and muscle action potentials for the purpose of evaluating nerve and muscle function.

electromyography (EMG) Strictly defined, the recording and study of insertion, spontaneous, and voluntary electric activity of muscle. It is commonly used to refer to nerve conduction studies as well. See also *clinical electromyography* and *electroneuromyography*.

electroneurography (ENG) The recording and study of the action potentials of peripheral nerves. Synonymous with *nerve conduction studies*.

electroneuromyography (ENMG) The combined studies of *electromyography* and *electroneurography*. Synonymous with *clinical electromyography*.

EMG See *electromyography*.

*end-plate activity Spontaneous electric activity recorded with a needle electrode close to muscle end-plates. May be either of two forms:

1. *Monophasic:* Low-amplitude (10–20 μV), short-duration (0.5–1 msec), monophasic (negative) potentials that occur in a dense, steady pattern and are restricted to a localized area of the muscle. Because of the multitude of different potentials occurring, the exact frequency, although appearing to be high, cannot be defined. These nonpropagated potentials probably are miniature end-plate potentials recorded extracellularly. This form of end-plate activity has been referred to as *end-plate noise* or *sea shell sound (sea shell noise* or *roar)*.

2. *Biphasic:* Moderate-amplitude (100–300 μV), short-duration (2–4 msec), biphasic (negative-positive) spike potentials that

occur irregularly in short bursts with a high frequency (50–100 Hz), restricted to a localized area within the muscle. These propagated potentials are generated by muscle fibers excited by activity in nerve terminals. These potentials have been referred to as *biphasic spike potentials, end-plate spikes,* and, incorrectly, *nerve potentials.*

end-plate noise   See *end-plate activity (monophasic).*

end-plate potential (EPP)   The graded nonpropagated membrane potential induced in the postsynaptic membrane of the muscle fiber by the action of acetylcholine released in response to an action potential in the presynaptic axon terminal.

end-plate spike   See *end-plate activity (biphasic).*

end-plate zone   The region in a muscle where the neuromuscular junctions of the skeletal muscle fibers are concentrated.

ENG   See *electroneurography.*

ENMG   See *electroneuromyography.*

EPP   See *end-plate potential.*

EPSP   See *excitatory postsynaptic potential.*

evoked compound muscle action potential   See *compound muscle action potential.*

evoked potential   Electric waveform elicited by and temporally related to a stimulus, most commonly an electric stimulus delivered to a sensory receptor or nerve, or applied directly to a discrete area of the brain, spinal cord, or muscle. See *auditory evoked potential, brain stem auditory evoked potential, spinal evoked potential, somatosensory evoked potential, visual evoked potential, compound muscle action potential,* and *compound sensory nerve action potential.*

evoked potential studies   Recording and analysis of electric waveforms of biologic origin elicited in response to electric or physiologic stimuli. Generally used to refer to studies of waveforms generated in the peripheral and central nervous system, whereas *nerve conduction studies* refers to studies of waveforms generated in the peripheral nervous system. There are two systems for naming complex waveforms in which multiple components can be distinguished. In the first system, the different components are labeled PI or NI for the initial positive and negative potentials, respectively, and PII, NII, PIII,

NIII, etc., for subsequent positive and negative potentials. In the second system, the components are specified by polarity and average peak latency in normal persons to the nearest millisecond. The first nomenclature principle has been used in an abbreviated form to identify the seven positive components (I–VII) of the normal *brain stem auditory evoked potential*. The second nomenclature principle has been used to identify the positive and negative components of *visual evoked potentials* (N$\overline{75}$, P$\overline{100}$) and *somatosensory evoked potentials* (P$\overline{9}$, P$\overline{11}$, P$\overline{13}$, P$\overline{14}$, N$\overline{20}$, P$\overline{23}$). Regardless of the nomenclature system, it is possible under standardized conditions to establish normal ranges of amplitude, duration, and latency of the individual components of these *evoked potentials*. The difficulty with the second system is that the latencies of components of evoked potentials depend on the length of the pathways in the neural tissues. Thus, the components of an SEP recorded in a child have different average latencies from the same components of an SEP recorded in an adult. Despite this problem, there is no better system available for naming these components at this time. See *auditory evoked potentials, brain stem auditory evoked potentials, visual evoked potentials,* and *somatosensory evoked potentials.*

evoked response Tautology. Use of term discouraged. See preferred term, *evoked potential.*

excitability Capacity to be activated by or react to a stimulus.

excitatory postsynaptic potential (EPSP) A local, graded depolarization of a neuron in response to activation by a nerve terminal of a synapse. Contrast with *inhibitory postsynaptic potential.*

exploring electrode Synonymous with *active electrode*. See *recording electrode.*

F reflex See preferred term, *F wave.*

F response Synonymous with *F wave*. See preferred term, *F wave.*

***F wave** A *compound action potential* evoked intermittently from a muscle by a supramaximal electric stimulus to the nerve. Compared with the maximal amplitude *M wave* of the same muscle, the F wave has a smaller amplitude (1–5% of the *M wave*), variable configuration, and a longer, more variable latency. The F wave can be found in many muscles of the upper and lower extremities, and the latency is longer with more distal sites of stimulation. The F wave is due to antidromic activation of motor neurons. It was named by Magladery and McDougal in 1950. Compare the *H wave* and the *A wave*.

*facilitation Improvement of neuromuscular transmission that results in the activation of previously inactive muscle fibers. Facilitation may be identified in several ways:

1. *Incrementing response:* A reproducible increase in the amplitude associated with an increase in the area of successive electric responses *(M waves)* during *repetitive nerve stimulation.*

2. *Postactivation* or *posttetanic facilitation:* Nerve stimulation studies performed within a few seconds after a brief period (2–15 sec) of nerve stimulation producing *tetanus* or after a strong voluntary contraction may show changes in the configuration of the *M wave(s)* compared with the results of identical studies of the rested neuromuscular junction as follows:

   a. *Repair of the decrement:* A diminution of the decrementing response seen with slow rates (2–5 Hz) of *repetitive nerve stimulation.*

   b. *Increment after exercise:* An increase in the amplitude associated with an increase in the area of the M wave elicited by a single supramaximal stimulus.

Facilitation should be distinguished from pseudofacilitation. *Pseudofacilitation* occurs in normal persons with *repetitive nerve stimulation* at high (20–50 Hz) rates or after strong volitional contraction, and probably reflects a reduction in the temporal dispersion of the summation of a constant number of muscle fiber action potentials. *Pseudofacilitation* produces a response characterized by an increase in the amplitude of the successive M waves with a corresponding decrease in the duration of the M wave resulting in no change in the area of the negative phase of the successive M waves.

far-field potential Electric activity of biologic origin generated at a considerable distance from the recording electrodes. Use of the terms *near-field potential* and *far-field potential* is discouraged because all potentials in clinical neurophysiology are recorded at some distance from the generator and there is no consistent distinction between the two terms.

fasciculation The random, spontaneous twitching of a group of muscle fibers or a motor unit. This twitch may produce movement of the overlying skin (limb), mucous membrane (tongue), or digits. The electric activity associated with the spontaneous contraction is called the *fasciculation potential*. See also *myokymia*. Historically, the term *fibrillation* has been used to describe fine twitching of muscle fibers visible through the skin or mucous membrane, but this usage is no longer acceptable.

*fasciculation potential The electric potential often associated with a visible *fasciculation* that has the configuration of a *motor unit action potential* but that occurs spontaneously. Most commonly these potentials occur sporadically and are termed "single fasciculation potentials." Occasionally, the potentials occur as a grouped discharge and are termed a "brief repetitive discharge." The occurrence of repetitive firing of adjacent fasciculation potentials, when numerous, may produce an undulating movement of muscle (see *myokymia*). Use of the terms *benign fasciculation* and *malignant fasciculation* is discouraged. Instead, the configuration of the potentials, peak-to-peak amplitude, duration, number of phases, and stability of configuration, in addition to frequency of occurrence, should be specified.

fatigue Generally, a state of depressed responsiveness resulting from protracted activity and requiring an appreciable recovery time. Muscle fatigue is a reduction in the force of contraction of muscle fibers and follows repeated voluntary contraction or direct electric stimulation of the muscle.

fiber density (1) Anatomically, fiber density is a measure of the number of muscle or nerve fibers per unit area. (2) In *single fiber electromyography*, the fiber density is the mean number of *muscle fiber action potentials* fulfilling amplitude and rise time criteria belonging to one motor unit within the recording area of the *single fiber needle electrode* encountered during a systematic search in the weakly, voluntarily contracted muscle. See also *single fiber electromyography* and *single fiber needle electrode*.

fibrillation The spontaneous contractions of individual muscle fibers that are not visible through the skin. This term has been used loosely in electromyography for the preferred term, *fibrillation potential*.

*fibrillation potential The electric activity associated with a spontaneously contracting (fibrillating) muscle fiber. It is the action potential of a single muscle fiber. The action potentials may occur spontaneously or after movement of the needle electrode. The potentials usually fire at a constant rate, although a small proportion fire irregularly. Classically, the potentials are biphasic spikes of short duration (usually less than 5 msec) with an initial positive phase and a peak-to-peak amplitude of less than 1 mV. When recorded with concentric or monopolar needle electrodes, the firing rate has a wide range (1–50 Hz) and often decreases just before cessation of an individual discharge. A high-pitched regular sound is associated with the discharge of fibrillation potentials and has been described in the old literature as "rain on a tin roof." In addition to this classic form of fibrillation potentials, *positive sharp waves* also may be recorded from fibrillating muscle fiber when the potential arises from an area immediately adjacent to the needle electrode.

firing pattern Qualitative and quantitative descriptions of the sequence of discharge of potential waveforms recorded from muscle or nerve.

firing rate Frequency of repetition of a potential. The relationship of the frequency to the occurrence of other potentials and the force of muscle contraction may be described. See also *discharge frequency*.

frequency Number of complete cycles of a repetitive waveform in one second. Measured in *hertz* (Hz) or *cycles per second* (cps or c/sec).

frequency analysis Determination of the range of frequencies composing a potential waveform, with a measurement of the absolute or relative amplitude of each component frequency.

full interference pattern See *interference pattern*.

functional refractory period See *refractory period*.

G1, G2 Synonymous with *Grid 1, Grid 2,* and newer terms, *Input Terminal 1, Input Terminal 2*. See *recording electrode*.

"giant" motor unit action potential Use of term discouraged. It refers to a *motor unit action potential* with a peak-to-peak amplitude and duration much greater than the range recorded in corresponding muscles in normal persons of similar age. Quantitative measurements of amplitude and duration are preferable.

Grid 1 Synonymous with *G1, Input Terminal 1*, or *active* or *exploring electrode*. See *recording electrode*.

Grid 2 Synonymous with *G2, Input Terminal 2*, or *reference electrode*. See *recording electrode*.

ground electrode An electrode connected to the patient and to a large conducting body (such as the earth) used as a common return for an electric circuit and as an arbitrary zero potential reference point.

grouped discharge The term has been used historically to describe three phenomena: (1) irregular, voluntary grouping of *motor unit action potentials* as seen in a tremulous muscular contraction, (2) involuntary grouping of *motor unit action potentials* as seen in *myokymia,* (3) general term to describe repeated firing of *motor unit action potentials.* See preferred term, *repetitive discharge.*

H reflex Abbreviation for Hoffmann reflex. See *H wave.*

H response See preferred term, *H wave.*

*H wave A compound muscle action potential having a consistent latency evoked regularly, when present, from a muscle by an electric stimulus to the nerve. It is regularly found only in a limited group of physiologic extensors, particularly the calf muscles. The H wave is obtained most easily with the cathode positioned proximal to the anode. Compared with the maximum amplitude *M wave* of the same muscle, the H wave has a smaller amplitude, a longer latency, and a lower optimal stimulus intensity. The latency is longer with more distal sites of stimulation. A stimulus intensity sufficient to elicit a maximal amplitude M wave reduces or abolishes the H wave. The H wave is thought to be due to a spinal reflex, the Hoffmann reflex, with electric stimulation of afferent fibers in the mixed nerve to the muscle and activation of motor neurons to the muscle through a monosynaptic connection in the spinal cord. The reflex and wave are named in honor of Hoffmann's description (1918). Compare the *F wave.*

habituation Decrease in size of a reflex motor response to an afferent stimulus when the latter is repeated, especially at regular and recurring short intervals.

hertz (Hz) Unit of frequency equal to *cycles per second.*

Hoffmann reflex See *H wave.*

hyperpolarization See *polarization.*

Hz See *hertz.*

Increased insertion activity See *insertion activity.*

*increment after exercise See *facilitation.*

incremental response See preferred term, *incrementing response.*

*incrementing response   A reproducible increase in amplitude and/or area of successive responses (M wave) to *repetitive nerve stimulation*. The rate of stimulation and the number of stimuli should be specified. An incrementing response is commonly seen in two situations. First, in normal persons the configuration of the M wave may change with repetitive nerve stimulation so that the amplitude increases progressively as the duration decreases, but the area of the M wave remains the same. This phenomenon is termed *pseudofacilitation*. Second, in disorders of neuromuscular transmission, the configuration of the M wave may change with repetitive nerve stimulation so that the amplitude progressively increases as the duration remains the same or increases, and the area of the M wave increases. This phenomenon is termed *facilitation*. Contrast with *decrementing response*.

indifferent electrode   Synonymous with *reference electrode*. Use of term discouraged. See *recording electrode*.

inhibitory postsynaptic potential (IPSP)   A local graded hyperpolarization of a neuron in response to activation at a synapse by a nerve terminal. Contrast with *excitatory postsynaptic potential*.

injury potential   The potential difference between a normal region of the surface of a nerve or muscle and a region that has been injured; also called a *demarcation potential*. The injury potential approximates the potential across the membrane because the injured surface is almost at the potential of the inside of the cell.

Input Terminal 1   The input terminal of the differential amplifier at which negativity, relative to the other input terminal, produces an upward deflection on the graphic display. Synonymous with *active* or *exploring electrode* (or older term, *Grid 1*). See *recording electrode*.

Input Terminal 2   The input terminal of the differential amplifier at which negativity, relative to the other input terminal, produces a downward deflection on the graphic display. Synonymous with *reference electrode* (or older term, *Grid 2*). See *recording electrode*.

*insertion activity   Electric activity caused by insertion or movement of a needle electrode. The amount of the activity may be described as normal, reduced, and increased (prolonged), with a description of the waveform and repetitive rate.

interdischarge interval   Time between consecutive discharges of the same potential. Measurements should be made between the corresponding points on each waveform.

interference Unwanted electric activity arising outside the system being studied.

*interference pattern Electric activity recorded from a muscle with a needle electrode during maximal voluntary effort. A *full interference pattern* implies that no individual *motor unit action potentials* can be clearly identified. A *reduced interference pattern (intermediate pattern)* is one in which some of the individual MUAPs may be identified while other individual MUAPs cannot be identified because of overlap. The term *discrete activity* is used to describe the electric activity recorded when each of several different MUAPs can be identified. The term *single unit pattern* is used to describe a single MUAP, firing at rapid rate (should be specified) during maximum voluntary effort. The force of contraction associated with the interference pattern should be specified. See also *recruitment pattern.*

intermediate interference pattern See *interference pattern.*

International 10–20 System A system of electrode placement on the scalp in which electrodes are placed either 10% or 20% of the total distance between the nasion and inion in the sagittal plane, and between right and left preauricular points in the coronal plane.

interpeak interval Difference between the peak latencies of two components of a waveform.

interpotential interval Time between two different potentials. Measurement should be made between the corresponding parts on each waveform.

involuntary activity *Motor unit potentials* that are not under voluntary control. The condition under which they occur should be described, e.g., spontaneous or reflex potentials and, if elicited by a stimulus, the nature of the stimulus. Contrast with *spontaneous activity.*

IPSP See *inhibitory postsynaptic potential.*

irregular potential See preferred term, *serrated action potential.*

iterative discharge See preferred term, *repetitive discharge.*

*jitter Synonymous with single fiber electromyographic jitter. Jitter is the variability with consecutive discharges of the *interpotential interval* between two muscle fiber action potentials belonging to the same motor unit. It usually is expressed quantitatively as the mean value of the difference between the interpotential intervals of successive discharges (the mean consecutive difference, MCD). Under certain conditions, jitter is expressed as the mean value of the difference between interpotential intervals arranged in the order of decreasing interdischarge intervals (the mean sorted difference, MSD).

Jolly test A technique described by Jolly (1895), who applied an electric current to excite a motor nerve while recording the force of muscle contraction. Harvey and Masland (1941) refined the technique by recording the M wave evoked by repetitive, supramaximal nerve stimulation to detect a defect of neuromuscular transmission. Use of the term is discouraged. See preferred term, *repetitive nerve stimulation.*

late component (of a motor unit action potential) See preferred term, *satellite potential.*

late response A general term used to describe an evoked potential having a longer latency than the *M wave.* See *A wave, F wave, H wave,* and *T wave.*

latency Interval between the onset of a stimulus and the onset of a response. Thus, the term *onset latency* is a tautology and should not be used. The *peak latency* is the interval between the onset of a stimulus and a specified peak of the evoked potential.

latency of activation The time required for an electric stimulus to depolarize a nerve fiber (or bundle of fibers as in a nerve trunk) beyond threshold and to initiate a regenerative action potential in the fiber(s). This time usually is of the order of 0.1 msec or less. An equivalent term now rarely used in the literature is the ''utilization time.''

latent period See synonym, *latency.*

linked potential See preferred term, *satellite potential.*

long-latency SEP That portion of a *somatosensory evoked potential* normally occurring at a time greater than 100 msec after stimulation of a nerve in the upper extremity at the wrist, or the lower extremity at the knee or ankle.

M response See synonym, *M wave.*

*M wave A *compound action potential* evoked from a muscle by a single electric stimulus to its motor nerve. By convention, the M wave elicited by supramaximal stimulation is used for motor nerve conduction studies. Ideally, the recording electrodes should be placed so that the initial deflection of the evoked potential is negative. The *latency,* commonly called the *motor latency,* is the latency (msec) to the onset of the first phase (positive or negative) of the M wave. The amplitude (mV) is the baseline-to-peak amplitude of the first negative phase, unless otherwise specified. The *duration* (msec) refers to the duration of the first negative phase, unless otherwise specified. Normally, the configuration of the M wave (usually biphasic) is quite stable with repeated stimuli at slow rates (1–5 Hz). See *repetitive nerve stimulation.*

macro motor unit action potential   (macro MUAP)   The average electric activity of that part of an anatomic motor unit that is within the recording range of a *macro-EMG electrode.* The potential is characterized by its consistent appearance when the small recording surface of the macro-EMG electrode is positioned to record action potentials from one muscle fiber. The following parameters can be specified quantitatively: (1) maximal peak-to-peak amplitude, (2) area contained under the waveform, (3) number of phases.

macro MUAP   See *macro motor unit action potential.*

*macroelectromyography (macro-EMG)   General term referring to the technique and conditions that approximate recording of all *muscle fiber action potentials* arising from the same motor unit.

macro-EMG   See *macroelectromyography.*

macro-EMG needle electrode   A modified *single fiber electromyography* electrode insulated to within 15 mm from the tip and with a small recording surface (25 μm in diameter) 7.5 mm from the tip.

malignant fasciculation   Use of term discouraged to describe a firing pattern of fasciculation potentials. Historically, the term was used to describe large, polyphasic fasciculation potentials firing at a slow rate. This pattern has been seen in progressive motor neuron disease, but the relationship is not exclusive. See *fasciculation potential.*

maximal stimulus   See *stimulus.*

maximum conduction velocity   See *conduction velocity.*

MCD   Abbreviation for mean consecutive difference. See *jitter.*

mean consecutive difference (MCD)   See *jitter.*

membrane instability   Tendency of a cell membrane to depolarize spontaneously, with mechanical irritation, or after voluntary activation.

MEPP   Miniature end-plate potential.

microneurography   The technique of recording peripheral nerve action potentials in man by means of intraneural electrodes.

midlatency SEP   That portion of the waveforms of a *somatosensory evoked potential* normally occurring within 25–100 msec after stimulation of a nerve in the upper extremity at the wrist, within 40–100 msec after stimulation of a nerve in the lower extremity at the knee, and within 50–100 msec after stimulation of a nerve in the lower extremity at the ankle.

miniature end-plate potential (MEPP)   The postsynaptic muscle fiber potentials produced through the spontaneous release of individual quanta of acetylcholine from the presynaptic axon terminals. As recorded with conventional concentric needle electrodes inserted in the end-plate zone, such potentials are characteristically monophasic, negative, of relatively short duration (less than 5 msec), and generally less than 20 μV in amplitude.

MNCV   Abbreviation for *motor nerve conduction velocity*. See *conduction velocity*.

monophasic action potential   An *action potential* with one phase.

monophasic end-plate activity   See *end-plate activity (monophasic)*.

monopolar needle recording electrode   A solid wire, usually stainless steel, usually coated, except at its tip, with an insulating material. Variations in voltage between the tip of the needle (active or exploring electrode) positioned in a muscle and a conductive plate on the skin surface or a bare needle in subcutaneous tissue (reference electrode) are measured. By convention, this recording condition is referred to as a monopolar needle electrode recording. It should be emphasized, however, that potential differences are always recorded between two electrodes.

motor latency   Interval between the onset of a stimulus and the onset of the resultant *compound muscle action potential (M wave)*. The term may be qualified, as *proximal motor latency* or *distal motor latency,* depending on the relative position of the stimulus.

motor nerve conduction velocity (MNCV)   See *conduction velocity*.

motor point   The point over a muscle where a contraction of a muscle may be elicited by a minimal-intensity, short-duration electric stimulus. The motor point corresponds anatomically to the location of the terminal portion of the motor nerve fibers (end-plate zone).

motor response (1) The compound muscle action potential *(M wave)* recorded over a muscle with stimulation of the nerve to the muscle, (2) the muscle twitch or contraction elicited by stimulation of the nerve to a muscle, (3) the muscle twitch elicited by the muscle stretch reflex.

motor unit The anatomic unit of an anterior horn cell, its axon, the neuromuscular junctions, and all of the muscle fibers innervated by the axon.

*motor unit action potential (MUAP) Action potential reflecting the electric activity of a single anatomic motor unit. It is the compound action potential of those muscle fibers within the recording range of an electrode. With voluntary muscle contraction, the action potential is characterized by its consistent appearance with, and relationship to, the force of contraction. The following parameters should be specified, quantitatively if possible, after the recording electrode is placed so as to minimize the *rise time* (which by convention should be less than 0.5 msec):

1. Configuration
   a. *Amplitude,* peak-to-peak (μV or mV)
   b. *Duration,* total (msec)
   c. Number of *phases (monophasic, biphasic, triphasic, tetraphasic, polyphasic)*
   d. Sign of each *phase* (negative, positive)
   e. Number of *turns*
   f. Variation of shape, if any, with consecutive discharges
   g. Presence of *satellite (linked) potentials,* if any
2. *Recruitment* characteristics
   a. Threshold of activation (first recruited, low threshold, high threshold)
   b. *Onset frequency* (Hz)
   c. Recruitment frequency (Hz) or *recruitment interval* (msec) of individual potentials

Descriptive terms implying diagnostic significance are not recommended, e.g., *myopathic, neuropathic, regeneration, nascent, giant,*

BSAP, and *BSAPP*. See *polyphasic action potential* and *serrated action potential*.

motor unit fraction   See *scanning EMG*.

motor unit potential (MUP)   See synonym, *motor unit action potential*.

motor unit territory   The area in a muscle over which the muscle fibers belonging to an individual motor unit are distributed.

movement artifact   See *artifact*.

MSD   Abbreviation for mean sorted difference. See *jitter*.

MUAP   See *motor unit action potential*.

multielectrode   See *multilead electrode*.

multilead electrode   Three or more insulated wires inserted through a common metal cannula with their bared tips at an aperture in the cannula and flush with the outer circumference of the cannula. The arrangement of the bare tips relative to the axis of the cannula and the distance between each tip should be specified.

multiple discharge   Four or more *motor unit action potentials* of the same form and nearly the same amplitude occurring consistently in the same relationship to one another and generated by this same axon or muscle fiber. See *double* and *triple discharge*.

multiplet   See *multiple discharge*.

MUP   Abbreviation for *motor unit potential*. See preferred term, *motor unit action potential*.

muscle action potential   Term commonly used to refer to a *compound muscle action potential*.

muscle cramp   Most commonly, an involuntary, painful muscle *contraction* associated with electric activity. (See *cramp discharge*.) Muscle cramps may be accompanied by other types of *repetitive discharges*, and in some metabolic myopathies (McArdle's disease) the painful, contracted muscle may show *electric silence*.

muscle fiber action potential   Action potential recorded from a single muscle fiber.

muscle fiber conduction velocity   The speed of propagation of a single *muscle fiber action potential*, usually expressed as meters per second. The muscle fiber conduction velocity usually is less than most nerve conduction velocities, varies with the rate of discharge of the muscle fiber, and requires special techniques for measurement.

muscle stretch reflex Activation of a muscle that follows stretch of the muscle, e.g., by percussion of a muscle tendon.

myoedema Focal muscle contraction produced by muscle percussion and not associated with propagated electric activity; may be seen in hypothyroidism (myxedema) and chronic malnutrition.

myokymia Continuous quivering or undulating movement of surface and overlying skin and mucous membrane associated with spontaneous, repetitive discharge of *motor unit potentials*. See *myokymic discharge, fasciculation,* and *fasciculation potential.*

*myokymic discharge *Motor unit action potentials* that fire repetitively and may be associated with clinical myokymia. Two firing patterns have been described. Commonly, the discharge is a brief, repetitive firing of single units for a short period (up to a few seconds) at a uniform rate (2–60 Hz) followed by a short period (up to a few seconds) of silence, with repetition of the same sequence for a particular potential. Less commonly, the potential recurs continuously at a fairly uniform firing rate (1–5 Hz). Myokymic discharges are a subclass of *grouped discharges* and *repetitive discharges.*

myopathic motor unit potential Use of term discouraged. It has been used to refer to low-amplitude, short-duration, polyphasic *motor unit action potentials*. The term incorrectly implies specific diagnostic significance of a motor unit potential configuration. See *motor unit action potential.*

myopathic recruitment Use of term discouraged. It has been used to describe an increase in the number of and firing rate of *motor unit action potentials* compared with normal for the strength of muscle contraction.

mytonia The clinical observation of delayed relaxation of muscle after voluntary contraction or percussion. The delayed relaxation may be electrically silent or accompanied by propagated electric activity, such as *myotonic discharge, complex repetitive discharge,* or *neuromyotonic discharge.*

*myotonic discharge Repetitive discharge at rates of 20–80 Hz are of two types: (1) biphasic (positive-negative) spike potentials less than 5 msec in duration resembling *fibrillation potentials,* and (2) positive waves of 5–20 msec in duration resembling *positive sharp waves.*

Both potential forms are recorded after needle insertion, after voluntary muscle contraction, or after muscle percussion and are due to independent, repetitive discharges of single muscle fibers. The amplitude and frequency of the potentials must both wax and wane to be identified as myotonic discharges. This change produces a characteristic musical sound in the audio display of the electromyograph because of the corresponding change in pitch, which has been likened to the sound of a "dive bomber." Contrast with *waning discharge.*

myotonic potential   See preferred term, *myotonic discharge.*

NAP   Abbreviation for *nerve action potential.* See *compound nerve action potential.*

nascent motor unit potential   From the Latin *nascens,* to be born. Use of term is discouraged as it incorrectly implies diagnostic significance of a motor unit potential configuration. Term has been used to refer to very low-amplitude, long-duration, highly polyphasic motor unit potentials observed during early states of reinnervation of muscle. See *motor unit action potential.*

NCS   See *nerve conduction studies.*

NCV   Abbreviation for *nerve conduction velocity.* See *conduction velocity.*

near constant frequency trains   See preferred term, *complex repetitive discharge.*

near-field potential   Electric activity of biologic origin generated near the recording electrodes. Use of the terms *near-field potential* and *far-field potential* is discouraged because all potentials in clinical neurophysiology are recorded at some distance from the generator and there is no consistent distinction between the two terms.

needle electrode   An electrode for recording or stimulating, shaped like a needle. See specific electrodes: *bifilar (Bipolar) needle recording electrode, concentric needle electrode, macro-EMG needle electrode, monopolar needle electrode, multilead electrode, single fiber needle electrode,* and *stimulating electrode.*

nerve action potential (NAP)   Strictly defined, refers to an action potential recorded from a single nerve fiber. The term is commonly used to refer to the compound nerve action potential. See *compound nerve action potential.*

nerve conduction studies (NCS)   Synonymous with *electroneurogra-*

phy. Recording and analysis of electric *waveforms* of biologic origin elicited in response to electric or physiologic *stimuli*. Generally, *nerve conduction studies* refer to studies of waveforms generated in the peripheral nervous system, whereas *evoked potential studies* refer to studies of waveforms generated in both the peripheral and central nervous system. The waveforms recorded in *nerve conduction studies* are *compound sensory nerve action potentials* and *compound muscle action potentials*. The *compound sensory nerve action potentials* generally are referred to as *sensory nerve action potentials*. The *compound muscle action potentials* generally are referred to by letters that have historical origins: *M wave, F wave, H wave, T wave, A wave, R1 wave*, and *R2 wave*. It is possible under standardized conditions to establish normal ranges of amplitude, duration, and latencies of these *evoked potentials* and to calculate the maximum conduction velocity of sensory and motor nerves.

nerve conduction velocity (NCV)   Loosely used to refer to the maximum nerve conduction velocity. See *conduction velocity*.

nerve fiber action potential   Action potential recorded from a single nerve fiber.

nerve potential   Equivalent to *nerve action potential*. Also commonly, but inaccurately, used to refer to the biphasic form of *end-plate activity*. The latter use is incorrect because muscle fibers, not nerve fibers, are the source of these potentials.

nerve trunk action potential   See preferred term, *compound nerve action potential*.

neurapraxia   Failure of nerve conduction, usually reversible, due to metabolic or microstructural abnormalities without disruption of the axon. See preferred electrodiagnostic term, *conduction block*.

neuromyotonia   Clinical syndrome of continuous muscle fiber activity manifested as continuous muscle rippling and stiffness. The accompanying electric activity may be intermittent or continuous. Terms used to describe related clinical syndromes are *continuous muscle fiber activity, Isaac syndrome, Isaac–Merton syndrome, quantal squander syndrome, generalized myokymia, pseudomyotonia, normocalcemic tetany*, and *neurotonia*.

*neuromyotonic discharge   Bursts of *motor unit action potentials* that originate in the motor axons firing at high rates (150–300 Hz) for a few seconds, and that often start and stop abruptly. The amplitude of the response typically wanes. Discharges may occur spontaneously or be initiated by needle movement, voluntary effort, and ischemia or percussion of a nerve. These discharges should be distinguished from *myotonic discharges* and *complex repetitive discharges*.

neuropathic motor unit potential   Use of term discouraged. It was used to refer to abnormally high-amplitude, long-duration, polyphasic *motor unit action potentials*. The term incorrectly implies a specific diagnostic significance of a motor unit potential configuration. See *motor unit action potential*.

neuropathic recruitment   Use of terms discouraged. It has been used to describe a recruitment pattern with a decreased number of *motor unit action potentials* firing at a rapid rate. See preferred terms, *reduced interference pattern, discrete activity,* and *single unit pattern*.

neurotmesis   Partial or complete severance of a nerve, with disruption of the axons, their myelin sheaths, and the supporting connective tissue, resulting in degeneration of the axons distal to the injury site.

noise   Strictly defined, potentials produced by electrodes, cables, amplifier, or storage media and unrelated to the potentials of biologic origin. The term has been used loosely to refer to one form of *endplate activity*.

onset frequency   The lowest stable frequency of firing for a single *motor unit action potential* that can be voluntarily maintained by a person.

onset latency   Tautology. See *latency*.

order of activation   The sequence of appearance of different *motor unit action potentials* with increasing strength of voluntary contraction. See *recruitment*.

orthodromic   Propagation of an impulse in the direction the same as physiologic conduction, e.g., conduction along motor nerve fibers toward the muscle and conduction along sensory nerve fibers toward the spinal cord. Contrast with *antidromic*.

paired discharge   Two action potentials occurring consistently in the same relationship with each other. Contrast with *double discharge*.

paired response   Use of term discouraged. See preferred term, *paired discharge*.

paired stimuli   Two consecutive stimuli. The time interval between the two stimuli and the intensity of each stimulus should be specified. The first stimulus is called the *conditioning stimulus* and the second stimulus is the *test stimulus*. The *conditioning stimulus* may modify the tissue excitability, which can then be evaluated by the response to the test stimulus.

parasite potential   See preferred term, *satellite potential.*

peak latency   Interval between the onset of a stimulus and a specified peak of the evoked potential.

phase   That portion of a *wave* between the departure from, and the return to, the *baseline.*

polarization   As used in neurophysiology, the presence of an electric potential difference across an excitable cell membrane. The potential across the membrane of a cell when it is not excited by an input or spontaneously active is termed the *resting potential;* it is at a stationary nonequilibrium state with regard to the electric potential difference across the membrane. *Depolarization* describes a reduction in the magnitude of the polarization toward the zero potential whereas *hyperpolarization* refers to an increase in the magnitude of the polarization relative to the resting potential. *Repolarization* describes an increase in polarization from the depolarized state toward, but not above, the normal resting potential.

polyphasic action potential   An *action potential* having five or more phases. See *phase.* Contrast with *serrated action potential.*

*positive sharp wave   A biphasic, positive-negative *action potential* initiated by needle movement and recurring in a uniform, regular pattern at a rate of 1–50 Hz; the discharge frequency may decrease slightly just before cessation of discharge. The initial positive deflection is rapid (<1 msec), its duration usually is less than 5 msec, and the amplitude is up to 1 mV. The negative phase is of low amplitude, with a duration of 10–100 msec. A sequence of positive sharp waves is commonly referred to as a *train of positive sharp waves.* Positive sharp waves can be recorded from the damaged area of fibrillating muscle fibers. Its configuration may result from the position of the needle electrode, which is felt to be adjacent to the depolarized segment of a muscle fiber injured by the electrode. Note that the positive sharp waveform is not specific for muscle fiber damage. *Motor unit* *action potentials* and potentials in *myotonic discharges* may have the configuration of positive sharp waves.

positive wave   Loosely defined, the term refers to a positive sharp wave. See *positive sharp wave.*

*postactivation depression   A descriptive term indicating a reduction in the amplitude associated with a reduction in the area of the M wave(s) in response to a single *stimulus* or *train of stimuli* that occurs a few minutes after a brief (30–60 sec), strong voluntary contraction or a period of *repetitive nerve stimulation* that produces *tetanus.* *Postactivation exhaustion* refers to the cellular mechanisms responsible for the observed phenomenon of *postactivation depression.*

postactivation exhaustion   A reduction in the safety factor (margin) of neuromuscular transmission after sustained activity of the neuromuscular junction. The changes in the configuration of the M wave due to *postactivation exhaustion* are referred to as *postactivation depression.*

postactivation facilitation   See *facilitation.*

postactivation potentiation   Refers to the increase in the force of contraction (mechanical response) after *tetanus* or strong voluntary contraction. Contrast *postactivation facilitation.*

posttetanic facilitation   See *facilitation.*

posttetanic potentiation   The incrementing mechanical response of muscle during and after *repetitive nerve stimulation* without a change in the amplitude of the action potential. In spinal cord physiology, the term has been used to describe enhancement of excitability or reflex outflow of the central nervous system after a long period of high-frequency stimulation. This phenomenon has been described in the mammalian spinal cord, where it lasts minutes or even hours.

potential   A physical variable created by differences in charges, measurable in volts, that exists between two points. Most biologically produced potentials arise from the difference in charge between two sides of a cell membrane. See *polarization.*

potentiation   Physiologically, the enhancement of a response. Some authors use the term *potentiation* to describe the incrementing mechanical response of muscle elicited by *repetitive nerve stimulation,* i.e., *posttetanic potentiation,* and the term *facilitation* to describe the incrementing electric response elicited by *repetitive nerve stimulation,* i.e., *postactivation facilitation.*

prolonged insertion activity See *insertion activity.*

propagation velocity of a muscle fiber The speed of transmission of a muscle fiber action potential.

proximal latency See *motor latency* and *sensory latency.*

*pseudofacilitation See *facilitation.*

pseudomyotonic discharge Use of term discouraged. It has been used to refer to different phenomena, including (1) *complex repetitive discharges,* and (2) *repetitive discharges* that do not wax or wane in both frequency and amplitude, and end abruptly. These latter discharges may be seen in disorders such as polymyositis in addition to disorders with *myotonic discharges.* See preferred term, *waning discharge.*

pseudopolyphasic action potential Use of term discouraged. See preferred term, *serrated action potential.*

R1, R2 waves See *blink responses.*

recording electrode Device used to record electric potential difference. All electric recordings require two *electrodes.* The recording electrode close to the source of the activity to be recorded is called the *active* or *exploring electrode,* and the other recording electrode is called the *reference electrode.* Active electrode is synonymous with *Input Terminal 1* (or older terms, *Grid 1* and *G1*) and the reference electrode with *Input Terminal 2* (or older terms, *Grid 2* and *G2*).

In some recordings, it is not certain which electrode is closer to the source of the biologic activity, i.e., recording with a *bifilar (bipolar) needle electrode.* In this situation, it is convenient to refer to one electrode as Input Electrode 1 and the other electrode as Input Electrode 2.

By present convention, a potential difference that is negative at the active electrode (Input Terminal 1) relative to the reference electrode (Input Terminal 2) causes an upward deflection on the oscilloscope screen. The term ''monopolar recording'' is not recommended, because all recording requires two electrodes; however, it is commonly used to describe the use of an intramuscular needle exploring electrode in combination with a surface disk or subcutaneous needle reference electrode. A similar combination of needle electrodes has been used to record nerve activity and also has been referred to as "monopolar recording."

recruitment The successive activation of the same and additional motor units with increasing strength of voluntary muscle contraction. See *motor unit action potential.*

recruitment frequency Firing rate of a *motor unit action potential (MUAP)* when a different MUAP first appears with gradually increasing strength of voluntary muscle contraction. This parameter is essential to assessment of *recruitment pattern.*

recruitment interval The *interdischarge interval* between two consecutive discharges of a *motor unit action potential (MUAP)* when a different MUAP first appears with gradually increasing strength of voluntary muscle contraction. The reciprocal of the recruitment intervals is the *recruitment frequency.*

*recruitment pattern A qualitative and/or quantitative description of the sequence of appearance of *motor unit action potentials* with increasing strength of voluntary muscle contraction. The *recruitment frequency* and *recruitment interval* are two quantitative measures commonly used. See *interference pattern* for qualitative terms commonly used.

reduced insertion activity See *insertion activity.*

reduced interference pattern See *interference pattern.*

reference electrode See *recording electrode.*

reflex A stereotyped *motor response* elicited by a sensory *stimulus.*

refractory period The *absolute refractory period* is the period after an *action potential* during which no stimulus, however strong, evokes a further response. The *relative refractory period* is the period after an *action potential* during which a stimulus must be abnormally large to evoke a second response. The *functional refractory period* is the period after an *action potential* during which a second *action potential* cannot yet excite the given region.

regeneration motor unit potential Use of term discouraged. See *motor unit action potential.*

relative refractory period See *refractory period.*

*repair of the decrement See *facilitation.*

repetitive discharge General term for the recurrence of an *action potential* with the same or nearly the same form. The term may refer to recurring potentials recorded in muscle at rest, during voluntary contraction, or in response to single nerve stimulus. See *double discharge, triple discharge, multiple discharge, myokymic discharge, myotonic discharge,* and *complex repetitive discharge.*

*repetitive nerve stimulation The technique of repeated supramaximal stimulations of a nerve while recording M waves from muscles innervated by the nerve. The number of stimuli and the frequency of stimulation should be specified. Activation procedures performed before the test should be specified, e.g., sustained voluntary contraction or contraction induced by nerve stimulation. If the test was performed after an activation procedure, the time elapsed after the activation procedure was completed also should be specified. The technique is used commonly to assess the integrity of neuromuscular transmission. For a description of specific patterns of responses, see the terms *incrementing response, decrementing response, facilitation,* and *postactivation depression.*

repolarization See *polarization.*

residual latency Refers to the calculated time difference between the measured distal latency of a motor nerve and the expected distal latency, calculated by dividing the distance between the stimulus cathode and the active recording electrode by the maximum conduction velocity measured in a more proximal segment of a nerve. The residual latency is due in part to neuromuscular transmission time and to slowing of conduction in terminal axons due to decreasing diameter and the presence of unmyelinated segments.

response Used to describe an activity elicited by a *stimulus.*

resting membrane potential Voltage across the membrane of an excitable cell at rest. See *polarization.*

rheobase See *strength-duration curve.*

rise time The interval from the onset of a change of a potential to its peak. The method of measurement should be specified.

*satellite potential A small action potential separated from the main MUAP by an isoelectric interval and firing in a time-locked relationship to the main *action potential.* These potentials usually follow, but may precede, the main action potential. Also called *late component, parasite potential, linked potential,* and *coupled discharge* (less preferred terms).

scanning EMG   A technique by which an electromyographic electrode is advanced in defined steps through muscle while a separate SFEMG electrode is used to trigger both the oscilloscope-sweep and the advancement device. This recording technique provides temporal and spatial information about the motor unit. Distinct maxima in the recorded activity are considered to be generated by muscle fibers innervated by a common branch of the axon. These groups of fibers form a *motor unit fraction.*

sea shell sound (sea shell roar or noise)   Use of term discouraged. See *end-plate activity, monophasic.*

sensory delay   See preferred terms, *sensory latency* and *sensory peak latency.*

sensory latency   Interval between the onset of a stimulus and the onset of the *compound sensory nerve action potential.* This term has been used loosely to refer to the *sensory peak latency.* The term may be qualified as *proximal sensory latency* or *distal sensory latency,* depending on the relative position of the stimulus.

sensory nerve action potential (SNAP)   See *compound sensory nerve action potential.*

sensory nerve conduction velocity   See *conduction velocity.*

sensory peak latency   Interval between the onset of a *stimulus* and the peak of the negative phase of the *compound sensory nerve action potential.* Note that the term *latency* refers to the interval between the onset of a stimulus and the onset of a response.

sensory potential   Used to refer to the compound sensory nerve action potential. See *compound sensory nerve action potential.*

sensory response   Used to refer to a sensory evoked potential, e.g., *compound sensory nerve action potential.*

SEP   See *somatosensory evoked potential.*

serrated action potential   An action potential waveform with several changes in direction *(turns)* that do not cross the baseline. This term is preferred to the terms *complex action potential* and *pseudopolyphasic action potential.* See also *turn* and *polyphasic action potential.*

SFEMG   See *single fiber electromyography*.

shock artifact   See *artifact*.

***short-latency somatosensory evoked potential** (SSEP)   That portion of the waveforms of a *somatosensory evoked potential* normally occurring within 25 msec after stimulation of the median nerve in the upper extremity at the wrist, 40 msec after stimulation of the common peroneal nerve in the lower extremity at the knee, and 50 msec after stimulation of the posterior tibial nerve in the lower extremity at the ankle.

1. *Median nerve SSEPs:*   Normal short-latency response components to median nerve stimulation are designated P̄9, P̄1̄1̄, P̄1̄3̄, P̄1̄4̄, N̄2̄0̄, and P̄2̄3̄ in records taken between scalp and noncephalic reference electrodes, and N̄9̄, N̄1̄1̄, N̄1̄3̄, and N̄1̄4̄ in cervical spine-scalp derivation. It should be emphasized that potentials having opposite polarity but similar latency in spine-scalp and scalp-noncephalic reference derivations do not necessarily have identical generator sources.

2. *Common peroneal nerve SSEPs:*   Normal short-latency response components to common peroneal stimulation are designated P̄2̄7̄ and N̄3̄5̄ in records taken between scalp and noncephalic reference electrodes, and L3 and T12 from a cervical spine-scalp derivation.

3. *Posterior tibial nerve SSEPs:*   Normal short-latency response components to posterior tibial nerve stimulation are designated as the PF potential in the popliteal fossa, P̄3̄7̄ and N̄4̄5̄ waves in records taken between scalp and noncephalic reference electrode, and L3 and T12 potentials from a cervical spine-scalp derivation.

silent period   A pause in the electric activity of a muscle such as that seen after rapid unloading of a muscle.

***single fiber electromyography** (SFEMG)   General term referring to the technique and conditions that permit recording of a single *muscle fiber action potential*. See *single fiber needle electrode* and *jitter*.

single fiber EMG   See *single fiber electromyography*.

single fiber needle electrode   A needle *electrode* with a small recording surface (usually 25 μm in diameter) permitting the recording of single muscle fiber action potentials between the active recording surface and the cannula. See *single fiber electromyography*.

single unit pattern   See *interference pattern*.

SNAP   Abbreviation for *sensory nerve action potential*. See *compound sensory nerve action potential*.

somatosensory evoked potentials (SEPs)   Electric waveforms of biologic origin elicited by electric stimulation or physiologic activation of peripheral sensory fibers, e.g., the median nerve, common peroneal nerve, or posterior tibial nerve. The normal SEP is a complex waveform with several components that are specified by polarity and average peak latency. The polarity and latency of individual components depend on (1) patient variables, such as age and sex, (2) stimulus characteristics, such as intensity, rate of stimulation, and (3) recording parameters, such as amplifier time constants, electrode placement, and electrode combinations. See *short-latency SEPs*.

spike   (1) In cellular neurophysiology, a short-lived (usually in the range of 1–3 msec), all-or-none change in membrane potential that arises when a graded response passes a threshold; (2) The electric record of a nerve impulse or similar event in muscle or elsewhere; (3) In clinical EEG recordings, a wave with a duration less than 80 msec (usually 15–80 msec).

spinal evoked potential   Electric waveforms of biologic origin recorded over the sacral, lumbar, thoracic, or cervical spine in response to electric stimulation or physiologic activation of peripheral sensory fibers. See preferred term, *somatosensory evoked potential*.

spontaneous activity   Electric activity recorded from muscle or nerve at rest after insertion activity has subsided and when there is no voluntary contraction or external stimulus. Compare with *involuntary activity*.

SSEP   See *short-latency somatosensory evoked potential*.

staircase phenomenon   The progressive increase in the force of a muscle contraction observed in response to continued low rates of direct or indirect muscle stimulation.

stigmatic electrode   Of historic interest. Used by Sherrington for *active* or *exploring electrode*.

stimulating electrode   Device used to apply electric current. All electric stimulation requires two electrodes: the negative terminal is termed the *cathode* and the positive terminal, the *anode*. By convention, the stimulating electrodes are called *"bipolar"* if they are encased or attached together. Stimulating electrodes are called *"monopolar"* if they are not encased or attached together. Electric stimulation for *nerve conduction studies* generally requires application of the cathode to produce depolarization of the nerve trunk fibers. If the anode is placed inadvertently between the cathode and the recording electrodes, a focal block of nerve conduction *(anodal block)* may occur and cause a technically unsatisfactory study.

stimulus   Any external agent, state, or change that is capable of influencing the activity of a cell, tissue, or organisms. In clinical *nerve conduction studies,* an electric stimulus generally is applied to a nerve or a muscle. The electric stimulus may be described in absolute terms or with respect to the evoked potential of the nerve or muscle. In absolute terms, the electric stimulus is defined by a duration (msec), a waveform (square, exponential, linear, etc.), and a strength or intensity measured in voltage (V) or current (mA). With respect to the evoked potential, the stimulus may be graded as subthreshold, threshold, submaximal, maximal, or supramaximal. A *threshold stimulus* is that stimulus just sufficient to produce a detectable response. Stimuli less than the threshold stimulus are termed *subthreshold.* The *maximal stimulus* is the stimulus intensity after which a further increase in the stimulus intensity causes no increase in the amplitude of the evoked potential. Stimuli of intensity below this level but above threshold are *submaximal.* Stimuli of intensity greater than the maximal stimulus are termed *supramaximal.* Ordinarily, supramaximal stimuli are used for nerve conduction studies. By convention, an electric stimulus of approximately 20% greater voltage/current than required for the maximal stimulus may be used for supramaximal stimulation. The frequency, number, and duration of a series of stimuli should be specified.

stimulus artifact   See *artifact.*

strength-duration curve   Graphic presentation of the relationship between the intensity (Y axis) and various durations (X axis) of the threshold electric stimulus for a muscle with the stimulating cathode positioned over the *motor point.* The *rheobase* is the intensity of an electric current of infinite duration necessary to produce a minimal visible twitch of a muscle when applied to the motor point. In clinical practice, a duration of 300 msec is used to determine the rheobase. The *chronaxie* is the time required for an electric current twice the *rheobase* to elicit the first visible muscle twitch.

submaximal stimulus See *stimulus*.

subthreshold stimulus See *stimulus*.

supramaximal stimulus See *stimulus*.

surface electrode Conducting device for stimulating or recording placed on a skin surface. The material (metal, fabric), configuration (disk, ring), size, and separation should be specified. See *electrode (ground, recording, stimulating)*.

synchronized fibrillation See preferred term, *complex repetitive discharge*.

*T wave A compound action potential evoked from a muscle by rapid stretch of its tendon, as part of the muscle stretch reflex.

temporal dispersion Relative desynchronization of components of a compound action potential due to different rates of conduction of each synchronously evoked component from the stimulation point to the recording electrode.

terminal latency Synonymous with preferred term, *distal latency*. See *motor latency* and *sensory latency*.

test stimulus See *paired stimuli*.

tetanic contraction The contraction produced in a muscle through repetitive maximal direct or indirect stimulation at a sufficiently high frequency to produce a smooth summation of successive maximum twitches. The term also may be applied to maximum voluntary contractions in which the firing frequencies of most or all of the component motor units are sufficiently high that successive twitches of individual motor units fuse smoothly. Their tensions all combine to produce a steady, smooth maximum contraction of the whole muscle.

tetanus The continuous contraction of muscle caused by repetitive stimulation or discharge of nerve or muscle. Contrast *tetany*.

tetany A clinical syndrome manifested by muscle twitching, cramps, and carpal and pedal spasm. These clinical signs are manifestations of peripheral and central nervous system nerve irritability from several causes. In these conditions, *repetitive discharges (double discharge, triple discharge, multiple discharge)* occur frequently with voluntary activation of *motor unit action potentials* or may appear as *sponta-*

neous activity and are enhanced by systemic alkalosis or local ischemia.

tetraphasic action potential   *Action potential* with four phases.

threshold   The level at which a clear and abrupt transition occurs from
one state to another. The term generally is used to refer to the voltage
level at which an *action potential* is initiated in a single axon or a
group of axons. It also is operationally defined as the intensity that
produced a response in about 50% of equivalent trials.

threshold stimulus   See *stimulus*.

train of positive sharp waves   See *positive sharp wave*.

train of stimuli   A group of stimuli. The duration of the group or the
number of stimuli and the frequency of the stimuli should be specified.

triphasic action potential   *Action potential* with three phases.

triple discharge   Three *motor unit action potentials* of the same form
and nearly the same amplitude, occurring consistently in the same
relationship to one another and generated by this same axon or muscle fiber. The interval between the second and the third action potential often exceeds that between the first two, and both usually are in
the range of 2–20 msec.

triplet   See *triple discharge*.

turn   Point of change in direction in the waveform and the magnitude
of the voltage change after the turning point. It is not necessary that
the voltage change passes through the baseline. The minimal excur-
sion required to constitute a change should be specified.

unipolar needle electrode   See synonym, *monopolar needle recording
electrode*.

utilization time   See preferred term, *latency of activation*.

VEPs   See *visual evoked potentials*.

VERs   Abbreviation for *visual evoked responses*. See *visual evoked
potentials*.

*****visual evoked potentials** (VEPs)   Electric waveforms of biologic origin
are recorded over the cerebrum and elicited by light stimuli. VEPs
are classified by stimulus rate as transient or steady-state VEPs, and
can be divided further by presentation mode. The normal transient
VEP to checkerboard pattern reversal or shift has a major positive
occipital peak at about 100 msec (P$\overline{100}$), often preceded by a negative

peak ($\overline{N75}$). The precise range of normal values for the latency and amplitude of $\overline{P100}$ depends on several factors: (1) patient variables, such as age, sex, and visual acuity, (2) stimulus characteristics, such as type of stimulator, full-field or half-field stimulation, check size, contrast, and luminescence, and (3) recording parameters, such as placement and combination of recording electrodes.

visual evoked responses (VERs) See *visual evoked potentials.*

volitional activity See *voluntary activity.*

voltage Potential difference between two recording sites.

volume conduction Spread of current from a potential source through a conducting medium, such as the body tissues.

voluntary activity In electromyography, the electric activity recorded from a muscle with consciously controlled muscle contraction. The effort made to contract the muscle should be specified relative to that of a corresponding normal muscle, e.g., minimal, moderate, or maximal. If the recording remains isoelectric during the attempted contraction of the muscle and artifacts have been excluded, it can be concluded that there is no voluntary activity.

waning discharge General term referring to a *repetitive discharge* that gradually decreases in frequency or amplitude before cessation. Contrast with *myotonic discharge.*

wave An undulating line constituting a graphic representation of change, e.g., a changing electric potential difference. See *A wave, F wave, H wave,* and *M wave.*

waveform The shape of a *wave.* The term often is used synonymously with wave.

SECTION II:
ILLUSTRATIONS OF SELECTED WAVEFORMS

Figure 1. Compound sensory nerve action potentials

Figure 2. Short-latency SEPs of the median nerve

Figure 3. Short-latency SEPs of the common peroneal nerve

Figure 4. Short-latency SEPs of the posterior tibial nerve

Each illustration is accompanied by a complete explanation that is the same as that given in the glossary. The definitions have been repeated fully with the illustrations so that readers do not need to refer back and forth between the illustrations and the definitions.

The illustrations have been modified and adapted from material submitted by members of the AAEE. The illustrations of the short-latency somatosensory evoked potentials were reproduced from the *Journal of Clinical Neurophysiology* (1978; 1:41–53) with permission of the Journal editor and the authors.

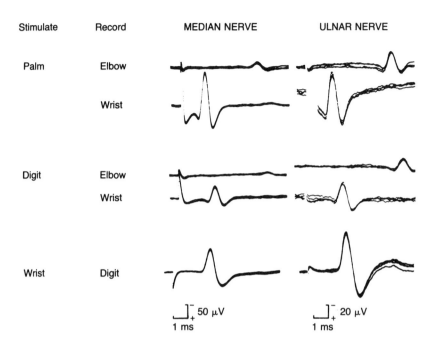

Figure 1. *Compound sensory nerve action potentials* recorded with surface electrodes in a normal person. A compound nerve action potential is considered to have been evoked from afferent fibers if the recording electrodes detect activity only in a sensory nerve or in a sensory branch of a mixed nerve, or if the electric stimulus is applied to a sensory nerve or a dorsal nerve root, or an adequate stimulus is applied synchronously to sensory receptors. The amplitude, latency, duration, and configuration should be noted. Generally, the amplitude is measured as the maximum peak-to-peak voltage, the latency as either the latency to the initial deflection or the peak latency to the negative peak, and the duration as the interval from the first deflection of the waveform from the baseline to its final return to the baseline. The compound sensory nerve action potential has been referred to as the *sensory response* or *sensory potential.*

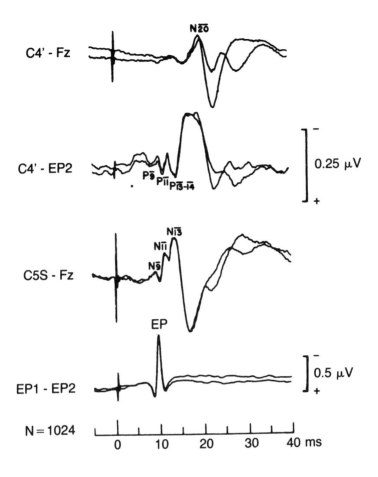

Figure 2. *Short-latency somatosensory evoked potentials* elicited by electric stimulation of the median nerve at the wrist (MN-SSEPs) occur within 25 msec of the stimulus in normal persons. Normal short-latency response components to median nerve stimulation are designated P$\overline{9}$, P$\overline{11}$, P$\overline{13}$, P$\overline{14}$, N$\overline{20}$, and P$\overline{23}$ in records taken between scalp and noncephalic reference electrodes, and N$\overline{9}$, N$\overline{11}$, N$\overline{13}$, and N$\overline{14}$ in cervical spine-scalp derivation. It should be emphasized that potentials having opposite polarity but similar latency in spine-scalp and scalp-noncephalic reference derivations do not necessarily have identical generator sources. The C4′ designation indicates that the recording scalp electrode was placed 2 cm posterior to the International 10–20 C4 electrode location.

435

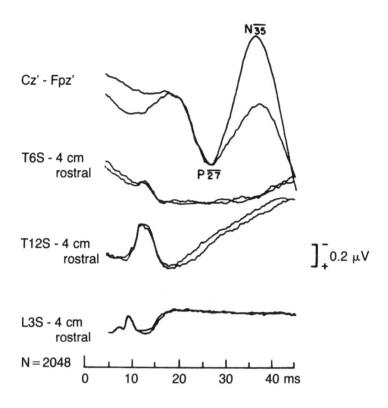

Figure 3. *Short-latency somatosensory evoked potentials* elicited by stimulation of the common peroneal nerve at the knee (CPN-SSEPs) occur within 40 msec of the stimulus in normal persons. It is suggested that individual response components be designated as follows: (1) spine components: L3 and T12 spine potentials, (2) scalp components: P27 and N35. The Cz' and Fpz' designations indicate that the recording scalp electrode was placed 2 cm posterior to the International 10–20 Cz and Fpz electrode locations.

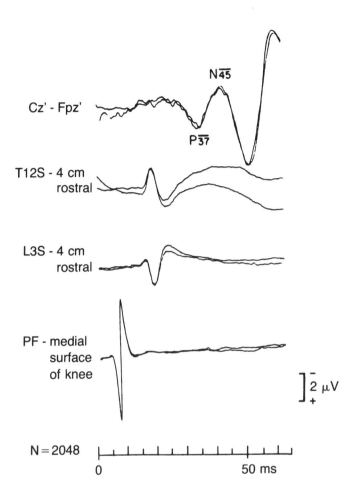

Figure 4. *Short-latency somatosensory evoked potentials* elicited by electric stimulation of the posterior tibial nerve (PTN-SSEPs) at the ankle occur within 50 msec of the stimulus in normal persons. It is suggested that individual response components be designated as follows: (1) nerve trunk (tibial nerve) component in the popliteal fossa: PF potential, (2) spine components: L3 and T12 potentials, (3) scalp components: P37 and N45 waves. The Cz' and Fpz' designations indicate that the recording scalp electrode was placed 2 cm posterior to the International 10–20 Cz and Fpz electrode locations.

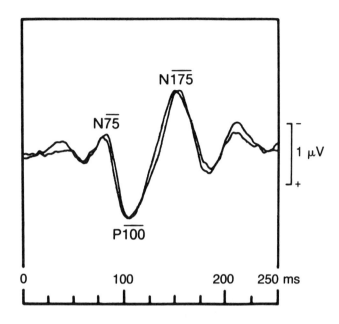

Figure 5. *Visual evoked potential (VEP).* Normal occipital VEP to checkerboard pattern reversal stimulation recorded between occipital (01) and vertex (Cz) electrodes showing N75, P100, and N175 peaks. VEPs are electric waveforms of biologic origin recorded over the cerebrum and elicited by light stimuli. VEPs are classified by stimulus rate as transient or steady-state VEPs, and can be divided further by presentation mode. The normal transient VEP to checkerboard pattern reversal or shift has a major positive occipital peak at about 100 msec (P100), often preceded by a negative peak (N75). The precise range of normal values for the latency and amplitude of P100 depends on several factors: (1) patient variables, such as age, sex, and visual acuity, (2) stimulus characteristics, such as type of stimulator, full-field or half-field stimulation, check size, contrast, and luminescence, and (3) recording parameters, such as placement and combination of recording electrodes.

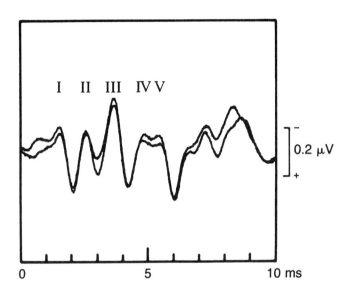

Figure 6. *Brain stem auditory evoked potential (BAEP).* Normal BAEP to stimulation of the left ear, recorded between left ear (A2) and vertex (Cz) electrodes. Brain stem auditory evoked potentials are electric waveforms of biologic origin elicited in response to sound stimuli. The normal BAEP consists of a sequence of up to seven waves, named I–VII, that occur during the first 10 msec after the onset of the stimulus and have positive polarity at the vertex of the head. In this recording, negativity in Input Terminal 1 or positivity in Input Terminal 2 causes an upward deflection.

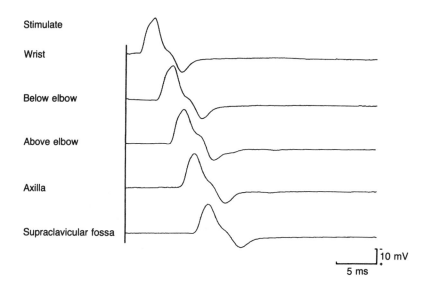

Figure 7. *M waves* recorded with surface electrodes over the abductor digiti quinti muscle elicited by electric stimulation of the ulnar nerve at several levels. The M wave is a compound action potential evoked from a muscle by a single electric stimulus to its motor nerve. By convention, the M wave elicited by supramaximal stimulation is used for motor nerve conduction studies. Ideally, the recording electrodes should be placed so that the initial deflection of the evoked potential is negative. The latency, commonly called the *motor latency,* is the latency (msec) to the onset of the first phase (positive or negative) of the M wave. The amplitude (mV) is the baseline-to-peak amplitude of the first negative phase, unless otherwise specified. The *duration* (msec) refers to the duration of the first negative phase, unless otherwise specified. Normally, the configuration of the M wave (usually biphasic) is quite stable with repeated stimuli at slow rates (1–5 Hz). See *repetitive nerve stimulation.*

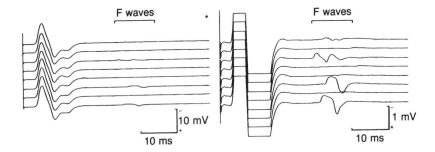

Figure 8. *F waves* recorded with surface electrodes over the abductor digiti quinti muscle elicited by electric stimulation of the ulnar nerve at the wrist with two different gain settings. The F wave is a compound action potential evoked intermittently from a muscle by a supramaximal electric stimulus to the nerve. Compared with the maximal amplitude M wave of the same muscle, the F wave has a smaller amplitude (1–5% of the M wave), variable configuration, and a longer, more variable latency. The F wave can be found in many muscles of the upper and lower extremities, and the latency is longer with more distal sites of stimulation. The F wave is due to antidromic activation of motor neurons. It was named by Magladery and McDougal in 1950. Compare the *H wave* and the *A wave.*

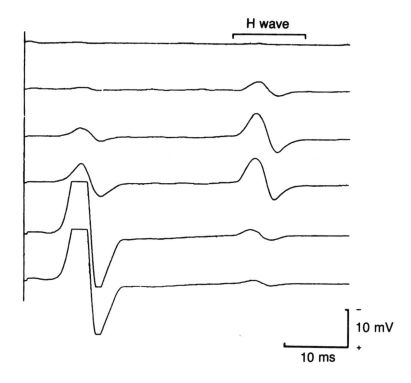

Figure 9. *H waves* recorded with surface electrodes over the soleus muscle elicited by electric stimulation of the posterior tibial nerve at the knee. The stimulus intensity was increased gradually (top tracing to bottom tracing). The H wave is a compound muscle action potential having a consistent latency evoked regularly, when present, from a muscle by an electric stimulus to the nerve. It is regularly found only in a limited group of physiologic extensors, particularly the calf muscles. The H wave is obtained most easily with the cathode positioned proximal to the anode. Compared with the maximum amplitude M wave of the same muscle, the H wave has a smaller amplitude, a longer latency, and a lower optimal stimulus intensity. The latency is longer with more distal sites of stimulation. A stimulus intensity sufficient to elicit a maximal amplitude M wave reduces or abolishes the H wave. The H wave is thought to be due to a spinal reflex, the Hoffmann reflex, with electric stimulation of afferent fibers in the mixed nerve to the muscle and activation of motor neurons to the muscle through a monosynaptic connection in the spinal cord. The reflex and wave are named in honor of Hoffmann's description in 1918. Compare the *F wave*.

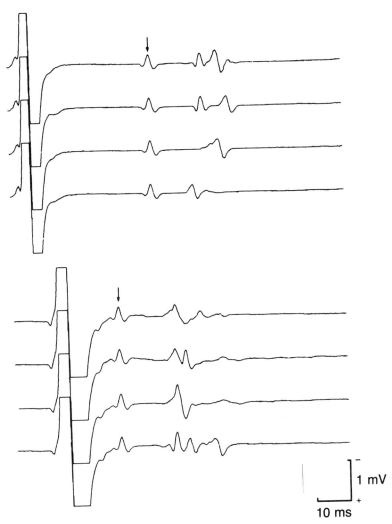

Figure 10. *A waves* (under arrow markers) recorded with surface electrodes over the abductor hallucis brevis elicited by electric stimulation of the posterior tibial nerve at the level of the ankle (top four traces) and at the level of the knee (bottom four traces). The A wave is a compound action potential evoked consistently from a muscle by submaximal electric stimuli to the nerve and frequently abolished by supramaximal stimuli. The amplitude of the A wave is similar to that of the F wave, but the latency is more constant. The A wave usually occurs before the F wave, but may occur afterward. The A wave is due to normal or pathologic axonal branching. Compare the *F wave*.

443

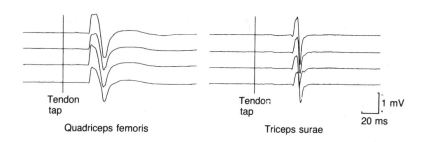

Figure 11. The *T wave* is a compound action potential evoked from a muscle by rapid stretch of its tendon, as part of the muscle stretch reflex. The T waves were recorded with surface electrodes over the quadriceps femoris (left tracings) and triceps surae (right tracings) and elicited by stretching the muscles by tapping the corresponding tendon.

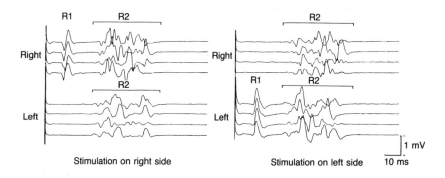

Figure 12. *Blink responses* recorded with surface electrodes over the right orbicularis oculi *(upper tracings)* and left orbicularis oculi *(lower tracings)* elicited by electric stimulation of the supraorbital nerve on the right *(left tracings)* and on the left *(right tracings)*. The blink responses are compound muscle action potentials evoked from orbicularis oculi muscles as a result of brief electric or mechanical stimuli to the cutaneous area innervated by the supraorbital (or less commonly, the infraorbital) branch of the trigeminal nerve. Typically, there is an early compound muscle action potential *(R1 wave)* ipsilateral to the stimulation site with a latency of about 10 msec and a bilateral late compound muscle action potential *(R2 wave)* with a latency of approximately 30 msec. Generally,

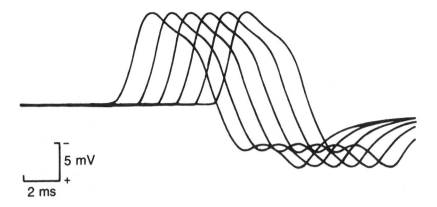

Figure 13. Study in a normal person. The successive M waves are displayed to the right. The M waves were recorded with surfaced electrodes over the hypothenar eminence (abductor digiti quinti) during ulnar nerve stimulation at a rate of 3 Hz. Note the configuration of the successive M waves is unchanged. *Repetitive nerve stimulation* is a technique of repeated supramaximal stimulations of a nerve while recording M waves from muscles innervated by the nerve. The number of stimuli and the frequency of stimulation should be specified. Activation procedures performed before the test should be specified, e.g., sustained voluntary contraction or contraction induced by nerve stimulation. If the test was performed after an activation procedure, the time elapsed after the activation procedure was completed also should be specified. The technique is used commonly to assess the integrity of neuromuscular transmission. For a description of specific patterns of responses, see the terms *incrementing response, decrementing response, facilitation,* and *postactivation depression.*

---

only the R2 wave is associated with a visible twitch of the orbicularis oculi. The configuration, amplitude, duration, and latency of the two components, along with the sites of recording and the sites of stimulation, should be specified. R1 and R2 waves probably are oligosynaptic and polysynaptic brain stem reflexes, respectively, together called the *blink reflex,* with the afferent arc provided by the sensory branches of the trigeminal nerve and the efferent arc provided by the facial nerve motor fibers.

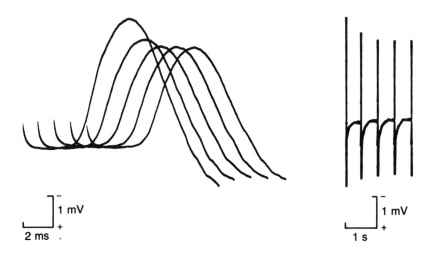

Figure 14. *Repetitive nerve stimulation* study in a patient with myasthenia gravis. Successive M waves were recorded with surface electrodes over the rested cheek (nasalis) muscle during repetitive facial nerve stimulation at a rate of 2 Hz, with a display to permit measurement of the amplitude and duration of the negative phase *(left)* or peak-to-peak amplitude *(right)*. A *decrementing response* is a reproducible decline in the amplitude and/or area of the M wave of successive responses to repetitive nerve stimulation. The rate of stimulation and the total number of stimuli should be specified. Decrementing responses with disorders of neuromuscular transmission are seen most reliably with slow rates (2–5 Hz) of nerve stimulation. A decrementing response with repetitive nerve stimulation commonly occurs in disorders of neuromuscular transmission, but also can be seen in some neuropathies, myopathies, and motor neuron disease. An artifact resembling a decrementing response can result from movement of the stimulating or recording electrodes during repetitive nerve stimulation. Contrast with *incrementing response.*

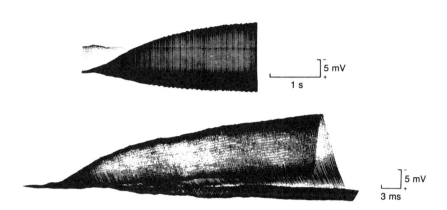

Figure 15. *Repetitive nerve stimulation* study in a patient with Lambert–Eaton myasthenic syndrome (LEMS). An *incrementing response* was recorded with surface electrodes over the hypothenar eminence *(abductor digiti quinti)* during repetitive ulnar nerve stimulation at a rate of 50 Hz with a display to permit measurement of the peak-to-peak amplitude *(top)* or amplitude and duration of the negative phase *(bottom).* An incrementing response is a reproducible increase in amplitude and/or area of successive responses (M wave) to repetitive nerve stimulation. The rate of stimulation and the number of stimuli should be specified. An incrementing response is commonly seen in two situations. First, in normal persons the configuration of the M wave may change with repetitive nerve stimulation so that the amplitude progressively increases as the duration decreases, but the area of the M wave remains the same. This phenomenon is termed *pseudofacilitation.* Second, in disorders of neuromuscular transmission, the configuration of the M wave may change with repetitive nerve stimulation so that the amplitude progressively increases as the duration remains the same or increases, and the area of the M wave increases. This phenomenon is termed *facilitation.* Contrast with *decrementing response.*

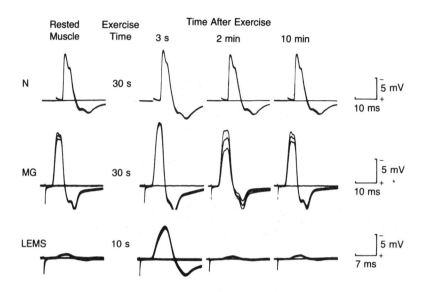

Figure 16. *Repetitive nerve stimulation* studies in a normal person (N) and patients with myasthenia gravis (MG) and Lambert–Eaton myasthenic syndrome (LEMS). Three successive M waves were elicited by repetitive nerve stimulation at a rate of 2 Hz. The three responses were superimposed. This method of display emphasizes a change in the configuration of successive responses, but does not permit identification of the order of the responses. In each superimposed display of three responses in which the configuration did change, the highest amplitude response was the first response, and the lowest amplitude response was the third response. After testing the rested muscle, the muscle was forcefully contracted for 10 to 30 sec (exercise time). The repetitive nerve stimulation was carried out again 3 sec, 2 min, and 10 min after the exercise ended. The results illustrate *facilitation* and *postactivation depression*. Facilitation is the improvement of neuromuscular transmission that

results in the activation of previously inactive muscle fibers. Facilitation may be identified in several ways:

1. *Incrementing response:* A reproducible increase in the amplitude associated with an increase in the area of successive electric responses (M waves) during repetitive nerve stimulation. (See Figure 15).

2. *Postactivation* or *posttetanic facilitation:* Nerve stimulation studies performed within a few seconds after a brief period (2–15 sec) of nerve stimulation producing tetanus or after a strong voluntary contraction may show changes in the configuration of the M wave(s) compared with the results of identical studies of the rested neuromuscular junction as follows:

   a. *Repair of the decrement:* A diminution of the decrementing response seen with slow rates (2–5 Hz) of repetitive nerve stimulation. This phenomenon is illustrated by the comparison of the results of the repetitive nerve stimulation of the MG patient before and 3 sec after exercise.

   b. *Increment after exercise:* An increase in the amplitude associated with an increase in the area of the M wave elicited by a single supramaximal stimulus. This phenomenon is illustrated by the repetitive nerve stimulation of the LEMS patient before and 3 sec after exercise.

Postactivation depression is a descriptive term indicating a reduction in the amplitude associated with a reduction in the area of the M wave(s) in response to a single stimulus or train of stimuli that occurs a few minutes after a brief (30–60 sec), strong, voluntary contraction or a period of repetitive nerve stimulation that produces tetanus. *Postactivation exhaustion* refers to the cellular mechanisms responsible for the observed phenomenon of postactivation depression. Postactivation depression is illustrated by comparison of the magnitude of the decrementing response to repetitive nerve stimulation in the MG patient before and 2 min after exercise.

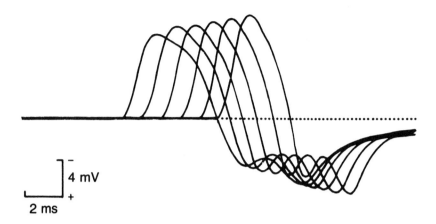

4 mV

2 ms

Figure 17. *Repetitive nerve stimulation* study in a normal person. The successive M waves were recorded with surface electrodes over the hypothenar eminence (abductor digiti quinti) during ulnar nerve stimulation at a rate of 30 Hz. Pseudofacilitation may occur in normal persons with repetitive nerve stimulation at high (20–50 Hz) rates or after strong volitional contraction, and probably reflects a reduction in the temporal dispersion of the summation of a constant number of muscle fiber action potentials because of increases in the propagation velocity of action potentials of muscle cells with repeated activation. *Pseudofacilitation* should be distinguished from *facilitation.* The recording shows an incrementing response characterized by an increase in the amplitude of the successive M waves with a corresponding decrease in the duration of the M wave resulting in no change in the area of the negative phase of the successive M waves.

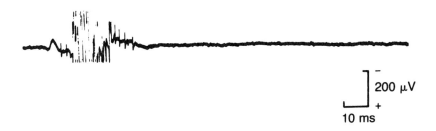

200 μV

10 ms

Figure 18. *Insertion activity* in a normal person. Insertion activity is the electric activity caused by insertion or movement of a needle electrode. The amount of the activity may be described as normal, reduced, increased (prolonged), with a description of the waveform and repetitive rate.

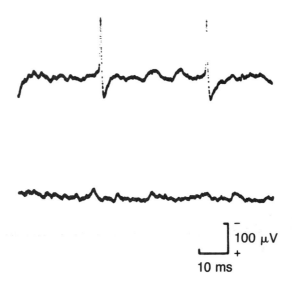

Figure 19. Spontaneous electric activity recorded with a needle electrode close to muscle end-plates. May be either of two forms:
1. *Monophasic (upper and lower traces):* Low-amplitude (10–20 μV), short-duration (0.5–1 msec), monophasic (negative) potentials that occur in a dense, steady pattern and are restricted to a localized area of the muscle. Because of the multitude of different potentials occurring, the exact frequency, although appearing to be high, cannot be defined. These nonpropagated potentials probably are miniature end-plate potentials recorded extracellularly. This form of end-plate activity has been referred to as *end-plate noise* or *sea shell sound (sea shell noise or roar).*
2. *Biphasic (upper trace):* Moderate-amplitude (100–300 μV), short-duration (2–4 msec), biphasic (negative-positive) spike potentials that occur irregularly in short bursts with a high frequency (50–100 Hz), restricted to a localized area within the muscle. These propagated potentials are generated by muscle fibers excited by activity in nerve terminals. These potentials have been referred to as *biphasic spike potentials, end-plate spikes,* and, incorrectly, *nerve potentials.*

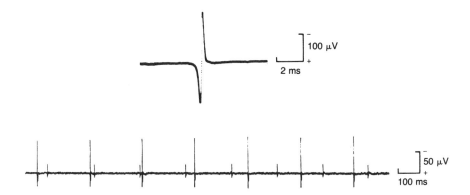

Figure 20. The *top trace* shows a single *fibrillation potential* waveform. The *bottom trace* shows the pattern of discharge of two other fibrillation potentials that differ with respect to amplitude and discharge frequency. A fibrillation potential is the electric activity associated with a spontaneously contracting (fibrillating) muscle fiber. It is the action potential of a single muscle fiber. The action potentials may occur spontaneously or after movement of the needle electrode. The potentials usually fire at a constant rate, although a small proportion fire irregularly. Classically, the potentials are biphasic spikes of short duration (usually less than 5 msec) with an initial positive phase and a peak-to-peak amplitude of less than 1 mV. When recorded with concentric or monopolar needle electrode, the firing rate has a wide range (1–50 Hz) and often decreases just before cessation of an individual discharge. A high-pitched regular sound is associated with the discharge of fibrillation potentials and has been described in the old literature as "rain on a tin roof." In addition to this classic form of fibrillation potentials, positive sharp waves also may be recorded from fibrillating muscle fibers when the potentials arises from an area immediately adjacent to the needle electrode.

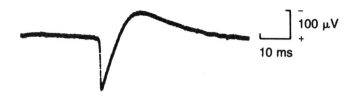

100 μV

10 ms

TRAIN OF POSITIVE SHARP WAVES

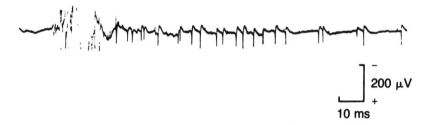

200 μV

10 ms

Figure 21. The *top trace* shows a single *positive sharp wave.* The *bottom trace* shows the pattern of initial discharge of a number of different positive sharp waves after movement of the recording needle electrode in denervated muscle. A positive sharp wave is a biphasic, positive-negative action potential initiated by needle movement and recurring in a uniform, regular pattern at a rate of 1–50 Hz; the discharge frequency may decrease slightly just before cessation of discharge. The initial positive deflection is rapid (<1 msec), its duration usually is less than 5 msec, and the amplitude is up to 1 mV. The negative phase is of low amplitude, with a duration of 10–100 msec. A sequence of positive sharp waves is commonly referred to as a *train of positive sharp waves.* Positive sharp waves can be recorded from the damaged area of fibrillating muscle fibers. Its configuration may result from the position of the needle electrode, which is felt to be adjacent to the depolarized segment of a muscle fiber injured by the electrode. Note that the positive sharp waveform is not specific for muscle fiber damage. Motor unit action potentials and potentials in myotonic discharges may have the configuration of positive sharp waves.

454

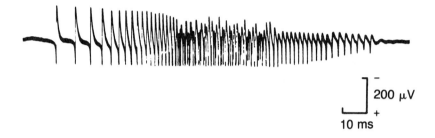

$$] \; \overset{-}{200 \; \mu V}$$
$$\underset{+}{\rule{0pt}{0pt}}$$
10 ms

Figure 22. Repetitive discharge at rates of 20–80 Hz are of two types: (1) biphasic (positive-negative) spike potentials less than 5 msec in duration resembling fibrillation potentials, (2) positive waves of 5–20 msec in duration resembling positive sharp waves. Both potential forms are recorded after needle insertion, after voluntary muscle contraction or after muscle percussion, and are due to independent, repetitive discharges of single muscle fibers. The amplitude and frequency of the potentials must both wax and wane to be identified as myotonic discharges. This change produces a characteristic musical sound in the audio display of the electromyograph due to the corresponding change in pitch, which has been likened to the sound of a "dive bomber." Contrast with *waning discharge*.

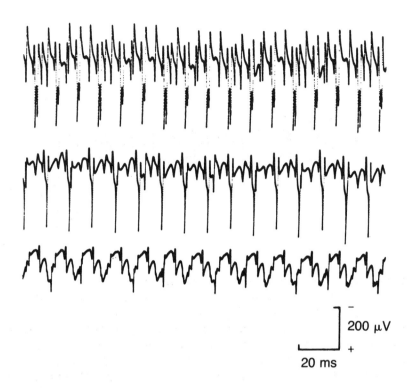

Figure 23. A *complex repetitive discharge* is a polyphasic or serrated action potential that may begin spontaneously or after a needle movement. They have a uniform frequency, shape, and amplitude, with abrupt onset, cessation, or change in configuration. Amplitude ranges from 100 μV to 1 mV and frequency of discharge from 5–100 Hz. This term is preferred to *bizarre high frequency discharge, bizarre repetitive discharge, bizarre repetitive potential, near constant frequency trains, pseudomyotonic discharge,* and *synchronized fibrillation.*

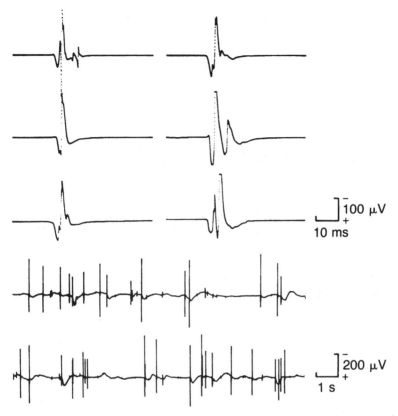

$$\overline{}100 \; \mu V$$
$$+$$
10 ms

$$\overline{}200 \; \mu V$$
$$+$$
1 s

Figure 24. Six different *fasciculation potentials* are displayed in the *top traces,* with a time scale to permit characterization of the individual waveforms. The *bottom two traces* display fasciculation potentials with a time scale to demonstrate the random discharge pattern. A fasciculation potential is the electric potential often associated with a visible fasciculation that has the configuration of a motor unit action potential but that occurs spontaneously. Most commonly these potentials occur sporadically and are termed *single fasciculation potentials.* Occasionally, the potentials occur as a grouped discharge and are termed a *brief repetitive discharge.* The occurrence of repetitive firing of adjacent fasciculation potentials, when numerous, may produce an undulating movement of muscle (see *myokymia*). Use of the terms *benign fasciculation* and *malignant fasciculation* is discouraged. Instead, the configuration of the potentials, peak-to-peak amplitude, duration, number of phases, and stability of configuration, in addition to frequency of occurrence, should be specified.

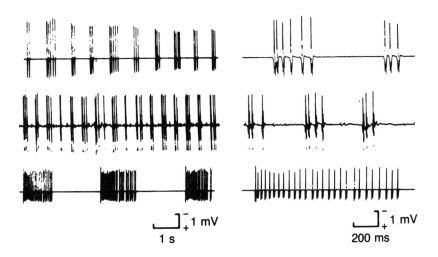

Figure 25. Tracings of three different *myokymic discharges* displayed with a time scale *(left)* to illustrate the firing pattern and with a different time scale *(right)* to illustrate that the individual potentials have the configuration of a motor unit action potential. A myokymic discharge is a group of motor unit action potentials that fire repetitively and may be associated with clinical myokymia. Two firing patterns have been described. Commonly, the discharge is a brief, repetitive firing of single units for a short period (up to a few seconds) at a uniform rate (2–60 Hz) followed by a short period (up to a few seconds) of silence, with repetition of the same sequence for a particular potential. Less commonly, the potential recurs continuously at a fairly uniform firing rate (1–5 Hz). Myokymic discharges are a subclass of grouped discharges and repetitive discharges.

First dorsal interosseous

Abductor digiti quinti

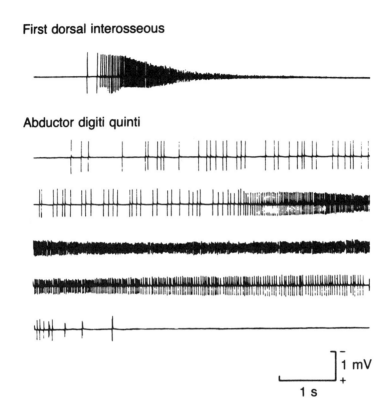

1 mV

1 s

Figure 26. The time scale was chosen to illustrate the characteristic firing pattern. A *neuromyotonic discharge* is a burst of motor unit action potentials that originate in the motor axons firing at high rates (150–300 Hz) for a few seconds, and often start and stop abruptly. The amplitude of the response typically wanes. Discharges may occur spontaneously or be initiated by needle movement, voluntary effort, and ischemia or percussion of a nerve. These discharges should be distinguished from *myotonic discharges* and *complex repetitive discharges*.

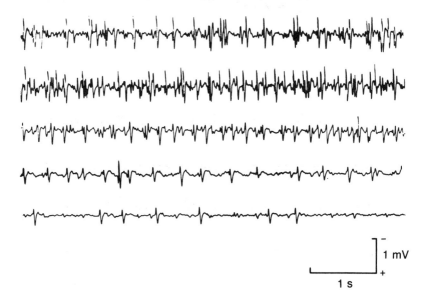

Figure 27. A *cramp discharge* arises from the involuntary repetitive firing of motor unit action potentials at high frequency (up to 150 Hz) in a large area of muscle, usually associated with painful muscle contraction. Both the discharge frequency and the number of motor unit action potentials firing increase gradually during development and both subside gradually with cessation. See *muscle cramp.*

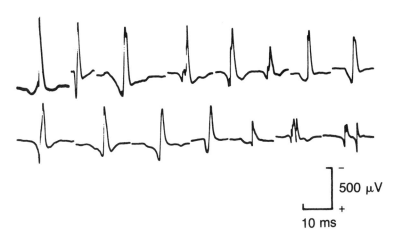

500 μV

10 ms

Figure 28. A *motor unit action potential (MUAP)* is the action potential reflecting the electric activity of a single anatomic motor unit. It is the compound action potential of those muscle fibers within the recording range of an electrode. With voluntary muscle contraction, the action potential is characterized by its consistent appearance with, and relationship to, the force of contraction. The following parameters should be specified, quantitatively if possible, after the recording electrode is placed so as to minimize the rise time (which by convention should be less than 0.5 msec).

1. Configuration
   a. Amplitude, peak-to-peak (μV or mV)
   b. Duration, total (msec)
   c. Number of phases (monophasic, biphasic, triphasic, tetraphasic, polyphasic)
   d. Sign of each phase (negative, positive)
   e. Number of turns
   f. Variation of shape, if any, with consecutive discharges
   g. Presence of satellite (linked) potentials, if any
2. Recruitment characteristics
   a. Threshold of activation (first recruited, low threshold, high threshold)
   b. Onset frequency (Hz)
   c. Recruitment frequency (Hz) or recruitment interval (msec) of individual potentials.

Descriptive terms implying significance are not recommended, e.g., myopathic, neuropathic, regeneration, nascent, giant, BSAP, and BSAPP. See *polyphasic action potential, serrated action potential.*

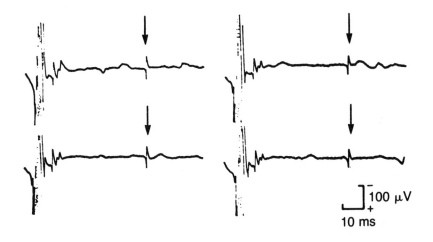

Figure 29.   Four tracings of the same motor unit action potential with the *satellite potential* indicated by the arrow. A satellite potential is a small action potential separated from the main MUAP by an isoelectric interval and firing in a time-locked relationship to the main action potential. These potentials usually follow, but may precede, the main action potential. Also called *late component, parasite potential, linked potential,* and *coupled discharge* (less preferred terms).

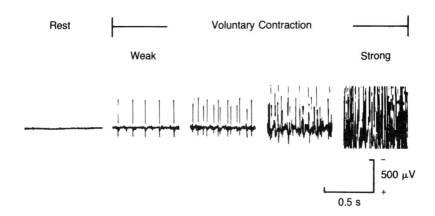

Figure 30. *Recruitment pattern* and interference pattern. Recruitment refers to the successive activation of the same and new motor units with increasing strength of voluntary muscle contraction. The recruitment pattern is a qualitative and/or quantitative description of the sequence of appearance of motor unit action potentials with increasing strength of voluntary muscle contraction. The recruitment frequency and recruitment interval are two quantitative measures commonly used. The interference pattern is the electric activity recorded from a muscle with a needle electrode during maximal voluntary effort. A full interference pattern implies that no individual motor unit action potential can be clearly identified (see tracing on *far right*). A reduced interference pattern (intermediate pattern) is one in which some of the individual MUAPs may be identified whereas other individual MUAPs cannot be identified because of overlap. The term *discrete activity* is used to describe the electric activity recorded when each of several different MUAPs can be identified. The term *single unit pattern* is used to describe a single MUAP, firing at rapid rate (should be specified) during maximum voluntary effort. The force of contraction associated with the interference pattern should be specified.

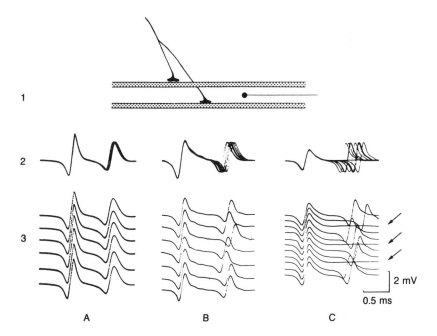

Figure 31. *Single fiber electromyography*—jitter. Schematic representation of the location of the recording surface of single fiber needle electrode recording from two muscle fibers innervated by the same motor neuron *(row 1)*. Consecutive discharges of a potential pair are shown in a superimposed display *(row 2)* and in a raster display *(row 3)*. The potential pairs were recorded from the extensor digitorum communis of a patient with myasthenia gravis and show normal jitter *(column A)*, increased jitter *(column B)*, and increased jitter and impulse blocking *(column C, arrows)*. Jitter is synonymous with "single fiber electromyographic jitter." Jitter is the variability with consecutive discharges of the interpotential interval between two muscle fiber action potentials belonging to the same motor unit. It usually is expressed quantitatively as the mean value of the difference between the interpotential intervals of successive discharges (the mean consecutive difference, MCD). Under certain conditions, jitter is expressed as the mean value of the difference between interpotential intervals arranged in the order of decreasing interdischarge intervals (the mean sorted difference, MSD).

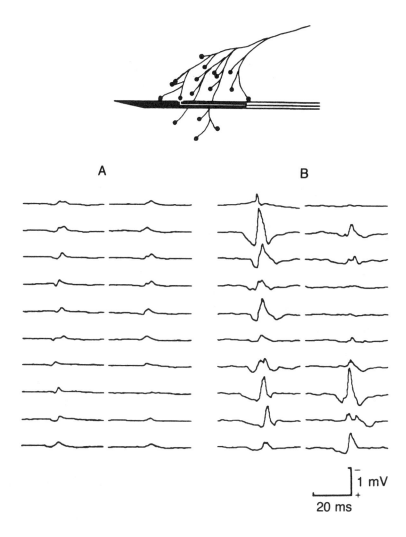

A **B**

]⁻ 1 mV
⌐____⌐ +
20 ms

Figure 32. *Macroelectromyography (macro-EMG).* Schematic representation of the location of the recording surface of the macroelectromyography electrode recording from all the muscle fibers innervated by the same motor neuron *(upper diagram).* Muscle fiber action potentials recorded by the technique of macroelectromyography *(lower traces)* from a healthy person *(column A)* and from a patient with amyotrophic lateral sclerosis *(column B).* Macroelectromyography is a general term referring to the technique and conditions that approximate recording of all muscle fiber action potentials arising from the same motor unit.

465

Bibliography

Abramson DI, Hlavova A, Rickert B, et al.: Effect of ischemia on median and ulnar motor nerve conduction velocities at various temperatures. *Arch Phys Med Rehabil* 51:463–470, 1970.

Abramson DI, Hlavova A, Rickert B, et al.: Effect of ischemia on latencies of the median nerve in the hand at various temperatures. *Arch Phys Med Rehabil* 51:471–480, 1970.

Ackermann H, Scholz E, Koehler W, Dichgans J: Influence of posture and voluntary background contraction upon compound muscle action potentials from anterior tibial and soleus muscle following transcranial magnetic stimulation. *Electroencephalogr Clin Neurophysiol* 81:71–80, 1991.

Ad Hoc Committee of the AAEM Special Interest Group on Single Fiber EMG, Gilchrist JM, Coordinator: Single fiber EMG reference values: A collaborative effort. *Muscle Nerve* 15:151–161, 1992.

Alfonsi E, Moglia A, Sandrini G, Pisoni MR, Arrigo A: Electrophysiological study of long thoracic nerve conduction in normal subjects. *Electromyogr Clin Neurophysiol* 26:63–67, 1986.

Amassian VE, Cracco RQ, Maccabee PJ: Focal stimulation of human cerebral cortex with the magnetic coil: a comparison with electrical stimulation. *Electroencephalogr Clin Neurophysiol* 74:401–416, 1989.

American Association of Electromyography and Electrodiagnosis. Nomenclature Committee: Glossary of terms in clinical electromyography. *Muscle Nerve* 10(85):G5–G60, 1987.

American Encephalographic Society: American Encephalographic Society Guidelines for intraoperative monitoring of sensory evoked potentials. *J Clin Neurophysiol* 4: 397–416, 1987.

Anziska B, Cracco RQ: Short latency somatosensory evoked potentials: Studies in patients with focal neurological disease. *Electroencephalogr Clin Neurophysiol* 49: 227–239, 1980.

Anziska BJ, Cracco RQ: Short latency SEPs to median nerve stimulation: Comparison of recording methods and origin of components. *Electroencephalogr Clin Neurophysiol* 52:531–539, 1981.

Arezzo JC, Schaumburg HH, Vaughan HG Jr, Spencer PS, Barna JA: Hind limb somatosensory evoked potentials in the monkey: The effects of distal axonopathy. *Ann Neurol* 12:24–32, 1982.

Baer RD, Johnson EW: Motor nerve conduction velocities in normal children. *Arch Phys Med Rehabil* 46:698–704, 1965.

Baran EM, Stagliano N, Whitenack S, Jaeger S, Kresch E: Sensory conduction abnormalities and brachial plexus lesions. *Muscle Nerve* 15:1186–1187, 1992.

Baran EM, Jacobs M, Kresch E, Odland J: Correlation coefficient analysis of somatosensory evoked potential waveforms. *Muscle Nerve* 7:571, 1984.

Baran EM, Grover W, Brown L: Stimulus-response characteristics of spinal evoked potentials. *Electroencephalogr Clin Neurophysiol* 52:108P, 1981. (Abstract)

Baran EM: Spinal cord responses to peripheral nerve stimulation in man. *Arch Phys Med Rehabil* 61:10–17, 1980.

Baran EM: Lumbar and thoracic spinal evoked potentials in man: Frontiers in engineering and health care. In: *Proceedings of the Fourth Annual Conference of IEEE Engineering in Medicine and Biology Society.* New York: IEEE, 1982;44–49.

Baran EM: Spinal and scalp somatosensory evoked potentials in spinal disorders. In: Course C: *Somatosensory Evoked Potentials.* Rochester, MN: American Association of Electromyography and Electrodiagnosis, 1983;57–66.

Baran EM, Daube J: Lower extremity somatosensory evoked potentials. An American Association of Electromyography and Electrodiagnosis Workshop. September 1984.

Behse F, Buchthal F: Normal sensory conduction in the nerves of the leg in man. *J Neurol Neurosurg Psychiatry* 34:404–414, 1971.

Bennett MH, Jannetta PJ: Trigeminal evoked potentials in humans. *Electroencephalogr Clin Neurophysiol* 48:517–526, 1980.

Bhala RP, Goodgold J: Motor conduction in the deep palmar branch of the ulnar nerve. *Arch Phys Med Rehabil* 49:460–466, 1968.

Bolton CF: AAEM #40: Clinical neurophysiology of the respiratory system. *Muscle Nerve* 16:809–818, 1993.

Booth KR, Streletz LJ, Raab VE, Kerrigan JJ, Alaimo MA, Herbison GJ: Motor evoked potentials and central motor conduction: Studies of transcranial magnetic stimulation with recording from the leg. *Electroencephalogr Clin Neurophysiol* 81:57–62, 1991.

Botelho SY, Deaterly CF, Austin S, Comroe JH Jr: Evaluation of the electromyogram of patients with myasthenia gravis. *AMA Arch Neurol Psychiatry* 67:441–450, 1952.

Braddom RL, Johnson EW: H reflex: Review and classification with suggested clinical uses. *Arch Phys Med Rehabil* 55:412–417, 1974.

Braddom RL, Johnson EW: Standardization of H reflex and diagnostic use in S1 radiculopathy. *Arch Phys Med Rehabil* 55:161–166, 1974.

Bridgers SL, Delaney RC: Transcranial magnetic stimulation: An assessment of cognitive and other cerebral effects. *Neurology* 39:417–419, 1989.

Brown RH, Nash CL Jr, Berilla JA, Amaddio MD: Cortical evoked potential monitoring: A system for intraoperative monitoring of spinal cord function. *Spine* 9:256–261, 1984.

Brown RH, Nash CL: Current status of spinal cord monitoring. *Spine* 4:466–470, 1979.

Buchthal F, Rosenfalck A: Sensory conduction from digit to palm and from palm to wrist in the carpal tunnel syndrome. *J Neurol Neurosurg Psychiatry* 34:243–252, 1971.

Buchthal F, Rosenfalck A, Trojaborg W: Electrophysiological findings in entrapment of the median nerve at wrist and elbow. *J Neurol Neurosurg Psychiatry* 37:340–360, 1974.

Buchthal F: Electromyography in the evaluation of muscle diseases. *Neurol Clin* 3: 573–598, 1985.

Buchthal F, Rosenfalck A: Evoked action potentials and conduction velocity in human sensory nerves. *Brain Res* 3:1–119, 1966.

Butler ET, Johnson EW, Kaye ZA: Normal conduction velocity in the lateral femoral cutaneous nerve. *Arch Phys Med Rehabil* 55:31–32, 1974.

Caldwell JW, Crane CR, Boland GL: Determinations of intercostal motor conduction time in diagnosis of nerve root compression. *Arch Phys Med Rehabil* 49:515–518, 1968.

Campbell WW, Pridgeon RM, Sahni KS: Short segment incremental studies in the evaluation of ulnar neuropathy at the elbow. *Muscle Nerve* 15:1050–1054, 1992.

Campbell WW, Ward LC, Swift TR: Nerve conduction velocity varies inversely with height. *Muscle Nerve* 4:520–523, 1981.

Celesia GG, Kaufman D, Cone S: Effects of age and sex on pattern electroretinograms and visual evoked potentials. *Electroencephalogr Clin Neurophysiol* 68:161–171, 1987.

Celesia GG, Daly RF: Effects of aging on visual evoked responses. *Arch Neurol* 34: 403–407, 1977.

Celesia GG: Steady-state and transient visual evoked potentials in clinical practice. *Ann NY Acad Sci* 388:290–307, 1982.

Celesia GG, Daly RF: Visual electroencephalographic computer analysis (VECA). *Neurology* 27:637–641, 1977.

Cerra D, Johnson EW: Motor conduction velocity in premature infants. *Arch Phys Med Rehabil* 43:160–164, 1962.

Chang CW, Lien IN: Comparison of sensory nerve conduction in the palmar cutaneous branch and first digital branch of the median nerve: A new diagnostic method for carpal tunnel syndrome. *Muscle Nerve* 14:1173–1176, 1991.

Checkles NS, Russakov AD, Piero DL: Ulnar nerve conduction velocity: Effect of elbow position on measurement. *Arch Phys Med Rehabil* 52:362–365, 1971.

Checkles NS, Bailey JA, Johnson EW: Tape and caliper surface measurements in determination of peroneal nerve conduction velocity. *Arch Phys Med Rehabil* 50:214–218, 1969.

Cherington M: Accessory nerve: Conduction studies. *Arch Neurol* 18:708–709, 1968.

Chiappa KH: Pattern shift visual, brainstem auditory, and short-latency somatosensory evoked potentials in multiple sclerosis. *Neurology* 30(7PT2):110–123, 1980.

Chiappa KH, Cros D, Day B, Fang JJ, Macdonell R, Mavroudakis N: Magnetic stimulation of the human motor cortex: Ipsilateral and contralateral facilitation effects. *Electroencephalogr Clin Neurophysiol* 43(Suppl):186–201, 1991.

Chiappa KH, Gladstone KJ, Young RR: Brain stem auditory evoked responses: Studies of waveform variations in 50 normal human subjects. *Arch Neurol* 36:81, 1979.

Chiappa KH: *Evoked Potentials in Clinical Medicine.* New York: Raven Press, 1983.

Chiappa KH, Choi SK, Young RR: Short latency somatosensory evoked potentials following median nerve stimulation in patients with neurological lesions. In: Desmedt, JE (ed): *Progress in Clinical Neurophysiology, Vol. 7: Clinical Uses of Cerebral Brainstem and Spinal Somatosensory Evoked Potentials.* Basel: Karger, 1980; 264–281.

Chiappa KH, Cros D, Cohen D: Magnetic stimulation: Determination of coil current flow direction. *Neurology* 41:1154–1155, 1991.

Chisholm RC, Karrer R: Movement-related potentials and control of associated movements. *Int J Neurosci* 42:131–148, 1988.

Chu NS: Motor evoked potentials with magnetic stimulation: Correlations with height. *Electroencephalogr Clin Neurophysiol* 74:481–485, 1989.

Chu-Andrews J, Johnson RJ: *Electrodiagnosis: An Anatomical and Clinical Approach.* Philadelphia: JB Lippincott, 1986.

Claus D: Magnetic stimulation: Technical aspects. *Electroencephalogr Clin Neurophysiol* 43(Suppl):249–254, 1991.

Clawson DR, Cardenas DD: Dorsal nerve of the penis nerve conduction velocity: A new technique. *Muscle Nerve* 14:845–849, 1991.

Clay SA, Ramseyer JC: The orbicularis oculi reflex in infancy and childhood. *Neurology* 26:521–524, 1976.

Counter SA, Borg E, Lofqvist L, Brismar T: Hearing loss from the acoustic artifact of the coil used in extracranial magnetic stimulation. *Neurology* 40:1159–1162, 1990.

Counter SA, Borg E: Analysis of the coil generated impulse noise in extracranial magnetic stimulation. *Electroencephalogr Clin Neurophysiol* 85:280–288, 1992.

Cracco JB, Bosch VV, Cracco RQ: Cerebral and spinal somatosensory evoked potentials in children with CNS degenerative disease. *Electroencephalogr Clin Neurophysiol* 49: 437–445, 1980.

Cracco RQ: Spinal evoked response: Peripheral nerve stimulation in man. *Electroencephalogr Clin Neurophysiol* 35:379–386, 1973.

Cracco JB, Cracco RQ: Spinal somatosensory evoked potentials: Maturational and clinical studies. *Ann NY Acad Sci* 388:526–537, 1982.

Cracco RQ, Anziska BJ, Cracco JB, Vas GA, Rossini PM, Maccabee PJ: Short-latency somatosensory evoked potentials to median and peroneal nerve stimulation: Studies in normal subjects and patients with neurologic disease. *Ann NY Acad Sci* 388:412–425, 1982.

Cracco JB, Cracco RQ: Somatosensory spinal and cerebral evoked potentials in children with occult spinal dysraphism. *Neurology* 29:543, 1979. (Abstract)

Craft S, Currier DP, Nelson RM: Motor conduction of the anterior interosseous nerve. *Phys Ther* 57:1143–1147, 1977.

Cros D, Gominak S, Shahani B, Fang J, Day B: Comparison of electric and magnetic coil stimulation in the supraclavicular region. *Muscle Nerve* 15:587–590, 1992.

Cros D, Chiappa KH, Gominak S, Fang J, Santamaria J, King PJ, Shahani BT: Cervical magnetic stimulation. *Neurology* 40:1751–1756, 1990.

Date M, Schmid UD, Hess CW, Schmid J: Influence of peripheral nerve stimulation on the responses in small hand muscles to transcranial magnetic cortex stimulation. *Electroencephalogr Clin Neurophysiol* 43(Suppl):212–223, 1991.

Daube JR: Needle examination in clinical electromyography (AAEM Minimonograph #11). *Muscle Nerve* 14:685–700, 1991.

Davis JN: Phrenic nerve conduction in man. *J Neurol Neurosurg Psychiatry* 30:420–426, 1967.

Del Toro DR, Park TA, Mandel JD, Wertsch JJ: Development of a nerve conduction study technique for the medical calcaneal nerve. *Muscle Nerve* 15:1194, 1992. (Abstract)

Delbeke J, McComas AJ, Kopec SJ: Analysis of evoked lumbosacral potentials in man. *J Neurol Neurosurg Psychiatry* 41:293–302, 1978.

Desmedt JE, Brunko E, Debecker J: Maturation of the somatosensory evoked potentials in normal infants and children, with special reference to the early N1 component. *Electroencephalogr Clin Neurophysiol* 40:43–58, 1976.

Desmedt JE, Borenstein S: Diagnosis of myasthenia gravis by nerve stimulation. *Ann NY Acad Sci* 274:174–188, 1976.

Desmedt JE: The neuromuscular disorder in myasthenia gravis. II. Presynaptic cholinergic metabolism, myasthenic-like syndromes and a hypothesis. In: Desmedt JE (ed): *New Developments in Electromyography and Clinical Neurophysiology, Vol 1*. Basel: Karger, 1973;305–342.

Desmedt JE: The neuromuscular disorder in myasthenia gravis: I Electrical and mechanical response to nerve stimulation in hand muscles. In: Desmedt JE (ed): *New Developments in Electromyography and Clinical Neurophysiology, Vol 1*. Basel: Karger, 1973; 241–304.

Devi S, Lovelace RE, Duarte N: Proximal peroneal nerve conduction velocity: Recording from anterior tibial and peroneal brevis muscles. *Ann Neurol* 2:116–119, 1977.

deVisser O, Schimsheimer RJ, Hart AAM: The H-reflex of the flexor carpi radialis muscle: A study in controls and radiation-induced brachial plexus lesions. *J Neurol Neurosurg Psychiatry* 47:1098–1101, 1984.

Dhuna A, Gates J, Pascual-Leone A: Transcranial magnetic stimulation in patients with epilepsy. *Neurology* 41:1067–1071, 1991.

DiBenedetto M: Sensory nerve conduction in lower extremities. *Arch Phys Med Rehabil* 51:253–286 (passim), 1970.

Dick HC, Bradley WE, Scott FB, Timm GW: Pudendal sexual reflexes. Electrophysiologic investigations. *Urology* 3:376–379, 1974.

Dimitrijevic MR, Larsson LE, Lehmkuhl D, Sherwood A: Evoked spinal cord and nerve root potentials in humans using a non-invasive recording technique. *Electroencephalogr Clin Neurophysiol* 45:331–340, 1978.

Donchin E, Calloway E, Cooper R et al.: Publication criteria for studies of evoked potentials (EP) in man. Report of a committee. In: Desmedt JH (ed): *Process in Clinical Neurophysiology, Vol 1: Attention Voluntary Contraction, and Event-Related Cerebral Potentials*. Basel: Karger, 1977;1–11.

Dumitru D, Nelson MR: Posterior femoral cutaneous nerve conduction. *Arch Phys Med Rehabil* 71:979–982, 1990.

Dvorak J, Herdmann J, Theiler R: Magnetic transcranial brain stimulation: Painless evaluation of central motor pathways. Normal values and clinical application in spinal cord diagnostics: Upper extremities. *Spine* 15:155–160, 1990.

Eisen A, Stevens JC: Upper limb somatosensory evoked potentials. An American Association of Electromyography and Electrodiagnosis Workshop. 1984;1–4.

Eisen A: *The Somatosensory Evoked Potential* (Minimonograph #19). Rochester, MN: American Association of Electromyography and Electrodiagnosis, 1982;1–19.

Eisen A, Siejka S, Schulzer M, Calne D: Age-dependent decline in motor evoked potential (MEP) amplitude: With a comment on changes in Parkinson's disease, *Electroencephalogr Clin Neurophysiol* 81:209–215, 1991.

Ekstedt J, Nilsson G, Stalberg E: Calculation of the electromyographic jitter. *J Neurol Neurosurg Psychiatry* 37:526–539, 1974.

Engler GL, Spielholz NI, Bernhard WN, Danziger F, Merkin H, Wolff T: Somatosensory evoked potentials during Harrington instrumentation. *J Bone Joint Surg* 60A:528–532, 1978.

Epstein CM, Schwartzberg DG, Davey KR, Sudderth DB: Localizing the site of magnetic brain stimulation in humans. *Neurology* 40:666–670, 1990.

Ertekin C: Saphenous nerve conduction in man. *J Neurol Neurosurg Psychiatry* 32: 530–540, 1969.

Feibel A, Foca FJ: Sensory conduction of radial nerve. *Arch Phys Med Rehabil* 55: 314–316, 1974.

Ferbert A, Mussmann N, Menne A, Buchner H, Hartje W: Short-term memory performance with magnetic stimulation of the motor cortex. *Eur Arch Psychiatry Clin Neurosci* 241:135–138, 1991.

Findler G, Feinsod M: Sensory evoked response to electrical stimulation of the trigeminal nerve in humans. *J Neurosurg* 56:545–549, 1982.

Fu R, DeLisa JA, Kraft GH: Motor nerve latencies through the tarsal tunnel in normal adult subjects: Standard determinations corrected for temperature and distance. *Arch Phys Med Rehabil* 61:243–248, 1980.

Furby A, Bourriez JL, Jacquesson JM, Mounier-Vehier F, Guieu JD: Motor evoked potentials to magnetic stimulation: Technical considerations and normative data from 50 subjects. *J Neurol* 239:152–156, 1992.

Gamstorp I: Normal conduction velocity of ulnar, median and peroneal nerves in infancy, childhood, and adolescence. *Acta Paediatr Scand* 146(Suppl):68–76.

Gamstorp I, Shelburne SA: Peripheral sensory conduction in ulnar and median nerves of normal infants, children and adolescents. *Acta Paediatr Scand* 54:309–313, 1965.

Gassel MM: A study of femoral nerve conduction time. *Arch Neurol* 9:607–614, 1963.

Gates JR, Dhuna A, Pascual-Leone A: Lack of pathologic changes in human temporal lobes after transcranial magnetic stimulation. *Epilepsia* 33:504–508, 1992.

Ghezzi A, Callea L, Zaffaroni M, Montanini R, Tessera G: Motor potentials of bulbocavernosus muscle after transcranial and lumbar magnetic stimulation: Comparative study with bulbocavernosus reflex and pudendal evoked potentials. *J Neurol Neurosurg Psychiatry* 1991;54:524–526.

Ghezzi A, Callea L, Zaffaroni M, Zibetti A, Montanini R: Study of central and peripheral motor conduction in normal subjects. *Acta Neurol Scand* 84:503–506, 1991.

Ginzburg M, Lee M, Ginzburg J, Alba A: Median and ulnar nerve conduction determinations in the Erb's point-axilla segment in normal subjects. *J Neurol Neurosurg Psychiatry* 41:444–448, 1978.

Goldberg G: Supplementary motor area structure and function: Review and hypothesis. *Behav Brain Sci* 8:567–616, 1985.

Goldie WD, Chiappa KH, Young RR, Brooks EB: Brainstem auditory and short-latency somatosensory evoked responses in brain death. *Neurology* 31:248–256, 1981.

Goodgold J, Moldaver J: Changes in electromyographic wave forms in relation to variation in type and position of electrode. *Arch Phys Med Rehabil* 36:627–630, 1955.

Green RF, Brien M: Accessory nerve latency to the middle and lower trapezius. *Arch Phys Med Rehabil* 66:23–24, 1985.

Grundy BL, Nash CL Jr, Brown RH: Deliberate hypotension for spinal fusion: Prospective randomized study with evoked potential monitoring. *Can Anaesth Soc J* 29: 452–462, 1982.

Grundy BL, Nash CL Jr, Brown RH: Arterial pressure manipulation alters spinal cord function during correction of scoliosis. *Anesthesiology* 54:249–253, 1981.

Guld C, Rosenfalck A, Willison RG: Report of the committee on EMG instrumentation: Technical factors in recording electrical activity of muscle and nerve in man. *Electroencephalogr Clin Neurophysiol* 28:399–413, 1970.

Gupta PR, Dorfman LJ: Spinal somatosensory conduction in diabetes. *Neurology* 31: 841–845, 1981.

Gutmann L: Atypical deep peroneal neuropathy. In presence of accessory deep peroneal nerve. *J Neurol Neurosurg Psychiatry* 33:453–456, 1970.

Halar EM, DeLisa JA, Soine TL: Nerve conduction studies in upper extremities: Skin temperature corrections. *Arch Phys Med Rehabil* 64:412–416, 1983.

Halar EM, DeLisa JA, Brozovich FV: Nerve conduction velocity: Relationship of skin, subcutaneous, and intramuscular temperatures. *Arch Phys Med Rehabil* 61:199–203, 1980.

Halar EM, DeLisa JA, Brozovich FV: Peroneal nerve conduction velocity: The importance of temperature correction. *Arch Phys Med Rehabil* 62:439–443, 1981.

Haldeman S, Bradley WE, Bhatia NN: Evoked responses from the pudendal nerve. *J Urol* 128:976–980, 1982.

Haldeman S, Bradley WE, Bhatia NN, Johnson BK: Pudendal evoked responses. *Arch Neurol* 39:280–283, 1982.

Halliday AM: The visual evoked potential in healthy subjects. In: Halliday AM (ed): *Evoked Potentials in Clinical Testing*. New York: Churchill Livingstone, 1982.

Halliday AM, McDonald WI, Mushin J: Delayed visual evoked response in optic neuritis. *Lancet* 1:982–985, 1972.

Harvey AM, Masland RL: A method for the study of neuromuscular transmission in human subjects. *Bull Johns Hopkins Hosp* 68:81–93, 1941.

Haymaker W, Woodhall B: *Peripheral Nerve Injuries: Principles of Diagnosis*. Philadelphia: WB Saunders; 1953.

Hong CZ, Joynt RL, Lin JC, Lufty S, Causin P, Meltzer RJ: Axillary F-loop latency of ulnar nerve in normal young adults. *Arch Phys Med Rehabil* 62:565–569, 1981.

Hrbek A, Karlberg P, Kjellmer I, Olsson T, Riha M: Clinical application of evoked electroencephalographic responses in newborn infants: I. Perinatal asphyxia. *Dev Med Child Neurol* 19:34–44, 1977.

Hufnagel A, Elger CE, Marx W, Ising A: Magnetic motor-evoked potentials in epilepsy: Effects of the disease and of anticonvulsant medication. *Ann Neurol* 28:680–686, 1990.

Hufnagel A, Jaeger M, Elger CE: Transcranial magnetic stimulation: Specific and non-specific facilitation of magnetic motor evoked potentials. *J Neurol* 237:416–419, 1990.

Hughes JR, Stone JL, Fino JJ, Hart LA: Usefulness of different stimuli in visual evoked potentials. *Neurology* 37:656–662, 1987.

Hume AL, Cant BR, Shaw NA: Central somatosensory conduction time in comatose patients. *Ann Neurol* 5:379–384, 1979.

Hume AL, Cant BR: Conduction time in central somatosensory pathways in man. *Electroencephalogr Clin Neurophysiol* 45:361–375, 1978.

Izzo KL, Sridhara CR, Rosenholtz H, Lemont H: Sensory conduction studies of the branches of the superficial peroneal nerve. *Arch Phys Med Rehabil* 62:24–27, 1981.

Jabre JF: Ulnar nerve lesions at the wrist: New technique for recording from the sensory dorsal branch of the ulnar nerve. *Neurology* 30:873–876, 1980.

Jabre JF: Surface recording of the H-reflex of the flexor carpi radialis. *Muscle Nerve* 4: 435–438, 1981.

Jaeger S, Baran E, Mandel S, Whitenack S, Kresch E, Bess H, Odland JD: Mid-latency somatosensory evoked potential abnormalities in proximal sensory neuropathies. *Muscle Nerve* 8:618, 1985. (Abstract)

Jebsen RH: Motor conduction velocity of distal radial nerve. *Arch Phys Med Rehabil* 47:12–16, 1966.

Jebsen RH: Motor conduction velocity in proximal and distal segments of the radial nerve. *Arch Phys Med Rehabil* 47:597–602, 1966.

Jerger J, Hall J: Effects of age and sex on auditory brainstem response. *Arch Otolaryngol* 106:387–391, 1980.

Jimenez J, Easton JKM, Redford JB: Conduction studies of the anterior and posterior tibial nerves. *Arch Phys Med Rehabil* 51:164–179 (passim), 1970.

Johnson EW, Kukla RD, Wongsam PE, Piedmont A: Sensory latencies to the ring finger: Normal values and relation to carpal tunnel syndrome. *Arch Phys Med Rehabil* 62: 206–208, 1981.

Johnson EW, Ortiz PR: Electrodiagnosis of tarsal tunnel syndrome. *Arch Phys Med Rehabil* 47:776–780, 1966.

Johnson EW, Melvin JL: Sensory conduction studies of median and ulnar nerves. *Arch Phys Med Rehabil* 48:25–30, 1967.

Johnson EW, Wood PK, Powers JJ: Femoral nerve conduction studies. *Arch Phys Med Rehabil* 49:528–532, 1968.

Jones SJ: Short latency potentials recorded from the neck and scalp following median nerve stimulation in man. *Electroencephalogr Clin Neurophysiol* 43:853–863, 1977.

Jones SJ, Edgar MA, Ransford AO: Sensory nerve conduction in the human spinal cord: Epidural recordings made during scoliosis surgery. *J Neurol Neurosurg Psychiatry* 45:446–451, 1982.

Jones SJ, Edgar MA, Ransford AO, Thomas NP: A system for the electrophysiological monitoring of the spinal cord during operations for scoliosis. *J Bone Joint Surg* 65B: 134–139, 1983.

Kanakamedala RV, Hong CZ: Peroneal nerve entrapment at the knee localized by short segment stimulation. *Am J Phys Med Rehabil* 68:116–122, 1989.

Kanakamedala RV, Simons DG, Porter RW, Zucker RS: Ulnar nerve entrapment at the elbow localized by the short segment stimulation. *Arch Phys Med Rehabil* 69:959–963, 1988.

Kaplan PE: Electrodiagnostic confirmation of long thoracic nerve palsy. *J Neurol Neurosurg Psychiatry* 43:50–52, 1980.

Kasai T, Hayes KC, Wolfe DL, Allatt RD: Afferent conditioning of motor evoked potentials following transcranial magnetic stimulation of motor cortex in normal subjects. *Electroencephalogr Clin Neurophysiol* 85:95–101, 1992.

Kaufman D, Celesia GG: Simultaneous recording of pattern electroretinogram and visual evoked responses in neuro-opthalmologic disorders. *Neurology* 35:644–651, 1985.

Kelly JJ, Stolov WC: Motor Unit Potential Quantitation. An American Association of Electromyography and Electrodiagnosis Workshop. September 1984.

Kim DJ, Kalantri A, Guha S, Wainapel SF: Dorsal cutaneous nerve conduction: Diagnostic aid in ulnar neuropathy. *Arch Neurol* 38:321–322, 1981.

Kimura J: F-wave velocity in the central segment of the median and ulnar nerves. A study in normal subjects and in patients with Charcot-Marie-Tooth disease. *Neurology* 24:539–546, 1974.

Kimura J, Powers JM, Van Allen MW: Reflex response of orbicularis oculi muscle to supraorbital nerve stimulation: Study in normal subjects and in peripheral facial paresis. *Arch Neurol* 21:193–199, 1969.

Kimura J, Giron LT, Young SM: Electrophysiological study of Bell palsy. *Arch Otolaryngol* 102:140–143, 1976.

Kimura I, Seki H, Sasao S, Ayyar DR: The great auricular nerve conduction study: A technique, normative data and clinical usefulness. *Electromyogr Clin Neurophysiol* 27:39–43, 1987.

Kimura J: Collision technique: Physiologic block of nerve impulses in studies of motor nerve conduction velocity. *Neurology* 26:680–682, 1976.

Kimura J, Bosch P, Lindsay GM: F·wave conduction velocity in the central segment of the peroneal and tibial nerves. *Arch Phys Med Rehabil* 56:492–497, 1975.

Kimura J: The carpal tunnel syndrome: Localization of conduction abnormalities within the distal segment of the median nerve. *Brain* 102:619–635, 1979.

Kimura J: Principles and pitfalls of nerve conduction studies. *Ann Neurol* 16:415–429, 1984.

Kimura J, Bodensteiner J, Yamada T: Electrically elicited blink reflex in normal neonates. *Arch Neurol* 34:246–249, 1977.

Kjaer M: Visual evoked potentials in normal subjects and patients with multiple sclerosis. *Acta Neurol Scand* 62:1–13, 1980.

Kjaer M: Recognizability of brain stem auditory evoked potential components. *Acta Neurol Scand* 62:20–33, 1980.

Knezevic W, Bajada S: Peripheral autonomic surface potential: A quantitative technique for recording sympathetic conduction in man. *J Neurol Sci* 67:239–251, 1985.

Kornhuber HH: Attention, readiness for action, and stages of decision—Some electrophysiological correlates in man. *Exp Brain Res* (Suppl 9):420–429, 1984.

Kornhuber HH, Deecke L: Hirnpotentialanderungen beim Menschen vor und nach Willkurbewegungen, dargestellt mit Magnetbandspeicherung und Ruckwartsanalyze. *Pflugers Arch Physiol Gesamte Menschen Tiere* 281:52, 1964. (Abstract)

Kraft GH: Axillary, musculocutaneous and suprascapular nerve latency studies. *Arch Phys Med Rehabil* 53:383–387, 1972.

Kraft GH, Johnson EW: Proximal Motor Nerve Conduction and Late Responses. An American Association of Electromyography and Electrodiagnosis Workshop. September 1986.

Kresch EN, Baran EM, Mandel S, Whitenack S, Betz RR, Bess HL: Correlation analysis of somatosensory evoked potential waveforms. *Arch Phys Med Rehabil* 73:829–834, 1992.

Kristeva R, Cheyne D, Lang W, Lindinger G, Deecke L: Movement-related potentials accompanying unilateral and bilateral finger movements with different inertial loads. *Electroencephalogr Clin Neurophysiol* 75:410–418, 1990.

Kritchevsky M, Wiederholt WC: Short-latency somatosensory evoked potentials. *Arch Neurol* 35:706–711, 1978.

Krumholtz A, Weiss HD, Goldstein PJ, Harris KC: Evoked responses in vitamin B12 deficiency. *Ann Neurol* 9:407–409, 1981.

Lambert EH, Rooke ED: Myasthenic state and lung cancer. In: Brain WR, Norris FH (eds): *Remote Effects of Cancer on the Nervous System.* Orlando: Grune and Stratton, 1965;67–80.

Lambert EH: Diagnostic value of electrical stimulation of motor nerves. *Electroencephalogr Clin Neurophysiol* 14 (Suppl 22):9–16, 1962.

Lambert EH: The accessory deep peroneal nerve. A common variation in innervation of extensor digitorum brevis. *Neurology* 19:1169–1176, 1969.

Lee HJ, Bach JR, DeLisa JA: Deep personal sensory nerve: Standardization in nerve conduction study. *Am J Phys Med Rehabil* 69:202–204, 1990.

Lee HJ, Bach JR, DeLisa JA: Lateral dorsal cutaneous branch of the sural nerve: Standardization in nerve conduction study. *Am J Phys Med Rehabil* 71:318–320, 1992.

Liberson WT, Gratzer M, Zalis A, Grabinski B: Comparison of conduction velocities of motor and sensory fibers determined by different methods. *Arch Phys Med Rehabil* 47:17–23, 1966.

Lim CL, Yiannikas C: Motor evoked potentials: A new method of controlled facilitation using quantitative surface EMG. *Electroencephalogr Clin Neurophysiol* 85:38–41, 1992.

Livingstone EF, DeLisa JA, Halar EM: Electrodiagnostic values through the thoracic outlet using C-8 root needle studies, F waves, and cervical somatosensory evoked potentials. *Arch Phys Med Rehabil* 65:726–730, 1984.

LoMonaco M, DiPasqua PG, Tonali P: Conduction studies along the accessory, long thoracic, dorsal scapular, and thoracodorsal nerves. *Acta Neurol Scand* 68:171–176, 1983.

Lovelace RE, Myers SJ, Zablow L: Sensory conduction in peroneal and posterior tibial nerves using averaging techniques. *J Neurol Neurosurg Psychiatry* 36:942–950, 1973.

Lueders H, Gurd A, Hahn J, Andrish J, Weiker G, Klem G: A new technique for intraoperative monitoring of spinal cord function: Multichannel recording of spinal cord and subcortical evoked potentials. *Spine* 7:110–115, 1982.

Lum PB, Kanakamedala R: Conduction of the palmar cutaneous branch of the median nerve. *Arch Phys Med Rehabil* 67:805–806, 1986.

Maccabee PJ, Levine DB, Pinkhasov EI, Cracco RQ, Tsairis P: Evoked potentials recorded from scalp and spinous processes during spinal column surgery. *Electroencephalogr Clin Neurophysiol* 56:569–582, 1983.

MacDonell RA, Cros D, Shahani BT: Lumbosacral nerve root stimulation comparing electrical with surface magnetic coil techniques. *Muscle Nerve* 15:885–890, 1992.

Mackenzie K, DeLisa JA: Distal sensory latency measurement of the superficial radial nerve in normal adult subjects. *Arch Phys Med Rehabil* 62:31–34, 1981.

MacLean IC: Nerve root stimulation to evaluate conduction across the brachial and lumbosacral plexus. Recent advances in clinical electromyography. *AAEE Third Annual Continuing Education Course* 1980;51–55.

MacLean IC: *Spinal Nerve Stimulation.* Rochester, MN: American Association of Electromyography and Electrodiagnosis, 1988.

MacLean IC, Mattioni TA: Phrenic nerve conduction studies: A new technique and its application in quadriplegic patients. *Arch Phys Med Rehabil* 62:70–73, 1981.

Magladery JW, Porter WE, Park AM, Teasdall RD: Electrophysiological studies of nerve and reflex activity in normal man: IV. The two-neurone reflex and identification of certain action potentials from spinal roots and cord. *Bull Johns Hopkins Hosp* 88:499–519, 1952.

Markand ON, Kincaid JC, Pourmand RA, et al.: Electrophysiologic evaluation of diaphragm by transcutaneous phrenic nerve stimulation. *Neurology* 34:604–614, 1984.

Maskill D, Murphy K, Mier A, Owen M, Guz A: Motor cortical representation of the diaphragm in man. *J Physiol* 443:105–121, 1991.

Masur H, Ludolph AC, Hilker E, et al.: Transcranial magnetic stimulation: Influence on plasma levels of hormones of the anterior pituitary gland and of cortisol? *Funct Neurol* 6:59–63, 1991.

Matsumiya Y, Yamamoto T, Yarita M, Miyauchi S, Kling JW: Physical and physiological specification of magnetic pulse stimuli that produce cortical damage in rats. *J Clin Neurophysiol* 9:278–287, 1992.

Maynard FM, Stolov WC: Experimental error in determination of nerve conduction velocity. *Arch Phys Med Rehabil* 53:362–372, 1972.

McClelland RJ, McCrea RS: Intersubject variability of the auditory-evoked brain stem potentials. *Audiology* 18:462–471, 1979.

Melvin JL, Harris DH, Johnson EW: Sensory and motor conduction velocities in the ulnar and median nerves. *Arch Phys Med Rehabil* 47:511–519, 1966.

Melvin JL, Schuchmann JA, Lanese RR: Diagnostic specificity of motor and sensory nerve conduction variables in the carpal tunnel syndrome. *Arch Phys Med Rehabil* 54:69–74, 1973.

Michalewski HJ, Thompson LW, Patterson JV, Bowman TE, Litzelman D: Sex differences in the amplitudes and latencies of the human auditory brain stem potential. *Electroencephalogr Clin Neurophysiol* 48:351–356, 1980.

Morioka T, Tobimatsu S, Fujii K, et al.: Direct spinal versus peripheral nerve stimulation as monitoring techniques in epidurally recorded spinal cord potentials. *Acta Neurochir* 108:122–127, 1991.

Mysiw WJ, Colachis SC III: Electrophysiologic study of the anterior interosseous nerve. *Am J Phys Med Rehabil* 67:50–54, 1988.

Nainzadeh NK, Neuwirth MG, Bernstein R, Cohen LS: Direct recording of spinal evoked potentials to peripheral nerve stimulation by a specially modified electrode. In Ducker TB, Brown RH (eds): *Neurophysiology and Standards of Spinal Cord Monitoring.* New York: Springer-Verlag, 1988;234–244.

Nakano KK, Lundergan C, Okihiro MM: Anterior interosseous nerve syndromes. *Arch Neurol* 34:477–480, 1977.

Nash CL Jr, Lorig RA, Schatzinger LA, Brown RH: Spinal cord monitoring during operative treatment of the spine. *Clin Orthop* 126:100–105, 1977.

Nilsson J, Panizza M, Roth BJ, et al.: Determining the site of stimulation during magnetic stimulation of a peripheral nerve. *Electroencephalogr Clin Neurophysiol* 85:253–264, 1992.

Noel P, Desmedt JE: Somatosensory cerebral evoked potentials after vascular lesions of the brainstem and diencephalon. *Brain* 98:113–128, 1975.

Odderson IR, Halar EM: Localization of nerve depolarization with magnetic stimulation. *Muscle Nerve* 15:711–715, 1992.

Oh SJ, Sarala PK, Kuba T, Elmore RS: Tarsal tunnel syndrome: Electrophysiological study. *Ann Neurol* 5:327–330, 1979.

Oh SJ: Botulism: Electrophysiological studies. *Ann Neurol* 1:481–485, 1977.

Oh SJ: *Electromyography: Neuromuscular Transmission Studies.* Baltimore: Williams & Wilkins, 1988.

Olney RK, Wilbourn AJ: Ulnar nerve conduction study of the first dorsal interosseous muscle. *Arch Phys Med Rehabil* 66:16–18, 1985.

Olsen PZ: Prediction of recovery in Bell's palsy. *Acta Neurol Scand* 52 (Suppl 61):1–121, 1975.

Opsomer RJ, Caramia MD, Zarola F, Pesce F, Rossini PM: Neurophysiological evaluation of central-peripheral sensory and motor pudendal fibres. *Electroencephalogr Clin Neurophysiol* 74:260–270, 1989.

Palliyath SK: A technique for studying the greater auricular nerve conduction velocity. *Muscle Nerve* 7:232–234, 1984.

Panayiotopoulos CP, Scarpalezos S, Nastas PE: F-wave studies on the deep peroneal nerve. Part I. Control subjects. *J Neurol Sci* 31:319–329, 1977.

Panayiotopoulos CP, Scarpalezos S, Nastas PE: Sensory (1a) and F-wave conduction velocity in the proximal segment of the tibial nerve. *Muscle Nerve* 1:181–189, 1978.

Panizza M, Nilsson J, Roth BJ, Basser PJ, Hallett M: Relevance of stimulus duration for activation of motor and sensory fibers: Implications for the study of H-reflexes and magnetic stimulation. *Electroencephalogr Clin Neurophysiol* 85:22–29, 1992.

Pascual-Leone A, Valls-Sole J, Brasil-Neto JP, Cohen LG, Hallett M: Seizure induction and transcranial magnetic stimulation. *Lancet* 339:997, 1992. (Letter)

Pascual-Leone A, Cohen LG, Shotland LI, et al.: No evidence of hearing loss in humans due to transcranial magnetic stimulation. *Neurology* 42:647–651, 1992.

Pascual-Leone A, Dhuna A, Roth BJ, Cohen L, Hallett M: Risk of burns during rapid-rate magnetic stimulation in presence of electrodes. *Lancet* 336:1195–1196, 1990. (Letter)

Pathak KS, Brown RH, Cascorbi HF, Nash CL Jr: Effects of fentanyl and morphine on intraoperative somatosensory cortical-evoked potentials. *Anaesth Analg* 63:833–837, 1984.

Pavot AP, Ignacio DR, Lightfoote WF II: Diagnostic value of multimodality evoked potentials in stroke. *Arch Phys Med Rehabil* 64:492–493, 1983. (Abstract)

Pedersen L, Trojaborg W: Visual, auditory, and somatosensory pathway involvement in hereditary cerebellar ataxia, Friedreich's ataxia, and familial spastic paraplegia. *Electroencephalogr Clin Neurophysiol* 52:283–297, 1981.

Phillips LH II, Daube JR: Lumbosacral spinal evoked potentials in humans. *Neurology* 30:1175–1183, 1980.

Pitt MC, Daldry SJ: The use of weighted quadratic regression for the study of latencies of the P100 component of the visual evoked potential. *Electroencephalogr Clin Neurophysiol* 71:150–152, 1988.

Porter R: The Kugelberg Lecture: Brain mechanisms of voluntary motor commands—a review. *Electroencephalogr Clin Neurophysiol* 76:282–293, 1990.

Posas HN, Rivner MH: Nerve conduction studies of the medial branch of the deep peroneal nerve. *Muscle Nerve* 13:862, 1990. (Abstract)

Pradhan S, Taly A: Intercostal nerve conduction study in man. *J Neurol Neurosurg Psychiatry* 52:763–766, 1989.

Prevec TS: Effect of Valium on the somatosensory evoked potential. In: Desmedt JH (ed): *Progress in Clinical Neurophysiology, Vol 7: Clinical Uses of Cerebral Brainstem and Spinal Somatosensory Evoked Potentials*. Basel: Karger, 1980;311–318.

Pribyl R, You SB, Jantra P: Sensory nerve conduction velocity of the medial antebrachial cutaneous nerve. *Electromyogr Clin Neurophysiol* 19:41–46, 1979.

Ravnborg M, Blinkenberg M, Dahl K: Standardization of facilitation of compound muscle action potentials evoked by magnetic stimulation of the cortex. Results in healthy volunteers and in patients with multiple sclerosis. *Electroencephalogr Clin Neurophysiol* 81:195–201, 1991.

Ravnborg M, Knudsen GM, Blinkenberg M: No effect of pulsed magnetic stimulation on the blood-brain barrier in rats. *Neuroscience* 38:277–280, 1990.

Ravnborg M, Dahl K: Examination of central and peripheral motor pathways by standardized magnetic stimulation. *Acta Neurol Scand* 84:491–497, 1991.

Redmond MD, DiBenedetto M: Hypoglossal nerve conduction in normal subjects. *Muscle Nerve* 11:447–452, 1988.

Redmond MD, DiBenedetto M: Electrodiagnostic evaluation of the hypoglossal nerve. *Arch Phys Med Rehabil* 65:633, 1984. (Abstract)

Rossini PM, Cracco RQ, Cracco JB, House WJ: Short latency somatosensory evoked potentials to peroneal nerve stimulation: Scalp topography and the effect of different frequency filters. *Electroencephalogr Clin Neurophysiol* 52:540–552, 1981.

Roth BJ, Cohen LG, Hallett M, Friauf W, Basser PJ: A theoretical calculation of the electric field induced by magnetic stimulation of a peripheral nerve. *Muscle Nerve* 13: 734–741, 1990.

Rowe MJ III: Normal variability of the brain-stem auditory evoked response in young and old adult subjects. *Electroencephalogr Clin Neurophysiol* 44: 459–470, 1978.

Rowed DW, McLean JAG, Tator CH: Somatosensory evoked potentials in acute spinal cord injury: Prognostic value. *Surg Neurol* 9:203–210, 1978.

Roy EP III, Gutmann L, Riggs JE, Jones ET, Byrd JA, Ringel RA: Intraoperative somatosensory evoked potential monitoring in scoliosis. *Clin Orthop* 229:94–98, 1988.

Saeed MA, Gatens PF: Compound nerve action potentials of the medial and lateral plantar nerves through the tarsal tunnel. *Arch Phys Med Rehabil* 63:304–307, 1982.

Sanders DB: Single Fiber Electromyography. An American Association of Electromyography and Electrodiagnosis Workshop. October 1988.

Sanders DB, Phillips LH: Single Fiber Electromyography. An American Association of Electromyography and Electrodiagnosis Workshop. October 1984.

Sarala PK, Nishihara T, Oh SJ: Meralgia paresthetic: Electrophysiologic study. *Arch Phys Med Rehabil* 60:30–31, 1979.

Schuchmann JA: Sural nerve conduction: A standardized technique. *Arch Phys Med Rehabil* 58:166–168, 1977.

Schumm F, Stohr M: Accessory nerve stimulation in the assessment of myasthenia gravis. *Muscle Nerve* 7:147–151, 1984.

Shankar K, Means KM: Accessory nerve conduction in neck dissection subjects. *Arch Phys Med Rehabil* 71:403–405, 1990.

Shaw NA, Cant BR: Age-dependent changes in the latency of the pattern visual evoked potential. *Electroencephalogr Clin Neurophysiol* 48:237–241, 1980.

Sherwood AM: Characteristics of somatosensory evoked potentials recorded over the spinal cord and brain of man. *IEEE Trans Biomed Eng* 28:481–487, 1981.

Shibasaki H, Barrett G, Halliday E, Halliday AM: Components of the movement-related cortical potential and their scalp topography. *Electroencephalogr Clin Neurophysiol* 49:213–226, 1980.

Shibasaki H: Movement-associated cortical potentials in unilateral cerebral lesions. *J Neurol* 209:189–198, 1975.

Similowski T, Fleury B, Launois S, Cathala HP, Bouche P, Derenne JP: Cervical magnetic stimulation: A new painless method for bilateral phrenic nerve stimulation in conscious humans. *J Appl Physiol* 67:1311–1318, 1989.

Simpson JA: Fact and fallacy in measurement of conduction velocity in motor nerves. *J Neurol Neurosurg Psychiatry* 27:381–385, 1964.

Siroky MB, Sax DS, Krane RJ: Sacral signal tracing: The electrophysiology of the bulbocavernosus reflex. *J Urol* 122:661–664, 1979.

Slomic A, Rosenfalck A, Buchthal F: Electrical and mechanical response of normal and myasthenic muscle. With particular reference to the staircase phenomenon. *Brain Res* 10:1–78, 1968.

Spielholz NI, Benjamin MV, Engler GL, Ransohoff J: Somatosensory evoked potentials during decompression and stabilization of the spine: Methods and findings. *Spine* 4:500–505, 1979.

Spindler HA, Felsenthal G: Sensory conduction in the musculocutaneous nerve. *Arch Phys Med Rehabil* 59:20–23, 1978.

Stagliano N, Baran E, Kresch E, Freedman W: Correlation analysis of movement-related potentials. *Muscle Nerve* 14:895, 1991. (Abstract)

Stagliano N, Baran E, Kresch E, Freedman W: Quantitative analysis of the Bereitschaftspotential. *Muscle Nerve* 14:895–896, 1991. (Abstract)

Stalberg E, Trontelj JV: *Single Fibre Electromyography.* Old Working, Surrey U.K.: Mirvalle Press; 1979.

Stalberg E, Thiele B: Motor unit fibre density in the extensor digitorum communis muscle. *J Neurol Neurosurg Psychiatry* 38:874–880, 1975.

Stalberg E, Thiele B: Transmission block in terminal nerve twigs: A single fibre electromyographic finding in man. *J Neurol Neurosurg Psychiatry* 35:52–59, 1972.

Stalberg E, Ekstedt J: Single fibre EMG and microphysiology of the motor unit in normal and diseased human muscle. In: Desmedt JE (ed): *New Developments in Electromyography and Clinical Neurophysiology. VI: New concepts of the Motor Unit.* Basel: Karger, 1973;113–129.

Stalberg E, Andreassen S, Falck B, Lang H, Rosenfalck A, Trojaborg W: Quantitative analysis of individual motor unit potentials: A proposition for standardized terminology and criteria for measurement. *J Clin Neurophysiol* 3:313–348, 1986.

Starr A, Achor LJ: Auditory brain stem responses in neurological disease. *Arch Neurol* 32:761–768, 1975.

Stockard JJ, Sharbrough FW, Tinker JA: Effects of hypothermia on the human brainstem auditory response. *Ann Neurol* 3:368–370, 1978.

Stohr M, Shumm F, Ballier R: Normal sensory conduction in the saphenous nerve in man. *Electroencephalogr Clin Neurophysiol* 44:172–178, 1978.

Stohr M, Petruch F, Scheglmann K: Somatosensory evoked potentials following trigeminal nerve stimulation in trigeminal neuralgia. *Ann Neurol* 9:63–66, 1981.

Stolov WC, Slimp JC: Intraoperative monitoring of the vertebral canal. Rochester, MN: American Association of Electromyography and Electrodiagnosis. *Twelfth Annual Continuing Education Courses, 1989. Course B: Intraoperative Monitoring* 1989: 27–38.

Synek VM, Cowan JC: Saphenous nerve evoked potentials and the assessment of intraabdominal lesions of the femoral nerve. *Muscle Nerve* 6:453–456, 1983.

Tassinari CA, Michelucci R, Forti A, et al.: Transcranial magnetic stimulation in epileptic patients: Usefulness and safety. *Neurology* 40:1132–1133, 1990.

Taylor MJ, Davis CM: The Bereitschaftspotential before voluntary and instructed serial movements. In: EEG Suppl. 38. *Cerebral Psychophysiology: Studies in Event-Related Potentials*.

Taylor N, Jebsen RH, Tenckhoff HA: Facial nerve conduction latency in chronic renal insufficiency. *Arch Phys Med Rehabil* 51:259–263, 1970.

Thomas S, Merton WL, Boyd SG: Pituitary hormones in relation to magnetic stimulation of the brain. *J Neurol Neurosurg Psychiatry* 54:89–90, 1991. (Letter)

Thompson PD, Day BL, Rothwell JC, Dressler D, Maertens de Noordhout A, Marsden CD: Further observations on the facilitation of muscle responses to cortical stimulation by voluntary contraction. *Electroencephalogr Clin Neurophysiol* 81:397–402, 1991.

Tofts PS: The distribution of induced currents in magnetic stimulation of the nervous system. *Phys Med Biol* 35:1119–1128, 1990.

Toleikis JR, Sloan TB, Ronai AK: Optimal transcranial magnetic stimulation sites for the assessment of motor function. *Electroencephalogr Clin Neurophysiol* 81:443–449, 1991.

Tonzola RF, Ackil AA, Shahani BT, Young RR: Usefulness of electrophysiological studies in the diagnosis of lumbosacral root disease. *Ann Neurol* 9:305–308, 1981.

Trojaborg W: Motor and sensory conduction in the musculocutaneous nerve. *J Neurol Neurosurg Psychiatry* 39:890–899, 1976.

Trojaborg W, Sindrup EH: Motor and sensory conduction in different segments of the radial nerve in normal subjects. *J Neurol Neurosurg Psychiatry* 32:354–359, 1969.

Trojaborg W, Petersen E: Visual and somatosensory evoked cortical potentials in multiple sclerosis. *J Neurol Neurosurg Psychiatry* 42:323–330, 1979.

Truong XT, Russo FI, Vagi I, Rippel DV: Conduction velocity in the proximal sural nerve. *Arch Phys Med Rehabil* 60:304–308, 1979.

Uncini A, Lange DJ, Solomon M, Soliven B, Meer J, Lovelace RE: Ring finger testing in carpal tunnel syndrome: A comparative study of diagnostic utility. *Muscle Nerve* 12:735–741, 1989.

Uozumi T, Tsuji S, Murai Y: Motor potentials evoked by magnetic stimulation of the motor cortex in normal subjects and patients with motor disorders. *Electroencephalogr Clin Neurophysiol* 81:251–256, 1991.

Veilleux M, Daube JR, Cucchiara RF: Monitoring of cortical evoked potentials during surgical procedures on the cervical spine. *Mayo Clin Proc* 62:256–264, 1987.

Wagner AL, Buchthal F: Motor and sensory conduction in infancy and childhood: Reappraisal. *Dev Med Child Neurol* 14:189–216, 1972.

Wainapel SF, Kim DJ, Ebel A: Conduction studies of the saphenous nerve in healthy subjects. *Arch Phys Med Rehabil* 59:316–319, 1978.

Waylonis GW, Johnson EW: Facial nerve conduction delay. *Arch Phys Med Rehabil* 45:539–547, 1964.

Weber RJ, Piero DL: F wave evaluation of thoracic outlet syndrome: A multiple regression derived F wave latency predicting technique. *Arch Phys Med Rehabil* 59:464–469, 1978.

Wiederholt WC: Stimulus intensity and site of excitation in human median nerve sensory fibres. *J Neurol Neurosurg Psychiatry* 33:438–441, 1970.

Wilbourn AJ, Lambert E: The forearm median-to-ulnar nerve communication: Electrodiagnostic aspects. *Neurology* 26:368, 1976. (Abstract)

Wongsam PE, Johnson EW, Weinerman JD: Carpal tunnel syndrome: Use of palmar stimulation of sensory fibers. *Arch Phys Med Rehabil* 64:16–19, 1983.

Wu Y, Kunz RM, Putnam TD, Stratigos JS: Axillary F central latency: Simple electrodiagnostic technique for proximal neuropathy. *Arch Phys Med Rehabil* 64:117–120, 1983.

Yamada T, Machida M, Kimura J: Far-field somatosensory evoked potentials after stimulation of the tibial nerve. *Neurology* 32:1151–1158, 1982.

Yap C-B, Hirota T: Sciatic nerve motor conduction velocity study. *J Neurol Neurosurg Psychiatry* 30:233–239, 1967.

Young AW, Redmond MD, Hemler DE, Belandres PV: Radial motor nerve conduction studies. *Arch Phys Med Rehabil* 71:399–402, 1990.

Subject Index